Statistics for Biology

Series Editors:
M. Gail
K. Krickeberg
J. Samet
A. Tsiatis
W. Wong

For further volumes:
http://www.springer.com/series/2848

Daniel O. Stram

Design, Analysis, and Interpretation of Genome-Wide Association Scans

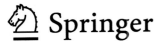 Springer

Daniel O. Stram
Department of Preventive Medicine
University of Southern California
Keck School of Medicine
Los Angeles, CA, USA

ISSN 1431-8776
ISBN 978-1-4614-9442-3   ISBN 978-1-4614-9443-0 (eBook)
DOI 10.1007/978-1-4614-9443-0
Springer New York Heidelberg Dordrecht London

Library of Congress Control Number: 2013954411

Printed on acid-free paper

Springer is part of Springer Science+Business Media (www.springer.com)

To Pavlova, Alex, and Douglas

Acknowledgments

Acknowledgments are due to Malcolm Pike, Larry Kolonel, and Brian Henderson for their vision in initiating the Multiethnic Cohort Study in Hawaii and Los Angeles. My work on genetic association studies began with a 6-month sabbatical spent at the Whitehead Institute/MIT Center for Genome Research in 2002 which was itself an offshoot of the early collaborations developed between the MEC and the Brave New World of twenty-first-century human genetics. Thanks to David Altshuler, Mark Daly, David Reich, Nick Patterson, Noel Burtt, Itsik Pe'er, and the many others from whom I learned enormously at that time. Additional sabbatical support in 2010 initiated the development of the material presented here into its current form. Special thanks to valued colleagues including Chris Haiman, Loic Le Marchand, Iona Cheng, Leigh Pearce, Peter Kraft and Duncan Thomas, as well as many students, with whom it has been a pleasure to work with during hugely exciting times.

Jianqi Zhang helped assess the text and homework problems from a student's point of view. Diane Lemasters assisted me with graphics and charts.

Contents

Chapter 1
Introduction

Abstract This chapter provides an elementary introduction to some of the basic biology and technology that underlies genetic association studies that rely on dense genotyping of nominally unrelated individuals to discover genetic variants related to risk of disease and other outcomes, phenotypes, or traits. This chapter discusses relevant aspects of DNA and RNA architecture, coding of amino acids, describes chromosomal organization, gives an overview of the most common types of sequence variation, and provides an overview of genotyping methods. It introduces concepts, databases, analysis programs, and example data that will be used in later portions of the book.

1.1 Historical Perspective

Many important ideas about genetics were discovered long before there was any biochemical knowledge of the way in which traits are transmitted from parents to offspring. By 1953, when Watson and Crick [1, 2] published their discoveries about the molecular structure of DNA (*deoxyribonucleic acid*), a great deal of knowledge about the nature of inheritance in plant, animal, and human species had been worked out from a long process of experiment and observation. Arguably the most important single researcher whose work led most directly to the field that is now called genetics was Charles Darwin whose theory of evolution [3] was published nearly 100 years before Watson and Crick. His work emphasized the fundamental ideas of within-species inheritable variation and natural selection as the driving force of evolution, so that while all members of a given species shared distinctions between other species, within-species inheritable variation could be selected for either naturally or by human breeding of animals and plants. Darwin's theory posited that accumulation of variation selected for within a given group of living organisms could eventually lead to new species when breeding populations of organisms became isolated geographically or by their habits of life. Natural selection for traits favorable to survival either in existing or new environments was

D.O. Stram, *Design, Analysis, and Interpretation of Genome-Wide Association Scans*,
Statistics for Biology and Health, DOI 10.1007/978-1-4614-9443-0_1,
© Springer Science+Business Media New York 2014

recognized as both imposing constraints on the type of differences that could be successfully passed on, but also as a force leading to increasing diversity and complexity of organisms' characteristics and behavior. Darwin came to his conclusions through his great knowledge of the geographical variation of similar species and of the practice of animal breeding. Especially important ideas of Darwin's were that novel inheritable trait variation could unpredictably appear in a single individual and that the most frequent cause of variability may be attributed to the male and female reproductive "elements" having been affected prior to the act of conception. Today we know that this is due to unpredictable, essentially random, de novo mutations due to errors in DNA replication during gamete formation causing DNA changes that affect protein properties and/or regulation.

Unknown to Darwin but fundamental to the emergence of modern genetics was the discovery by Gregor Mendel in 1866 of the general rules of inheritance in pairs that underlie the phenomenon of genetic dominance, equal segregation, and independent assortment, which today are known to apply to the transmission of chromosomes from parental generation to offspring, from diploid individuals (parents), through meiosis, to haploid gametes which then unite during conception to regain diploidy, with independent assortment applying to genes on different chromosomes. While the importance of "Mendel's Laws" was not recognized immediately, they were later rediscovered (by de Vries, Correns, and Tschermak), with the chromosomal theory of inheritance proposed by Sutton in 1902 and confirmed in 1910 by T. H. Morgan explaining why some traits are inherited independently from each other, while others (as previously discovered by Bateson and Punnett) are partly or fully linked. The linearity of chromosomes leads to a concept of genetic distance in terms of recombination probabilities as formalized by the first genetic maps (of traits in *Drosophila melanogaster*). Recombination was later identified (by Creighton and McClintok) to be due to the physical exchange of chromosome pieces. Other notable discoveries were of the mutagenic nature of ionizing radiation (Hermann Muller [4]) and the general relationship between mutations in a single gene and loss of specific enzymes [5].

Attempts to merge the work of Darwin (contributing the concepts of selection, isolation, formation of new inheritable mutation, and speciation) together with the observations of Mendel and his rediscoverers led to the foundations of quantitative, population, and statistical genetics principally through the work of Sewall Wright, J.B.S. Haldane, and R. A. Fisher. Their interests lay in understanding the quantitative implications of Mendelian inheritance on basic evolutionary phenomenon including natural selection, genetic drift, and gene flow. As we will see in Chaps. 2 and 4, genetic drift and gene flow between isolated groups lead to correlation patterns between individual's phenotypes that affect the statistical properties of the genetic association studies that are the topic of this book. Other important statistical concepts developed include the infinite sites model (Kimura and Crow [6]) with its implication of a single origin for most mutations—a fundamental concept in linkage disequilibrium-based association studies—and the resulting distribution of the number and frequency of genetic variants under neutral evolution [7] or selection.

1.2   DNA Basics

The discovery of the structure of DNA by Watson and Crick and its immediate implications on the biological basis for Mendelian inheritance as well as the discoveries, by H.G. Khorana, M. Nirenberg, and others, of the relationship between DNA codon (triples of letters of DNA) order and amino acid order in proteins revolutionized all areas of genetics. While the focus of this book is emphatically not devoted to molecular biology, a number of fundamental concepts concerning the nature of DNA are required in order for a statistician to effectively communicate with molecular biologists and epidemiologists, clinicians, and the like in the conduct of large-scale genetic association studies.

DNA is carried in almost all human cells in both the nucleus of a cell—where the DNA is organized into pairs of homologous chromosomes and in the mitochondria. Generally speaking, throughout this book we will be discussing only nuclear DNA variants, although we give a brief introduction to mitochondrial variants at the end of the next section.

1.2.1   Organization of Chromosomes

The human genome is composed of 22 *autosomes and 2 sex chromosomes* (X or Y). In normal individuals most body cells contain two copies of the genome and are said to be *diploid*. A normal diploid cell contains a total 46 chromosomes, 22 *homologous pairs* of autosomes, and either two X chromosomes (females) or an X and Y chromosome (males). Cells that contain one copy of the genome, such as sperm and unfertilized egg cells, are said to be *haploid*.

All chromosomes have a *centromere* which becomes evident during chromosomal duplication prior to cell division (the duplicated chromosomes are joined at the centromere). The centromere divides the chromosome into two arms. The shorter of the two is the *p (petite)* arm and the longer the *q* arm. Staining of duplicated chromosomes produces distinct bands, grouped together into regions, by which chromosomes can be visibly identified, and these bands are counted outward from the centromere; for example, 8q24 is the 4th band of the 2nd region of the long arm of chromosome 8. These can be further distinguished into sub-bands (8q24.1, 8q24.2, etc.) or sub-sub-bands (8q24.11, 8q24.12, etc.).

Chromosomes are duplicated during both *meiosis* and *mitosis*. Gametes (sperm and egg cells) are formed during meiosis from germ-line stem cells through a process involving an initial chromosomal duplication and two subsequent cell divisions which together results in a reduction of chromosome number of the gametes from diploid to haploid (with four gametes produced by each germ cell) so that each haploid gamete contains just one copy of each chromosome. It is during the first cell division that duplicated homologous chromosomes pair up and form physical connections called *chiasmata*, and meiotic recombination or *crossing-over* occurs at the chiasmata. Specific enzymes break the DNA strands and repair the break in a way that swaps material from one homologous chromosome with material from another. Two alleles that are on the same chromosome in the parent may not be on the same chromosome in the gametes. During meiosis in most organisms, at least one recombination takes place for each pair of homologous chromosomes [8–10]. This implies that the gametes receive contributions from both homologs of each chromosome pair (thus from both grandparents). Another process that also (although much less commonly than recombination) can alter homologous chromosomes during meiosis is that of gene conversion in which, rather than having the two homologs trade DNA evenly, the DNA from one (the donor) is simply copied into and replaces that of the other (recipient).

Haploid gametes unite during conception to form a fertilized diploid egg and thereafter grow through a process of mitotic duplication and cell differentiation. In mitosis there is no reduction in chromosome number since only one cell division takes place after chromosomal duplication, and each daughter cell receives identical genomic material. DNA copying errors can result in mutations during mitosis, but these only affect specific cell lineages and thus are not generally inherited by further generations. One important event that takes place early in mitotic development in females is the inactivation of one of the pair of X chromosomes. In random X inactivation, one of the X chromosomes is randomly chosen to be *methylated* (by addition of a methyl group to cytosine and adenine nucleotides) during mitosis, and gene expression from that chromosome is silenced for all descendant (daughter) cells. Random X inactivation occurs in the early female embryo where both the maternal and paternal X chromosome have an equal chance of becoming inactivated. This has two implications, the first is that the gene dose of the products of the X chromosome is similar in males (with only one copy) and in females (with two). However, in females different cells (derived from different early lineages) will have different (maternal or paternal derived) X chromosomes silenced, so that effects of genetic variants appearing on only one X chromosome will not be universally exhibited as they are in males. This is why such sex-linked recessive genetic traits as hemophilia and colorblindness remain much less common in females (where only homozygotes show the trait) than in males inheriting a single X chromosome. In other species X inactivation is not random, for example, in mice, where the paternal X chromosome is preferentially inactivated in all developing cells of the female embryo [11].

1.2.2   Organization of DNA

Each chromosome is made up of two *strands* of *deoxyribonucleic acid (DNA)* coiled into a double helix (see Fig. 1.1). Each strand has a *deoxyribose* backbone consisting of deoxyribose sugars bound together into a long chain, with each sugar having a 3' carbon linked, by a phosphate group, to the 5' carbon of the next sugar in the chain. The terminal sugar at one end of the DNA strand has a free 5' carbon, and the terminal sugar at the other end has a free 3' carbon. Attached to each sugar is a

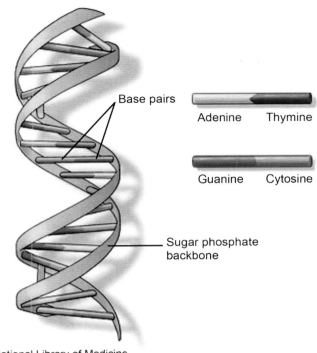

Fig. 1.1 Basic DNA structure (from http://static.ddmcdn.com/gif/dna-2.jpg)

base. Four different bases are found in DNA: two purines, *adenine* (A) and *guanine* (G), and two pyrimidines, *cytosine (C)* and *thymine (T)*. The two strands of double-stranded DNA are held together by bonding between opposing bases. Bonding occurs specifically between A and T and between G and C: thus the two strands must be *complimentary* (so that, e.g., a 5′-ACTGGGCA-3′ on one strand binds with 3′-TGACCCGT-5′ on the other). By convention sequences are usually specified by writing only a single strand (choosing by convection the 5′–3′ direction, which is also the direction of DNA synthesis). RNA is a very similar molecule to DNA except that it has a ribose backbone, generally exists only as single strands, and substitutes the base *uracil* (U) for thymine (T).

1.2.3   DNA and Protein

Less than 2 % of the human genome codes directly for the amino acid chains that make up protein molecules through a three-letter code (*codon*) that maps the

64 possible combinations of codes of form, AAA, AAC, AAT, . . ., TTT,[1] to one of the 20 amino acids or to one of the 3 STOP codons. Since there are more possible codons than amino acids, each *amino acid* is coded for by from 1 to 6 different codons. The linear order of the letter codes directly to the order of amino acids in the target protein. Generally, the *coding sequence* for a protein is separated in the DNA into several *exons* interspersed with noncoding *introns*. Transfer of information from DNA to *messenger RNA* involves transcription factors that recognize specific noncoding DNA regulatory sequences, physical separation through *RNA polymerase* of the two DNA strands over a short region to expose it for RNA base binding, and the copying of information from one of the strands (the template strand) to its complementary RNA. During transcription DNA is read from the template in the $3'-5'$ direction (so that RNA is assembled in the $5'-3'$ direction with respect to its own orientation) from the start of the first exon (the transcription start site), through all exons and introns, to the end of the last exon. The introns are immediately removed by a process called RNA splicing to form a mature mRNA. Many genes exhibit *alternative splicing* with certain exons being spliced out in certain tissues, so that several distinct proteins can be created from a different gene.

Translation involves migration of mature mRNA to the cell cytoplasm, for binding to ribosomal RNA/protein complexes called *ribosomes*. At the ribosome, the messenger RNA interacts with transfer RNAs (tRNA) that recognize the codons (through an *antisense* sequence complementary to the mRNA codons), each of which recruits specific amino acids for attachment to the growing polypeptide chain.

As mentioned above, less than 2 % of the 3 billion base pairs that make up a single copy of the human genome are thought to code directly for proteins. Other parts of DNA molecule code for different kinds of RNA including tRNA, ribosomal RNA (rRNA), and microRNAs (miRNA) (which block mRNA). Many other DNA elements are involved in gene regulation including the promoter sequences that RNA polymerase binds to as described briefly above. It is only recently that the *Encyclopedia of DNA Elements* project, ENCODE, has provided information implying that most of the genome contains elements that are linked to biochemical functions [12].

1.3 Types of Genetic Variation

1.3.1 Single-Nucleotide Variants and Polymorphisms

The most common type of genetic variant, which is ubiquitous throughout the human genome, is the *single-nucleotide variant* or SNV. An SNV consists of a single base variation at a specific position on a given strand (chromosome) of DNA with the change measured relative to some existing consensus sequence. A new

---

[1] These are DNA codons; RNA codons (translated from DNA for the purpose of interaction with the *ribosome* in protein formation) substitute thymine (T) with *uracil* U since T is replaced by U in RNA molecules.

SNV originates as a chance copying error during the process of meiosis (production of sperm or egg cells) or as a result of DNA damage in the subsequent sperm or egg cell, but the occurrence of a new variant at any given chromosomal location is a rare event, i.e., the vast majority of DNA base pairs are copied with complete fidelity during any one meiosis, and most subsequent DNA damage is completely repaired. Because of this rarity of de novo mutations, by far the vast majority of single-copy variants carried in the DNA of a given person have been inherited from one (or both) of their biological parents, who in turn inherited the variant from one or both of their parents, etc. all the way back to the original ancestral mutation.

Single-copying errors can occur during DNA replication prior to mitosis (ordinary cell division), or DNA damage can occur in ordinary (non-sex cell) cells as well, but the errors occurring during mitosis are not inherited from generation to generation and are only present in what is usually the very small number of direct descendant cells (an exception is when a variant originates in a cell of an early embryo, leading to mosaicism). Inherited variants are therefore present in either one or two copies in all typical cells (there are ~1 trillion cells per person) depending upon whether the variant was inherited from one or both parents.

In order to be denoted a *single-nucleotide polymorphism* (SNP) an SNV is (by tradition) required to be present at a frequency of at least 1 % or more of all chromosomes. The distinction between SNV and SNP, however, is somewhat arbitrary since SNV frequency is generally population dependent. The *1000 Genomes Project* maps more than 38 million SNPs [13] in the human genome with somewhat more SNPs seen in people of African ancestry than in people of the other two major continental groupings—Europeans and Asians. This difference in SNP numbers is likely because of population history since large African populations have been in existence longer than large European or Asian populations. Because of this complication, this book generally refers to both single-nucleotide polymorphisms and single-nucleotide variants as simply SNPs. More about the relationship between population history, population genetics, and SNP numbers and frequency is presented in Chap. 2.

While every SNP originated as an ancestral de novo variant, only a very small fraction of all de novo single base pair changes ever became frequent enough to be detectable in a population. For the vast majority of today's common SNPs, it is assumed that it was simply a matter of luck that they became frequent; in fact, it was far more likely that a de novo variant became extinct than it became frequent. The statistics of allele frequency distributions under various assumptions about population history and selective pressure are an important topic in population genetics theory; this book describes some relevant findings in the following chapter.

In certain cases selection in favor of a given SNP may have occurred—if that SNP altered some phenotypic characteristic in a way that increased reproductive fitness of the carriers of that SNP. Despite their importance in speciation and evolution, it is generally regarded that de novo occurrence of favorable mutations are very rare occurrences at least on quotidian time scales, and generally speaking the vast majority of SNPs are considered to be neutral with regard to reproductive fitness; this is especially true for common SNPs (since variants which decreased fitness

Table 1.1 DNA codons. The left rows refer to the first nucleotide, the columns to the second, and last to the third

Second nucleotide				
	T	C	A	G	
T	TTT Phenylalanine (Phe)	TCT Serine (Ser)	TAT Tyrosine (Tyr)	TGT Cysteine (Cys)	T
	TTC Phe	TCC Ser	TAC Tyr	TGC Cys	C
	TTA Leucine (Leu)	TCA Ser	TAA STOP	TGA STOP	A
	TTG Leu	TCG Ser	TAG STOP	TGG Tryptophan (Trp)	G
C	CTT Leucine (Leu)	CCT Proline (Pro)	CAT Histidine (His)	CGT Arginine (Arg)	T
	CTC Leu	CCC Pro	CAC His	CGC Arg	C
	CTA Leu	CCA Pro	CAA Glutamine (Gln)	CGA Arg	A
	CTG Leu	CCG Pro	CAG Gln	CGG Arg	G
A	ATT Isoleucine (Ile)	ACT Threonine (Thr)	AAT Asparagine (Asn)	AGT Serine (Ser)	T
	ATC Ile	ACC Thr	AAC Asn	AGC Ser	C
	ATA Ile	ACA Thr	AAA Lysine (Lys)	AGA Arginine (Arg)	A
	ATG Methionine (Met) or START	ACG Thr	AAG Lys	AGG Arg	G
G	GTT Valine Val	GCT Alanine (Ala)	GAT Aspartic acid (Asp)	GGT Glycine (Gly)	T
	GTC (Val)	GCC Ala	GAC Asp	GGC Gly	C
	GTA Val	GCA Ala	GAA Glutamic acid (Glu)	GGA Gly	A
	GTG Val	GCG Ala	GAG Glu	GGG Gly	

would be selected against and would be less likely to have become common). Thus by and large it is chance alone that leads to an initial single base pair variant originating in the formation of a single sperm or egg to be common in today's population. Common SNPs (and other common variants) may of course cause diseases of late adulthood without having significant effects on reproductive fitness.

The coding regions of genes directly code for proteins using a coding scheme that is universal throughout all living things on earth. Proteins are polypeptides that are synthesized as a linear combination of amino acids; each amino acid is coded by one or more three-letter sequences called codons, and the order of the codons specifies the order of the amino acids in the protein. Table 1.1 shows the DNA triplicate codon sequences for each of the 20 amino acids; note that there is considerable redundancy, i.e., there are a possible $4^3 = 64$ possible codons to code for 20 peptides. Several possible codons code for a *stop sequence* rather than amino acids, and all but two amino acids are mapped to by more than one codon. SNPs within exons that change codons without changing amino acids are called *synonymous SNPs*, and SNPs that do change codons from one to another amino acid are called *missense SNPs*. Because of coding redundancy (and undoubtedly also because of selection), the majority of SNPs in exons are synonymous, and the vast majority of SNPs in humans lie either in intronic DNA or completely outside the transcribed regions for genes. In some cases SNPs within exons can change amino acid codons to become STOP codons (known as *nonsense* changes), resulting in early termination of the gene's protein product; other times STOP codons can be affected by single base mutations leading to a loss of the stop codon, and a consequent gain in protein length. Deletions or insertions in the exons can result in frameshift mutations in which the entire protein sequence is modified. Frameshift mutations are an important source of deleterious mutations in the BRCA1 and BRCA2 cancer genes, for example [14]. The prediction of the consequence of amino acid changes on protein characteristics and function is an important biological and informatics problem, and computer programs and databases have been constructed to try to classify the significance of such changes, e.g., SIFT [15] and Polyphen [16].

Note that there is an inherent ambiguity in the identification of the alleles of an SNP due to the complementary nature of the double strands making up the DNA molecule. For example, suppose that on one strand the sequence at a particular location on a given chromosome was originally ATGAC, with its complement TACTG, and because of a copying error the G in the third position on the first strand is replaced by a T and hence C on the second strand replaced by an A so that the new strands ATTAC and TAATG remain (as they must) complementary; then if a probe (see Sect. 1.2) is designed for the first strand, it must be designed to detect a G/T polymorphism at the third position, while a probe designed for the other strand must detect a C/A polymorphism. This strand issue is one of the common problems that crop up when comparing SNP data from different genotyping platforms used in different studies in post-GWAS analysis (see Chap. 8). For our example if one platform uses probes for one strand and another uses the reverse probes, the difference (one study reporting a G/T polymorphism and the other a C/A polymorphism) will be readily apparent when comparing the two sets of data. Note however that if the ancestral G on one strand had been replaced by its complement C and (hence) the C on the opposite strand by a G, then both the probes would show the same polymorphism denoted as either G/C or C/G (with the allele in the second position being the "minor" or less frequent allele).

In order to avoid such ambiguities, the strand that an SNP is on can be identified. The approach (at least for human DNA) is to define "plus" (+) strand for a given chromosome as the strand of DNA for which the 5' end is the nearest to the centromere. Since bases in the human genome consensus sequence are numbered starting from the furthermost end of the p arm from the centromere to the furthermost end of the q arm, another way of defining the plus strand is as the strand for which moving from the 5' to the 3' end moves in increasing base position order. The minus strand is of course the other complementary strand to the plus strand. See Fig. 1.2.

The plus strand is sometimes called the *forward strand* and the minus strand the *reverse strand*, but this usage actually conflicts with an older terminology related to the particular probes used to originally definitively define the SNP as reported to the dbSNP database [17].

Ideally the SNP array and assay manufacturers all report the direction (plus or minus) of all probes used. One difficulty is that this has been a moving target, since

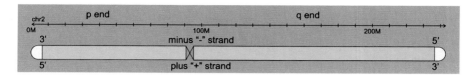

Fig. 1.2 Definition of the plus and minus strands of human DNA. As shown the plus strand is the strand for which the 5′ end of the molecule is closest to the centromere, the minus is its complement. Downloaded as image from http://hapmap.ncbi.nlm.nih.gov/

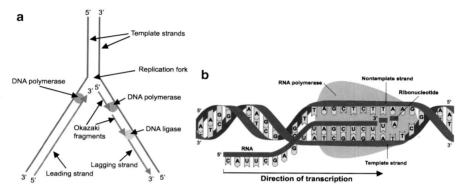

Fig. 1.3 DNA and RNA replication. During replication the direction of growth of the DNA molecule is from the 5′–3′ end. For the leading strand, the replication is continuous as a polymerase "reads" the DNA and adds nucleotides continuously; on the lagging strand, DNA replication still proceeds in the 5′–3′ direction but in short separated segments called Ozaki fragments. RNA synthesis copies the template strand (which could be either of the two strands) as the DNA is opened up with RNA polymerase and then closed. The direction of RNA synthesis (growth of the RNA molecule) is again 5′–3′, but the template could be either the plus or minus strand of DNA. Images downloaded from http://users.rcn.com/jkimball.ma.ultranet/BiologyPages / R/ReplicationFork.gif and http://1.bp.blogspot.com/_g5xPw_PeY0U/TJRnD0sfhFI/AAAAAAA AAQQ/Ylvd8d2yLgY/s1600/rna+synthesis.gif

early genome builds were quite unstable (base sequences could switch strands as more information was generated). With the much greater stability of later builds, this is in turn much less of a problem now than it once was.

Note that the plus strand is not necessarily either the coding or antisense strand for a particular gene, i.e., while RNA synthesis always proceeds in the 5′–3′ direction along a given strand, the template strand will be different (i.e., either plus or minus) for different genes (i.e., the reading direction could be either in the short arm to long arm direction or the long to short). DNA synthesis during replication also proceeds in the 5′–3′ direction (as the base pairs on each of the two template strands are read in the 3′–5′ direction). DNA synthesis proceeds continuously on one strand (the leading strand) which is the template strand of the DNA molecule where the replication fork moves in the 3′–5′ direction. Synthesis occurs in short separated segments (Ozaki fragments) along the other (lagging) strand as shown in Fig. 1.3.

Substitutions of a purine with another purine, i.e., C ↔ T, or a pyrimidine for another pyrimidine (A ↔ G) are termed *transitions*, while substitutions of a *purine ↔ pyrimidine* (C ↔ A, C ↔ G, T ↔ A, T ↔ G) are *transversions*. Although the possible transversions outnumber the possible transitions, transitions are approximately twice as frequent in the human genome. Manufacturers of genotype arrays often avoid choosing ambiguous T ↔ A and C ↔ G transversion SNPs altogether in an effort to allow the identification and immediate resolution of strand problems when comparing datasets with a minimum of effort. For example, the gene allele list for the *Illumina Omni SNP array* only lists A ↔ G and A ↔ C SNPs, but where the listed strand may be plus or minus. This corresponds, when strand is changed to correspond to the plus strand only, to having each of the four unambiguous possibilities: A ↔ G, C ↔ T, A ↔ C, and G ↔ T SNPs. Since the ambiguous transversions are much less common than the remaining unambiguous SNPs, little loss of coverage (see next chapter) is expected because of this.

1.3.2   Insertions/Deletions

Small insertions or deletions of DNA, *indels*, are also quite common over the human genome; they are thought to originate most commonly as deletions of existing DNA sequence [18] by a factor of about 3–1, compared to de novo insertions. About 1.4 million of them were found by phase 1 of the 1000 Genomes Project, sequencing of 1,092 genomes from diverse populations [13]. This may be compared to approximately 37 million SNPs found in the same project. When indels occur in coding regions, they will result in frameshift mutations unless the number of inserted or deleted bases is evenly divisible by three, since they disturb the reading of all subsequent codons during DNA translation. Such frameshift mutations can be very damaging to protein function and are implicated in many heritable diseases and syndromes.

1.3.3   Larger Structural Variants

Larger structural variants including deletions, insertions, and duplications of segments of DNA that are 1 kb or greater in extent are termed *copy number variants* or *CNVs*. It is only in the last 10 years or so that it has been discovered that such variants are present in relatively large numbers [19–21]. Other types of structural variants include *inversions* and *translocations*. Inversions are segments of DNA that are reversed in orientation compared to the rest of the chromosome, while translocations involve a change in the position of a chromosomal segment within a genome that involves no change in the total DNA content. Translocations can be intra- or inter-chromosomal. The largest structural variants involve entire chromosomes, e.g., the aneuploidies (abnormal chromosome number) such as trisomy 21 (resulting in Down syndrome) in which three copies of chromosome 21 are present. Aneuploidies of the sex chromosomes are the most common; these include both loss and gains of X or Y chromosomes, the most serious of which is the loss of one X chromosome in females resulting in Turner's syndrome.

1.3.4   Exonic Variation and Disease

The genetic basis for a large number of highly heritable phenotypes and diseases is now understood. The so-called "Mendelian" traits or disorders are most often due to protein changes in specific genes. A well-known example (and the most common Mendelian disorder in humans) is neurofibromatosis type I which is due to either deletions, missense, or nonsense mutations in the neurofibromin 1 gene (NF1), a gene which acts as a tumor suppressor. People with neurofibromatosis have tumors of the nerve tissue that can be benign or damaging. It is inherited in an autosomal dominant fashion, i.e., people carrying one or more copies of a damaged NF1 gene will have the disease, since the ability to suppress these tumors is attenuated. Interestingly about half of the NF1 cases are sporadic, i.e., neither parent has the disease; these cases are due to de novo mutations in the NF1 gene occurring during meiosis [22]. Children of sporadic neurofibromatosis cases can then inherit the new mutations and have the disease.

Many other examples of protein coding mutations and disease are cataloged in the OMIM database (Online Mendelian Inheritance in Man database, http://www.ncbi.nlm.nih.gov).

1.3.5   Non-exonic SNPs and Disease

While a large proportion of Mendelian disorders are due to protein-altering changes in one or a few genes, this is apparently not true of the vast majority of common disorders especially those which have onset late in life including common cancers, cardiovascular disease, and stroke. While protein changes in high-risk genes such as BRCA1 and BRCA2 are involved in a certain number of highly familial cases, the vast majority of common variants associated with late-onset complex disease do not seem to be directly related to alterations in protein sequence. Often the strongest associations are found with SNPs that are either in introns (intronic) or outside of the transcribed regions entirely (intergenic). It is sometimes found that a noncoding SNP association may be a surrogate for an underlying protein coding variant, but this does not appear to be very often the case [23]; it is assumed that the variants that underlie most such associations have functions that are regulatory in nature. At present for most associations

with complex disease risk, the underling causal variant is yet to be determined
as is its mode of action.

1.3.6 SNP Haplotypes

An SNP *haplotype* is a combination of from several to many SNPs on the same
chromosomal segment of DNA. *Haplotype blocks* are regions of a given chromosome for which little recombination (chromosomal shuffling) has yet to take place
(see discussion of recombination in Chap. 2). Thus the SNPs in a haplotype block
are inherited in distinct patterns. Conventional SNP genotyping does not directly
yield haplotype information, and thus the two haplotypes (one for each of the two
homologous chromosomes inherited from each parent) carried by an individual
must be inferred based on the genotypes (number of copies, 0, 1, or 2, of each SNP).
This inference can be highly accurate within haplotype blocks where there are few
recombinant haplotypes actually present, especially when genotypes from close
relatives, such as siblings, parents, or offspring, are available. Haplotypes are of
interest for two reasons; first, haplotype estimation is the key to SNP prediction for
missing or ungenotyped SNPs (or other variants), and in addition haplotypes
themselves may be the risk variants, i.e., it may matter whether SNPs alleles are
inherited on the same chromosome or not in terms of their direct effects [24]. Considerable discussion of haplotype estimation and SNP prediction is given in
Chaps. 5 and 6.

1.3.7 Microsatellites

Microsatellites, also called simple sequence repeats or short tandem repeats, are
repeating sequences of 2–6 base pairs of DNA, in which the number of copies
of the repeated sequence varies from individual to individual. They are often
highly variable between individuals since they appear to be especially susceptible to errors in duplication or during recombination. Microsatellites have
been used as markers in many linkage studies and their high degree of variability
makes them very informative about parental origin of linked disease loci in
these studies.

A variable CAG repeat within the coding region of the *HUNTINGTIN* gene is the
cause of Huntington's disease; repeat lengths equal to 40 or above are associated
with fully penetrant disease, while repeat lengths of 36–39 are associated with
increased risk.

The diversity of microsatellites also has led to their use in DNA fingerprinting
and in paternity testing. About 30,000 microsatellites are known in the human
genome. Some authors have proposed use of microsatellite markers rather than or in
addition to SNPs in GWAS studies [25].

1.3.8   Mitochondrial Variation

Mitochondria are organelles found in most eukaryotic cells, they are involved in the production of ATP used as a source of chemical energy, and in other cellular processes. In animals mitochondria are the only location of extrachromosomal DNA within the cell (in plants, chloroplasts also contain DNA). Each cell has 1 or (sometimes many) more mitochondria, each mitochondria has its own genome, and the DNA in the mitochondria is termed mtDNA. Mitochondria are inherited maternally; the mitochondrial genome consists of 16,600 base pairs arranged in a circle, coding for 37 genes; and each mitochondria has from 2 to 10 copies of the mtDNA. Despite the multiple copies most individuals are *homoplastic*, meaning that all copies are identical in sequence (or at least not detectably *heteroplastic*) [26]. Mitochondria interact with many genes that are coded in the nuclear DNA so that a comprehensive study of the effect of inherited variation and mitochondrial-related disease involves both the nuclear and mtDNA. A fairly large number of quite heterogeneous disorders [26, 27] are attributed to deletions of muscle-related mtDNA. Some common diseases (e.g., diabetes) also may be affected by such mitochondrial mutations, but the fraction of patients so affected is probably small.

Human populations can be divided into several mtDNA haplogroups that are based on specific SNPs, reflecting mutations accumulated by a discrete maternal linkage. Attempts to relate haplogroup to diseases such as Alzheimer's and Parkinson's have been made [26]; these efforts are complicated by the need to control for population differences in these diseases. Furthermore, because linkage disequilibrium (see Chap. 2) between mitochondrial SNPs is universal, localization of SNP associations within the mtDNA is difficult.

1.4   Overview of Genotyping Methods

The general idea of using *DNA hybridization* provides the approach used for SNP interrogation using very large-scale SNP arrays sold commercially by such companies as *Illumina* and *Affymetrix*. The binding of complementary DNA to sample DNA after *denaturation* (separation of two-stranded DNA into two one-stranded molecules by heating) is utilized. Allele-specific hybridization-based genotyping requires creation of probes that are specific for a certain portion of the genome containing an SNP, i.e., will be complementary only to DNA around that SNP. Generally two probes are required, which are different only at one base pair, namely, the SNP position, with one probe complementary for one allele of the SNP and the other probe complementary to the other allele. Note that a probe of length 20 has 4^{20} or approximately 10^{12} different possible probe sequences. Assuming that (to a first approximation) human DNA sequence is random with each base (A,T,G, or C) having equal frequency, then there is only approximately a 1 in 1,000 chance that the same 20 base sequence will occur more than once in the

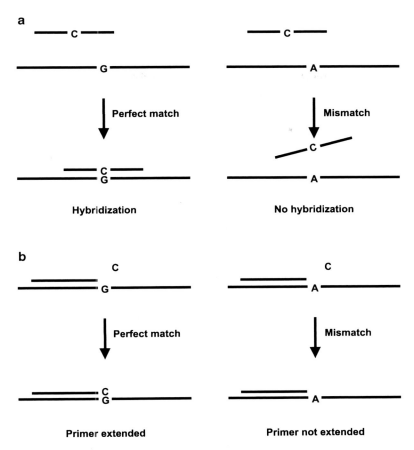

Fig. 1.4 Depiction of (**a**) DNA hybridization and single base extension and (**b**) allele-specific extension. Used with permission from Kwok [61]

human genome (of length 3×10^9 base pairs). Probe lengths typically are longer than this to allow for nearly similar sequences. The very basic idea (see Fig. 1.4) is that a probe that completely matches the target DNA will be more chemically stable than a probe that is even one base pair different (i.e., because of the SNP) than the target DNA. Each probe will be labeled, typically with a florescent dye of a specific color, so that the intensity of the expression of each dye will indicate whether a specific sample is homozygous for one or the other SNP allele (so that only one color dye will be expressed) or is heterozygous (both dyes will be expressed). A slightly different approach than having two different probes is to use (as in the Illumina Omni chip released commercially in 2009) a single probe that stops just before the base (SNP) to be interrogated. Then a single labeled base is added with the base complementary to the target sequence at that position. Again two different dyes are used as labels so that the two possible alleles may be identified. This method is termed single base pair extension. The Illumina Omni chip uses a 50 bp length probe and single base pair extension to interrogate each of approximately 1 million SNPs.

There are some regions of the genome that are highly repetitive, for example, for *acrocentric* chromosomes (those with the centromere positioned away from the center of the chromosome) such as chromosome 21, much of the short arm consists of many different types of repetitive sequence and is highly homologous to the short arms of other acrocentrics. Thus it would be essentially impossible to design probes that detect SNPs on the short arm of chromosome 21. Less radical repetition occurs in many other portions of the genome as well, and if the repetition is great enough, then it may be impossible to design a probe that will hybridize to just the one target region. Other problems in probe design occur when there are two SNPs that are very close to each other, so that there is less chemical stability than anticipated between the probe and target sequence. The chemical stability between probe and target can also depend upon base content. A length of double-stranded DNA with high G+C content is more chemically stable (e.g., denaturizes at a higher temperature) than does a length of DNA with high A+T content. This means that SNPs in high G+C regions can be difficult to detect because a single mismatch (i.e., the wrong SNP allele) may still produce a strong binding between probe and target so that differences in dye intensities may be much less distinctive for high G+C regions than desirable.

1.4.1 SNP Calling

When only small numbers of SNPs are being interrogated for a study, human assistance in calling all SNPs was often possible. Ideally a plot of dye intensities (Y vs. X with X the intensity of one dye and Y the intensity of the other) would reveal clusters that could be called easily by eye as in Fig. 1.5a [28]. When hundreds of thousands of SNPs are to be called for a study using a large-scale SNP array, human "curation" of each SNP is impossible, and we must rely upon automated algorithms to call SNPs. Once a set of interesting SNPs (i.e., those associated with the disease or outcome) is found, then the *cluster plots* for those SNPs should be examined carefully before getting too excited; almost all researchers in this area have had the experience that certain results that seemed at first glance to be extremely promising were upon examination found to have been artifacts of poor genotype calling. Cluster plots often are based upon a *polar transformation* of the X and Y intensities (e.g., as $\theta = \arctan(A/B)$, $R = A + B$) as in Fig. 1.5b. A typical example of a bad cluster plot (Fig. 1.5c) also is provided. A considerable number of algorithms for automatic genotyping calling using raw dye intensities have been described [28–35]. The interest here is not really in the details of these algorithms but rather to acquaint the reader with the kinds of typical output produced by genotyping platforms. Poor quality DNA for a sample is one common cause of poor genotype calling; genotype calling is complicated by other factors as well.

Fig. 1.5 Cluster plots on
(**a**) orthogonal and (**b**) polar
scale for SNPs with easily
called genotypes and (**c**) for
more problematic SNP.
Taken from [28]

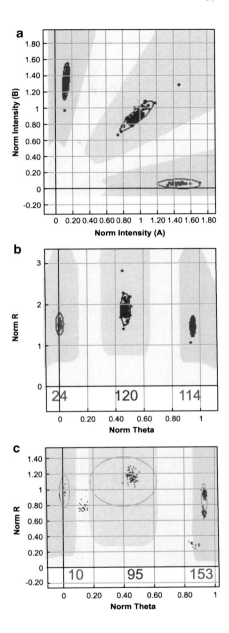

Generally it is more difficult to call rare SNPs than common SNPs since this
requires identification of the one or two clusters which are either very small or
completely absent. Copy number variation at a particular SNP site can produce very
difficult to interpret cluster plots, since intensities of samples exhibiting multiple
copies of the surrounding sequence will be unexpectedly amplified.

1.5   Overview of GWAS Genotype Arrays

At most arrays used in GWAS studies to date genotype approximately 500,000 to 1 million SNPs per sample, with an average spacing between SNPs of 3,000–6,000 base pairs (kb). This number of SNPs provides surrogates for (based on linkage disequilibrium, see Chap. 2) not only of most common SNPs but also of most common variants of other types, such as insertion/deletion polymorphisms and copy number variants. As described above, some portions of the genome contain too many repetitive elements to be amenable to probe design so that a certain fraction of the genome necessarily remains uncovered by GWAS arrays. Here the term *common variant* generally refers to alleles between 5 and 95 % in frequency in large human populations. The actual alleles that are common vary between populations and GWAS arrays targeting all variants common in African-origin populations require more SNPs since large populations have been in existence in Africa longer than in other portions of the world, allowing more time for recombination to have taken place (see Chap. 2). Until recently the focus of GWAS studies has been on common variation, partly because common variation is easier to interrogate than rare variation, but also because of theoretical arguments that common variation ought to contribute much more than rare variation to the risk of most common diseases (see Chap. 2). At present there is increased focus on rare variation, and certain GWAS arrays now have increased the number of SNPs present up to several million. General purpose GWAS arrays are produced by two main companies, Illumina based in San Diego and Affymetrix based in Santa Clara. In addition to these general purpose arrays, a number of custom arrays have been used widely in the GWAS community; these include fine-mapping chips designed to follow up GWAS associations in cancer (ICOGS chip) [36] and metabolic diseases (Metabochip) [37] and arrays targeting (the generally rare) nonsynonymous variation in exons (Exome chip) [23]. Additional chips of this type will undoubtedly continue to be developed and genotyped in large numbers.

1.6   Software and Data Resources

Some of the most important software and data resources helpful in the design, analysis, and interpretation of genome-wide association studies include:

1. *PLINK* [38] for manipulation, summarization, and cleaning of large-scale genetic marker datasets composed of diallelic variants, i.e., SNPs; in addition, PLINK can be used for many types of association analysis (note that the name PLINK is pronounced to rhyme with "blink"). This program is freely downloadable and the download point can easily be located by a web search using the keywords PLINK (current URL is *pngu.mgh.harvard.edu/~purcell/plink/*).
2. *EIGENSTRAT* [39] for principal components analysis (see Chaps. 2 and 4).
3. *MACH* [40], *SHAPEIT* [41], *BEAGLE* [42], and *IMPUTE2* [43] for haplotype phasing and genotype imputation (see Chaps. 5 and 6).

4. *QUANTO* [44] for sample size calculations.
5. *EMMAX* [45] for mixed model analysis of population stratification (see Chap. 4).
6. *GCTA* [46] for heritability analysis (see Chap. 8).

In addition to these stand-alone programs, there are a large number of *R* packages that have been developed for various aspects of genetic analysis, and it is assumed that the reader of this book is generally familiar with the *R* system (*R* is also freely downloadable from The Comprehensive R Archive Network cran.r-project.org). This book illustrates many concepts using simple simulations and analyses in *R*; *R* itself however is awkward for genome-wide analyses primarily because of weaknesses in input and output of very large files. However, *R* can be very useful in manipulating the output from the special purpose programs mentioned above, for summarization and graphical display. Also of note are the bioconductor packages for various genomics tasks that run within *R*, one of which is described below.

Finally the use of SAS (Cary NC, a definitely not-free program) is worth mention. While not optimized for GWAS analysis, SAS is very capable of processing large data files quickly including interpretation of complex user statements and macros. There are many cases when analysts need to use methods not available in the stand-alone programs, and there are many more options for performing the association tests built into the flagship SAS analysis procedures such as PROC GLM, PROC LOGISTIC, and PROC PHREG (for linear, logistic, and time to event modeling) than in PLINK. With some programming work SAS macros can be developed for genome-wide association analyses and will run quite well.

1.7 Web Resources

A great deal of information about human genetics and GWAS studies is available on the web. A short list of some of the most important resources is provided here and others are introduced in additional chapters.

1.7.1 Basic Genomics

dbSNP database, http://www.ncbi.nlm.nih.gov/projects/SNP/. This very extensive repository began as and continues to be the place that SNPs and other variants are reported (after discovery), compiled, and officially named. It provides technical details and extensive SNP annotation and links to other related resources.

UCSC Genome Browser, http://genome.ucsc.edu/. This website contains many important tools and datasets compiling sequence information for many genomes. The *blat* tool which maps sequences to genome location and strand is available here.

The HapMap project website, http://hapmap.ncbi.nlm.nih.gov/. This website gives results of extensive genotyping (in phases 1 and 2 of the project) of a total of 270 individuals comprised of 90 Yoruba in Ibadan, Nigeria (abbreviation: YRI); 45 Japanese in Tokyo, Japan (JPT); 45 Han Chinese in Beijing, China (CHB); and 90 CEPH (Utah residents with ancestry from northern and western Europe, CEU). These participants were genotyped for a total of over 3.1 million SNPs selected from the dbSNP repository. The HapMap phase 1 + 2 data were the primary source of genotype frequency and linkage disequilibrium information (see Chap. 2) used to select SNPs for most of the current generation of general purpose GWAS chips. HapMap phase 3 used two of the GWAS chips to genotype approximately 1.6 million SNPs in samples from a total of 11 populations.

1000 Genomes Project website, http://www.1000genomes.org/. This website provides results of next-generation sequencing (see Chap. 8) of 1,092 individuals from a variety of racial ethnic groups of similar diversity as HapMap phase 3. An aim of the project is to find most SNPs of frequency 1 % or greater in the populations studied. The resulting datasets currently serve as a reference panel for a great deal of large-scale SNP imputation (see Chap. 6) and as a source of genetic information for GWAS and specialty chip development.

Exome Sequencing Project ESP [47] http://evs.gs.washington.edu/EVS/. The goal of the NHLBI GO Exome Sequencing Project (ESP) is to discover novel genes and mechanisms contributing to heart, lung, and blood disorders by pioneering the application of next-generation sequencing of the protein coding regions of the human genome across diverse, richly phenotyped populations and to share these datasets and findings with the scientific community to extend and enrich the diagnosis, management, and treatment of heart, lung, and blood disorders.

1.7.2   GWAS Associations

A Catalog of Published Genome-Wide Association Studies [48] http://www. genome.gov/gwastudies/. This easily accessed and downloaded database provides a list of the thousands of published GWAS associations (with associations meeting statistical criteria for global significance) in human diseases and disease-related traits that have been discovered to date. The database is currently being updated regularly.

1.7.3   Annotation

For most common diseases, the vast majority of GWAS associations are with SNPs outside of coding regions [48, 49], either in introns or in *intergenic* regions, and not in LD with protein-altering variants. There has been much effort placed on predicting the functional implications of coding variants, but attempts to annotate the kinds of noncoding variants mostly associated in GWAS studies are more recent. Several different approaches are embodied in the websites, programs, and databases described below. By analyzing global RNA expression within individual tissues and treating the expression levels of genes as quantitative traits, variations in gene expression that are highly correlated with genetic variation can be identified as *expression quantitative trait loci*, or *eQTLs*. SNPs that have been observed to be correlated with gene expression, especially in tissues related to a disease of interest, become candidate functional variants when they are in LD with a GWAS hit. Sequence conservation over species is another potential source of annotation information since highly conserved regions are thought to have functional importance. Sequence conservation is used extensively in analysis of the significance of coding variation but can also be applied to noncoding regions. Analysis of chromatin packaging of DNA in a number of different tissues has been a key part of the identification of functional regions by the ENCODE and other projects, as has the identification of DNA sequences that serve as protein binding sites. The following is a selection of some of the currently utilized tools for identifying causal variation underlying GWAS associations:

SIFT [15] http://sift.jcvi.org/. Provides predictions of whether protein amino acid substitutions affect protein function. SIFT prediction is based upon the conservation of amino acid residues in sequence alignments from closely related sequences across species.

Polyphen2 [16] http://genetics.bwh.harvard.edu/pph2/. Also provides predictions of the significance of amino acid substitutions on protein function; these predictions are based upon analysis of disease-causing variants in human Mendelian disorders as well as on between-species sequence conservation.

The Genotype-Tissue Expression Project [50] http://www.broadinstitute.org/gtex/. The Genotype-Tissue Expression (GTEx) correlates human gene expression in a variety of tissues to genetic variation. This ongoing project will collect and analyze multiple human tissues from donors who are also densely genotyped for discovery and cataloging of additional eQTLs.

Gene Expression Variation (Genevar) [51] http://www.sanger.ac.uk/resources/software/genevar/. Genevar provides a database and browser of SNP-gene associations in eQTL studies including studies of adipose, LCL, and skin tissues collected from 856 healthy female twins of the MuTHER resource [52, 53]; lymphoblastoid cell lines from 726 HapMap3 CEU, CHB, GIH, JPT, LWK, MEX, MKK, and YRI individuals [54]; and fibroblast, LCL, and T-cells derived from umbilical cords of 75 Geneva GenCord individuals [55].

Encyclopedia of DNA Elements (ENCODE) [12] http://genome.ucsc.edu/ENCODE/. This is an ambitious project and consortium dedicated to identifying all functional elements of the human genome sequence. The primary assays used in ENCODE are ChiP-seq used to identify binding sites of DNA-associated proteins,

DNase I hypersensitivity which identifies regions of exposed (and hence actively transcribed) DNA, RNA sequencing, and assays of DNA methylation. The ENCODE project currently archives data at the UCSC Genome Bioinformatics Site, and a comprehensive data portal for ENCODE is under construction.

RegulomeDB [56] http://regulome.stanford.edu. RegulomeDB is a database that annotates SNPs with known and predicted regulatory elements in the intergenic regions of the human genome. Known and predicted regulatory DNA elements include regions of DNAse hypersensitivity, binding sites of transcription factors, and promoter regions that have been biochemically characterized to regulation transcription. Source of these data include public datasets from GEO, the ENCODE project, and published literature.

FunciSNP [49] http://bioconductor.org/packages/2.12/bioc/html/FunciSNP. html. This R package integrates information from GWAS, 1000 Genomes, and chromatin marks to identify functional SNPs in coding or noncoding regions. It is especially useful in finding all variants in LD with a given marker (e.g., a GWAS hit) and screening them for overlaps with known or predicted functional features.

HaploReg [57] http://www.broadinstitute.org/mammals/haploreg/haploreg. php. This online tool uses LD information from the 1000 Genomes Project to find SNPs and indels that are linked to a user-supplied GWAS hit and display predicted chromatin state in nine cell types, sequence conservation across species, effect on regulatory motifs, and enrichment of cell type-specific enhancers.

1.8   Hardware and Operating Systems

Most analyses for GWAS studies can be performed on single-user single-"node" machines either running Windows or Unix/Linux/Mac based. This includes most QC work and simple association tests. However, there are several important analyses that require so much computation that they typically are best performed on a computer cluster which can allow many jobs to run simultaneously rather than sequentially. Examples of these analyses include relatedness checking (discussed in Chap. 2) and genome-wide SNP imputation (discussed in Chap. 6).

Because such clusters are important and because Linux is a de facto standard operating system for these clusters, we assume in the data analysis that the reader of this book has access to a Linux-based cluster. The structure of this cluster is assumed to be as follows. There is a login node with a relatively small amount of memory available. Accessible to the login node is a (large) number of other processors with a range of memory available (up to several gigabytes or more). All nodes including the login node have access (pending appropriate permission) to all files on a (large) file system suitable for storing GWAS-sized datasets (many gigabytes for each analysis) and for providing workspace for large temporary files. In order to run anything more than the simplest sort of Linux commands, one uses the Linux *Portable Batch System* (*PBS*) *qsub* or equivalent command to request one or more nodes for job processing. This command can be used interactively (qsub -I), in which case one node is made available for the user to run programs on that node, or (more commonly) in batch mode. In batch mode it is assumed that before issuing qsub commands the user develops one or more PBS files that contain the sequence of commands to be executed in the course of the computer run. These commands are then submitted (using the qsub *filename* command syntax). Many different jobs can be started using qsub and will be queued and run when resources are available.

1.9   Data Example

The primary example used in this book is based on the Japanese American Prostate Cancer (JAPC) study [58], a relatively small but quite interesting GWAS study of prostate cancer that used an Illumina.Human660W_Quad_v1 SNP array to genotype approximately 600,000 SNPs. We will illustrate some standard QC checks, basic (single SNP) analyses of these data, correction for population stratification, and use of the software packages above to manipulate and analyze these data. These data are chosen because of the author's familiarity with the data as well as the fact that these data may (with proper authorization) be downloaded from the dbGAP website. Note that basic association results for this study have been published by Cheng et al. [58].

In the analysis of these data, we assume that we are starting out with genotype calls rather than the raw intensity data that the scanning platform produces as its native output. In fact we assume that we have available PLINK-formatted files *japc. bim, japc.fam, japc.bed*, and *japc_variables.txt* for the JAPC study. In addition an SNP information file available from Illumina (Human660W-Quad_v1_H.csv) for this chip is assumed available.

Three of the four available files are "human readable." *japc.bed* on the other hand is a binary file (containing genotypes in compressed format). Let us consider each of the files.

japc.bim is an SNP information file that contains fields for *chromosome, rsnumber or snp identifier, genetic distance, and physical location* for each SNP with data. Note that the Illumina information file Human660W-Quad_v1_H.csv contains much more information than this for each SNP. We will discuss this file as well, but it is not used directly in PLINK.

japc.fam is a sample identification file that contains fields *family id, individual id, father's id, mother's id, sex* (1 for males 2 for females), and *status* (1 for unaffected 2 for affected).

japc_variables.txt is a file that contains covariates and disease status for each individual. The fields are *famid, iid, aff*, and *age*. The *famid* and *iid* variables must appear in the *japc.fam* file in order to match the covariates to the samples with genotypes. Note here that affection status *aff* is coded slightly differently than is *status* on the genotype file; here *0* means unaffected, while *1* means affected. When logistic regression is used in PLINK (see Chap. 3), the status variable used is *aff* from the *japc_variables.txt* file. Note that the data contained in the files *japc. bim, japc.fam, and japc.bed* are all strictly defined by PLINK. The additional file *japc_variables.txt* has variables which will depend upon the needs of specific analyses. For example, we wish to adjust by age in the analysis so age is included (as a dichotomous variable).

The following PLINK commands are worth practicing:

```
plink --bfile japc --missing
```

This will create files called plink.imiss and plink.lmiss which contain information about the fraction of SNPs genotypes that are missing either by subject (imiss) or by SNP (lmiss). To change the name of the output files from plink.imiss and plink.lmiss, simply assign a new name using an –out command as in

```
plink --bfile japc --missing -- out check1
```

Then the output files will be called check1.imiss and check1.lmiss, respectively. To calculate frequencies, running the command

```
plink --bfile japc --freq
```

will create a file plink.frq which lists the following for each SNP:

```
CHR        Chromosome
SNP        SNP identifier
A1         Allele 1 code (minor allele)
A2         Allele 2 code (major allele)
MAF        Minor allele frequency
NCHROBS    Non-missing allele count
```

While this book will not attempt to teach all of the PLINK commands, PLINK will be used in many examples to follow. Documentation is available online from the program's author (Sean Purcell) http://pngu.mgh.harvard.edu/~purcell/plink/.

1.9.1 Save Your Work

Data cleaning and association testing using GWAS data is (nearly) always a multi-step process. It is important to automate all processes, by writing shell scripts, both so they can be run again on similar data and also so as to keep records of exactly what analyses were done to achieve the results on a given dataset that are used in manuscripts, reports, papers, books, etc. The Linux system and other Unix-based systems have powerful scripting capabilities as well as many built-in programs that aid in developing an analysis pipeline.

Homework Problems/Projects

1. The SNP information file from Illumina for the GWAS chip used in the JAPC study lists surrounding sequence information for each SNP. One of these is given below (for SNP designated rs1008618). Use the *blat* utility found on the UCSC Genome Browser (http://genome.ucsc.edu/cgi-bin/hgBlat?command=start) to identify the chromosome and strand (plus or minus) that this sequence refers to. Select the Feb 2009 build 37 (GRCh37/hg19) genome assembly in the box provided. The SNP of interest immediately follows the last base sequence given.

   AGGAGAAACATTTGCAAAAACCTTCTATGGAGACAAGAGAGATGA-
   GAGAGACTATGATGA

   Do the same for SNP rs1008619 with flanking sequence

   CCTTTACTCCTTCAGATTAGTCCAAAATATGGCTGCCAGAAT-
   GAGCTTCCTGAAGCACAA

   If the SNP of interest follows immediately on the right, then what is the position number of each SNP? Check your results using dbSNP.
2. The following flanking sequence (around a C/T SNP)

   AGATGATCAACAATTCAACACTCTTA[C/T]CTGGAGTCAAACTGGGGTATGAAAT

   refers to a nonsynonymous SNP in a gene that may be related to prostate cancer risk.

   (a) Use the web resources above to find the gene this SNP is in as well as its rs-number, chromosome, and position.
   (b) Which strand (+ or −) is the coding strand for the gene?
   (c) What is the amino acid change coded for by this SNP? What is the amino acid position number within the protein where this change occurs?

3. What factors affect the probability that a new de novo SNV in an exon will be synonymous, nonsynonymous, or cause a STOP codon? Note that base position within the codon is important, i.e., from Table 1.1 changes in the last codon often do not affect the coded amino acid. Consider the codon TTT which codes for the amino acid Phenylalanine.

   (a) If transitions are twice as common as transversions, what is the distribution of resulting codons due to a single-nucleotide change?
   (b) What is the distribution of resulting amino acid or stop codons? Assume that the probability of a change at each of the three positions is equal.

4. Even when using interactive programs such as R for certain tasks, it is important to record all the steps used to produce results, for example, by saving and polishing or otherwise improving the job history logs (.RHistory files) produced by R and saving them for future reference. Is R able to run in batch mode? How would a PBS (qsub) file call R to execute a text file containing R code and return results?

5. Note that there are several individuals listed in the *japc.fam* file who do not have sex or status defined on the file, NA for sex and -9 for status. We assume that all JAPC participants are males, and affection status is available on the *japc_variables.txt* file. Read the description of the PLINK commands in the data management section of the PLINK online documentation to learn the recommended way of fixing these issues (i.e., inputting correct sex and affection status into the .fam file for those with missing data). Of course one could manually (or with a program like SAS) edit the *japc.fam* file outside of PLINK. What is wrong with the latter approach?

6. The ENCODE project has recently published information about the role of noncoding DNA claiming that at least 80 % of human DNA is "active and needed" [59]. Review the publications from ENCODE, what sorts of techniques are used to make this determination? For a counterview, try reading reference [60].

7. Using the databases above: a genome-wide association study (GWAS) of breast cancer was conducted using the Illumina 1M SNP array in 15,000 cases and 15,000 controls of European ancestry. In this study a novel risk variant, rs11196191 (A allele, frequency $= 0.52$, OR per A allele $= 1.25$, $p = 10^{-10}$), was identified.

(A) Where is the novel breast cancer risk variant located with respect to chromosome location, genome position?

(B) Where is the SNP according to gene (i.e., upstream of gene or in an exon or intron—what gene)?

(C) What are the two alleles and the global minor allele frequency according to 1000 Genomes Project?

(D) Has this region been previously associated with any other disease or trait from a GWAS? If so, which SNP and which disease in particular and where is the variant located with respect to rs11196191?

(E) Using the ESP database, determine how many missense, nonsense/frameshift variants with frequencies >1 % are in the coding region of the nearby gene. Are these SNPs likely to explain the association? Why or why not?

(F) What is the frequency of the risk allele in 1000 Genomes Project populations?

(G) Is the breast cancer risk SNP correlated with the SNP(s) in D (above). Provide R^2. Use FunciSNP or HaploReg.

(H) Determine whether the risk allele for breast cancer is correlated with the allele that is associated with increased risk for the other phenotype.

(I) What does the information in H (above) tell you about pathways or mechanisms of disease for these phenotypes? (Bonus: What is the term used to describe a genetic effect of a single gene or variant on multiple phenotypic traits?)

References

1. Watson, J. D., & Crick, F. H. (1953). Molecular structure of nucleic acids; a structure for deoxyribose nucleic acid. *Nature, 171,* 737–738.
2. Watson, J. D., & Crick, F. H. (1953). Genetical implications of the structure of deoxyribonucleic acid. *Nature, 171,* 964–967.
3. Darwin, C. (1859). *On the origin of species by means of natural selection, or, the preservation of favoured races in the struggle for life.* London: John Murray.
4. Muller, H. J. (1927). Artificial transmutation of the gene. *Science, 66,* 84–87.
5. Beadle, G. W., & Tatum, E. L. (1941). Genetic control of biochemical reactions in Neurospora. *Proceedings of the National Academy of Sciences USA, 27,* 499–506.
6. Kimura, M., & Crow, J. F. (1964). The number of alleles that can be maintained in a finite population. *Genetics, 49,* 725–738.
7. Kimura, M. (1983). Rare variant alleles in the light of the neutral theory. *Molecular Biology and Evolution, 1,* 84–93.
8. Baker, B. S., Carpenter, A. T., Esposito, M. S., Esposito, R. E., & Sandler, L. (1976). The genetic control of meiosis. *Annual Review of Genetics, 10,* 53–134.
9. Kabak, D. B. (1996). Chromosome-size dependent control of meiotic recombination in humans. *Nature Genetics, 13,* 20–21.
10. KabackD, B., Guacci, V., Barber, D., & Mahon, J. W. (1992). Chromosome size-dependent control of meiotic recombination. *Science, 256,* 228–232.
11. Okamoto, I., Otte, A. P., Allis, C. D., Reinberg, D., & Heard, E. (2004). Epigenetic dynamics of imprinted X inactivation during early mouse development. *Science, 303,* 644–649.
12. Ecker, J. R., Bickmore, W. A., Barroso, I., Pritchard, J. K., Gilad, Y., & Segal, E. (2012). Genomics: ENCODE explained. *Nature, 489,* 52–55.
13. Abecasis, G. R., Auton, A., Brooks, L. D., DePristo, M. A., Durbin, R. M., Handsaker, R. E., et al. (2012). An integrated map of genetic variation from 1,092 human genomes. *Nature, 491,* 56–65.
14. King, M. C., Marks, J. H., & Mandell, J. B. (2003). Breast and ovarian cancer risks due to inherited mutations in BRCA1 and BRCA2. *Science, 302,* 643–646.
15. Kumar, P., Henikoff, S., & Ng, P. C. (2009). Predicting the effects of coding non-synonymous variants on protein function using the SIFT algorithm. *Nature Protocols, 4,* 1073–1081.
16. Adzhubei, I. A., Schmidt, S., Peshkin, L., Ramensky, V. E., Gerasimova, A., Bork, P., et al. (2010). A method and server for predicting damaging missense mutations. *Nature Methods, 7,* 248–249.
17. Nelson, S. (2011, March 25). UW Genetics Coordinating Center: the + and – of DNA strand issues, p 21. University of Washington, Seattle, WA
18. Zhang, Z., & Gerstein, M. (2003). Patterns of nucleotide substitution, insertion and deletion in the human genome inferred from pseudogenes. *Nucleic Acids Research, 31,* 5338–5348.
19. Iafrate, A. J., Feuk, L., Rivera, M. N., Listewnik, M. L., Donahoe, P. K., Qi, Y., et al. (2004). Detection of large-scale variation in the human genome. *Nature Genetics, 36,* 949–951.
20. Sebat, J., Lakshmi, B., Troge, J., Alexander, J., Young, J., Lundin, P., et al. (2004). Large-scale copy number polymorphism in the human genome. *Science, 305,* 525–528.
21. Feuk, L., Carson, A. R., & Scherer, S. W. (2006). Structural variation in the human genome. *Nature Reviews. Genetics, 7,* 85–97.
22. Bunin, G. R., Needle, M., & Riccardi, V. M. (1997). Paternal age and sporadic neurofibromatosis 1: a case-control study and consideration of the methodologic issues. *Genetic Epidemiology, 14,* 507–516.
23. Haiman, C. A., Han, Y., Feng, Y., Xia, L., Hsu, C., Sheng, X., et al. (2013). Genome-wide testing of putative functional exonic variants in relationship with breast and prostate cancer risk in a multiethnic population. *PLoS Genetics, 9,* e1003419.

24. Nackley, A. G., Shabalina, S. A., Tchivileva, I. E., Satterfield, K., Korchynskyi, O., Makarov, S. S., et al. (2006). Human catechol-O-methyltransferase haplotypes modulate protein expression by altering mRNA secondary structure. *Science, 314*, 1930–1933.

25. Tamiya, G., Shinya, M., Imanishi, T., Ikuta, T., Makino, S., Okamoto, K., et al. (2005). Whole genome association study of rheumatoid arthritis using 27 039 microsatellites. *Human Molecular Genetics, 14*, 2305–2321.

26. Taylor, R. W., & Turnbull, D. M. (2005). Mitochondrial DNA mutations in human disease. *Nature Reviews. Genetics, 6*, 389–402.

27. Holt, I. J., Harding, A. E., & Morgan-Hughes, J. A. (1988). Deletions of muscle mitochondrial DNA in patients with mitochondrial myopathies. *Nature, 331*, 717–719.

28. Illumina. (2009). Improved cluster generation with Gentrain2, Illumina Inc, San Diego

29. Schillert, A., & Ziegler, A. (2012). Genotype calling for the Affymetrix platform. *Methods in Molecular Biology, 850*, 513–523.

30. Korn, J. M., Kuruvilla, F. G., McCarroll, S. A., Wysoker, A., Nemesh, J., Cawley, S., et al. (2008). Integrated genotype calling and association analysis of SNPs, common copy number polymorphisms and rare CNVs. *Nature Genetics, 40*, 1253–1260.

31. Giannoulatou, E., Yau, C., Colella, S., Ragoussis, J., & Holmes, C. C. (2008). GenoSNP: a variational Bayes within-sample SNP genotyping algorithm that does not require a reference population. *Bioinformatics, 24*, 2209–2214.

32. Carvalho, B., Bengtsson, H., Speed, T. P., & Irizarry, R. A. (2007). Exploration, normalization, and genotype calls of high-density oligonucleotide SNP array data. *Biostatistics, 8*, 485–499.

33. Browning, B. L., & Yu, Z. (2009). Simultaneous genotype calling and haplotype phasing improves genotype accuracy and reduces false-positive associations for genome-wide association studies. *American Journal of Human Genetics, 85*, 847–861.

34. AFFYMETRIX. (2006). BRLMM: an improved genotype calling method for the GeneChip Human Mapping 500K Array Set. Santa Clara, CA: Affymetrix.

35. Li, G., Gelernter, J., Kranzler, H. R., & Zhao, H. (2012). M(3): an improved SNP calling algorithm for Illumina BeadArray data. *Bioinformatics, 28*, 358–365.

36. Eeles, R. A., Olama, A. A. A., Benlloch, S., Saunders, E. J., Leongamornlert, D. A., Tymrakiewicz, M., Ghoussaini, M., et al. (2013) Identification of 23 novel prostate cancer susceptibility loci using a custom array (the iCOGS) in an international consortium, PRACTICAL. *Nature Genetics, 45*, 385–391.

37. Wu, Y., Waite, L. L., Jackson, A. U., Sheu, W. H. H., Buyske, S., Absher, D., et al. (2013). Trans-ethnic fine-mapping of lipid loci identifies population-specific signals and allelic heterogeneity that increases the trait variance explained. *PLoS Genetics, 9*, e1003379.

38. Purcell, S., Neale, B., Todd-Brown, K., Thomas, L., Ferreira, M. A., Bender, D., et al. (2007). PLINK: a tool set for whole-genome association and population-based linkage analyses. *American Journal of Human Genetics, 81*, 559–575.

39. Price, A. L., Patterson, N. J., Plenge, R. M., Weinblatt, M. E., Shadick, N. A., & Reich, D. (2006). Principal components analysis corrects for stratification in genome-wide association studies. *Nature Genetics, 38*, 904–909.

40. Li, Y., Willer, C. J., Ding, J., Scheet, P., & Abecasis, G. R. (2010). MaCH: using sequence and genotype data to estimate haplotypes and unobserved genotypes. *Genetic Epidemiology, 34*, 816–834.

41. Delaneau, O., Marchini, J., & Zagury, J.-F. (2011). A linear complexity phasing method for thousands of genomes. *Nature Methods, 9*, 179–181.

42. Browning, B. L., & Browning, S. R. (2009). A unified approach to genotype imputation and haplotype-phase inference for large data sets of trios and unrelated individuals. *American Journal of Human Genetics, 84*, 210–223.

43. Howie, B. N., Donnelly, P., & Marchini, J. (2009). Impute2: a flexible and accurate genotype imputation method for the next generation of genome-wide association studies. *PLoS Genetics, 5*, e1000529.

44. Gauderman, W., & Morrison, J. (2006). QUANTO 1.1: a computer program for power and sample size calculations for genetic-epidemiology studies. http://hydra.usc.edu/gxe

45. Kang, H. M., Sul, J. H., Service, S. K., Zaitlen, N. A., Kong, S. Y., Freimer, N. B., et al. (2010). Variance component model to account for sample structure in genome-wide association studies. *Nature Genetics, 42*, 348–354.

46. Yang, J., Lee, S. H., Goddard, M. E., & Visscher, P. M. (2011). GCTA: a tool for genome-wide complex trait analysis. *The American Journal of Human Genetics, 88*, 76–82.

47. Fu, W., O'Connor, T. D., Jun, G., Kang, H. M., Abecasis, G., Leal, S. M., et al. (2013). Analysis of 6,515 exomes reveals the recent origin of most human protein-coding variants. *Nature, 493*, 216–220.

48. Hindorff, L. A., Sethupathy, P., Junkins, H. A., Ramos, E. M., Mehta, J. P., Collins, F. S., et al. (2009). Potential etiologic and functional implications of genome-wide association loci for human diseases and traits. *Proceedings of the National Academy of Sciences USA, 106*, 9362–9367.

49. Coetzee, S. G., Rhie, S. K., Berman, B. P., Coetzee, G. A., & Noushmehr, H. (2012). FunciSNP: an R/bioconductor tool integrating functional non-coding data sets with genetic association studies to identify candidate regulatory SNPs. *Nucleic Acids Research, 40*, e139.

50. GTEx Consortium. (2013). The Genotype-Tissue Expression (GTEx) project. *Nature Genetics, 45*, 580–585.

51. Yang, T. P., Beazley, C., Montgomery, S. B., Dimas, A. S., Gutierrez-Arcelus, M., Stranger, B. E., et al. (2010). Genevar: a database and Java application for the analysis and visualization of SNP-gene associations in eQTL studies. *Bioinformatics, 26*, 2474–2476.

52. Nica, A. C., Parts, L., Glass, D., Nisbet, J., Barrett, A., Sekowska, M., et al. (2011). The architecture of gene regulatory variation across multiple human tissues: the MuTHER study. *PLoS Genetics, 7*, e1002003.

53. Grundberg, E., Small, K. S., Hedman, A. K., Nica, A. C., Buil, A., Keildson, S., et al. (2012). Mapping cis- and trans-regulatory effects across multiple tissues in twins. *Nature Genetics, 44*, 1084–1089.

54. Stranger, B. E., Montgomery, S. B., Dimas, A. S., Parts, L., Stegle, O., Ingle, C. E., et al. (2012). Patterns of cis regulatory variation in diverse human populations. *PLoS Genetics, 8*, e1002639.

55. Dimas, A. S., Deutsch, S., Stranger, B. E., Montgomery, S. B., Borel, C., Attar-Cohen, H., et al. (2009). Common regulatory variation impacts gene expression in a cell type-dependent manner. *Science, 325*, 1246–1250.

56. Boyle, A. P., Hong, E. L., Hariharan, M., Cheng, Y., Schaub, M. A., Kasowski, M., et al. (2012). Annotation of functional variation in personal genomes using RegulomeDB. *Genome Research, 22*, 1790–1797.

57. Ward, L. D., & Kellis, M. (2012). HaploReg: a resource for exploring chromatin states, conservation, and regulatory motif alterations within sets of genetically linked variants. *Nucleic Acids Research, 40*, D930–D934.

58. Cheng, I., Chen, G. K., Nakagawa, H., He, J., Wan, P., Lurie, C., et al. (2012). Evaluating genetic risk for prostate cancer among Japanese and Latinos. *Cancer Epidemiology, Biomarkers & Prevention, 21*(11), 2048–2058.

59. Kolata, G. (2012, September 15). Bits of mystery DNA, far from 'junk,' play crucial role. *New York Times*, New York, NY

60. Graur, D., Zheng, Y., Price, N., Azevedo, R. B. R., Zufall, R. A., & Elhaik, E. (2013). On the immortality of television sets: "function" in the human genome according to the evolution-free gospel of ENCODE. *Genome Biology and Evolution, 5*, 578–590.

61. Kwok, P. Y. (2001). Methods for genotyping single nucleotide polymorphisms. *Annual Review of Genomics and Human Genetics, 2*, 235–258.

Chapter 2
Topics in Quantitative Genetics

Abstract An understanding of the genetics of current world populations provides the conceptual basis upon which today's genetic association studies rest. This chapter focuses specifically on gaining a basic grounding in three general topics:

1. *Linkage disequilibrium* **(LD), the nonrandom associations of alleles**. A discussion on how linkage disequilibrium varies between populations due to multiple factors, such as random drift in allele frequencies in isolated populations, population migration, *admixture*, and population expansion.
2. **Population heterogeneity**. A discussion of the effects of population heterogeneity, including population stratification, admixture, and relatedness between subjects—specifically, the distribution of *marker alleles* and their apparent association with each other and with causal variants, using marker data for the empirical *estimation of relatedness* and *kinship coefficients* and of *identity by descent* probabilities.
3. **The common disease-common variant hypothesis**. Arguments in favor of the *common disease-common variant hypothesis* and a discussion of distributions of allele frequencies for both marker alleles and causal variants.

In addition to these concepts, several important tools for the investigation of linkage disequilibrium and of population heterogeneity are introduced: specifically data from the HapMap project and data manipulation and LD visualization tools which help to explore these data effectively. *Principal components analysis* (PCA) of large-scale genetic data for the purpose of examining population substructure and admixture is introduced and illustrated using a download of phase 3 HapMap data for 11 population samples; an example of some simple PLINK commands and a corresponding R script is provided. These illustrate the selection (in PLINK) of a subset of SNPs to be used in the computation and display, by R, of leading principal components that characterize global population structure.

D.O. Stram, *Design, Analysis, and Interpretation of Genome-Wide Association Scans*,
Statistics for Biology and Health, DOI 10.1007/978-1-4614-9443-0_2,
© Springer Science+Business Media New York 2014

Many parts of the broader field of population genetics are entirely ignored here. Notably we do not discuss, except parenthetically, natural selection as a force determining allele frequency distributions within modern populations or the differences seen between modern populations. Differences between populations in allele frequencies for marker alleles or causal variants are largely assumed here to be due to random drift or founder effects and population expansion.

Implicitly we are restricting interest, and this is part of topic (3), to common genetic causes of disease. The mere fact that the alleles are common indicates that the reproductive fitness of carriers of the alleles is not greatly impacted; even when looking at *diseases* that do affect reproductive fitness (such as fatal childhood diseases, early adult onset mental illnesses), the selective pressure against alleles that cause modest increases in risk of such disease may be very minor if the diseases themselves are rare.

2.1   Distribution of a Single Diallelic Variant in a Randomly Mixing Population

2.1.1   Hardy–Weinberg Equilibrium

The description in Chap. 1 of the mechanics of gamete formation provides the basis for a discussion of first the marginal distribution of allele counts for a single individual and secondly the joint distribution of these counts between related individuals. The *Hardy–Weinberg rule* states that under a number of assumptions, the marginal distribution of the number of copies of a given allele observed in a single individual will follow a binomial distribution with index (i.e., the "number of trials") equal to 2 and mean parameter equal to the frequency in the population of that allele. For example, if we have a diallelic marker taking the values A with frequency p and a with frequency $(1 - p)$, then the number of copies, n_A, of A that a given individual carries will take the values 0, 1, and 2 with probabilities equal to $(1 - p)^2$, $2p(1 - p)$, and p^2, respectively. If an allele count, n_A, follows this distribution, then we say that it is in *Hardy–Weinberg equilibrium* with the name being reflective of the independent derivation of this rule by Godfrey Hardy and Wilhelm Weinberg in 1908. This marginal distribution applies to all individuals sampled from a given population for which there has been at least one generation of random mating; additional assumptions are that there is no reproductive disadvantage to carrying one or two of the two alleles (e.g., the allele does not increase the risk of early mortality and infertility) and that the number of copies carried by males is the same as that carried by females, e.g., the rule does not apply to X chromosome variants in males. Violations of random mating include the interrelated concepts of inbreeding, population stratification, and admixture, each of which will be discussed in the following.

2.1.2   Random Samples of Unrelated Individuals

Large-scale genotyping technology frees genetic studies from needing closely related individuals with disease, allowing for the (generally much easier) sampling of unrelated subjects from within a given population. If we have a sample of size N from a population in which the allele of interest is in Hardy–Weinberg equilibrium, and if the N individuals sampled are unrelated to each other (which is a reasonable expectation so long as the number of individuals sampled is small relative to the size of the population being targeted), then the distribution of the sum $\sum_{i=1}^{N} n_{iA}$ of the allele counts of allele A for each individual i will follow a binomial distribution with index equal to $2N$ and frequency also equal to p. In this case we can estimate p as $\hat{p} = \frac{1}{2N} \sum_{i=1}^{N} n_{iA}$. The variance of this estimator is then equal to

$$\frac{1}{(2N)^2} \sum_{i=1}^{N} \mathrm{Var}(n_{iA}) = \frac{1}{(2N)^2} 2Np(1-p) = \frac{1}{2N} p(1-p).$$

For values of N and p which jointly meet the requirement that $\min(2Np, 2N(1-p))$ is "large," the estimator $\hat{p}$ can be approximated as a normal random variable with mean p and standard error equal to $\sqrt{\frac{1}{2N}\hat{p}(1-\hat{p})}$ so that an approximate $1 - \alpha$ level confidence interval for p is given by

$$\hat{p} - z_{1-\alpha/2}\sqrt{\frac{\hat{p}(1-\hat{p})}{2N}} < p < \hat{p} + z_{1-\alpha/2}\sqrt{\frac{\hat{p}(1-\hat{p})}{2N}}. \tag{2.1}$$

The accuracy of such a confidence interval depends importantly on the type I error rate α; for the "traditional" α level of 0.05 , a value of $2Np$ of around 5 or so is generally considered adequate for the approximation to be reliable; however, for more rigorous α levels such as those often employed in GWAS studies (e.g., $\alpha = 5 \times 10^{-8}$), $2Np$ should be considerably larger (at least five times as large for common alleles) before approximate confidence intervals (and equivalently tests) can be safely relied upon. See Chap. 7 for more information.

2.1.3   Joint Distribution Between Relatives of Allele Counts for a Single SNP

In the following we consider the joint distribution of the number of copies, n_{iA}, and n_{jA} of the same diallelic variant taking values a and A, for two related individuals drawn from a randomly mixing population. Since the population is randomly

Table 2.1 All possible transmissions and number of copies of chromosomal region shared identically by descent for two full siblings

	Sibling 2			
Sibling 1	MGM, PGM	MGM, PGF	MGF, PGM	MGF, PGF
MGM, PGM	2	1	1	0
MGM, PGF	1	2	0	1
MGF, PGM	1	0	2	1
MGF, PGF	0	1	1	2

mixing, the marginal distribution of both n_{iA} and n_{jA} will follow the Hardy–Weinberg equilibrium, with the same value of allele frequency p, but the probabilities that each take the values 0, 1, or 2 will not be independent of each other. For example, if we select a mother and one of her children, the child will always share exactly one of the alleles of the mother, and so if the mother has genotype AA (for example), then it is impossible (in the absence of a de novo mutation) that the child will have n_{jA} equal to 0. This is because one chromosome is always passed from each parent to each offspring.

2.1.3.1 Identity by Descent

If we assume that all mating is between unrelated individuals, i.e., that the population is "outbred," then the degree of relatedness between individuals for whom a pedigree structure is known can be summarized in terms of the expected numbers of alleles that are inherited identically by descent from the founders of the pedigree. In order to clarify what inheritance *identical by descent* (*IBD*) means, consider a simple nuclear family with two parents and two offspring and we will label the four founders (parents) copies of a short chromosomal region according to whether the copy originated from each of the maternal grandmother (MGM), maternal grandfather (MGF), paternal grandmother (PGM), or paternal grandfather (PGF). Table 2.1 considers all 16 (equally probable for neutral alleles) combinations that could be transmitted to the two offspring and gives the number of copies of this segment that are therefore shared identically by descent. Since each cell has probability 1/16, we see that the probability (call it z_0) that the two siblings share no alleles is 1/4; the probability, z_2, they share two alleles is also 1/4; and the probability, z_1, that they share 1 allele is 1/2. Thus the expected number of shared copies is equal to $0 \times z_0 + 1 \times z_1 + 2 \times z_2 = 1$; dividing this by two gives the expected fraction of shared alleles as $(1/2)z_1 + z_2 = (1/2)$. Similar calculations for parent-offspring pairs give the three IBD sharing probabilities as $z_0 = 0$, $z_1 = 1$, and $z_2 = 0$ with the fraction of shared alleles again equal to $(1/2)$.[1]

---

[1] If however the maternal and/or paternal grandparents were related to each other, then there is a nonzero probability that a parent–offspring pair will share 2 alleles IBD, i.e., $z_2 > 0$. For example, if the parents are siblings, then the three IBD probabilities will be $z_0 = 0$, $z_1 = 5/8$, and $z_2 = 3/8$; *see below*.

Table 2.2 Joint probability distribution for counts, n, of number of copies of allele A given number of alleles shared IBD

Unphased genotype	n_1	n_2	Number of alleles shared IBD		
			0	1	2
(aa, aa)	0	0	$(1-p)^4$	$(1-p)^3$	$(1-p)^2$
(Aa, aa)	1	0	$2p(1-p)^3$	$p(1-p)^2$	0
(AA, aa)	2	0	$p^2(1-p)^2$	0	0
(aa, Aa)	0	1	$2p(1-p)^3$	$p(1-p)^2$	0
(Aa, Aa)	1	1	$4p^2(1-p)^2$	$p(1-p)^2 + (1-p)p^2$	$2p(1-p)$
(AA, Aa)	2	1	$2p^3(1-p)$	$p^2(1-p)$	0
(aa, AA)	0	2	$p^2(1-p)^2$	0	0
(Aa, AA)	1	2	$2p^3(1-p)$	$p^2(1-p)$	0
(AA, AA)	2	2	p^4	p^3	p^2

Such calculations can be extended to more complex pedigrees, and it can readily be shown, for example, that both half siblings and grandparent–grandchild pairs are expected to share 1/4 of their alleles IBD.

Now let us consider the *correlation* between the counts, $n_{A,1}$ and $n_{A,2}$, of an SNP allele observed in two related individuals (numbers 1 and 2) with a known relationship. We can compute the covariance between $n_{A,1}$ and $n_{A,2}$ as a function of the probabilities (z_0, z_1, z_2) of sharing either 0, 1, or 2 alleles identically by descent. To show this, we first need to describe the joint probability distribution of the count of a marker allele conditional on IBD status.

Table 2.2 shows the joint probabilities of n_1 and n_2 conditional on the number of alleles shared identically by descent. These probabilities are computed by simple counting assuming that both the shared and unshared alleles are sampled independently from a population of possible alleles. For example, the conditional probability of the genotype (Aa, Aa) being sampled given that 1 allele is shared in common can be broken into a fraction with numerator equal to

$\Pr(Aa, Aa$ is sampled$|$1st and 3rd alleles shared IBD$) \times \Pr($1st and 3rd alleles shared IBD$)$
$+ \Pr(Aa, Aa$ is sampled$|$1st and 4th alleles shared IBD$) \times \Pr($1st and 4th alleles shared IBD$)$
$+ \Pr(Aa, Aa$ is sampled$|$2nd and 3rd alleles shared IBD$) \times \Pr($2nd and 3rd alleles shared IBD$)$
$+ \Pr(Aa, Aa$ is sampled$|$2nd and 4th alleles shared IBD$) \times \Pr($2nd and 4th alleles shared IBD$)$

and denominator

$\Pr($1st and 3rd alleles shared$) + \Pr($1st and 4th alleles shared$)$
$+ \Pr($2nd and 3rd alleles shared$) + \Pr($2nd and 4th alleles shared$)$.

Consider the first probability $\Pr(Aa, Aa$ is sampled|1st and 3rd alleles shared). Since genotypes Aa and aA are treated here as indistinguishable, this probability can be further broken into the probability of sampling first an A (for the first and third alleles), then an a (for the 2nd allele), and then another a for the fourth allele, plus the probability of sampling first an a (for the first and third alleles) and then two A s in sequence (for the 2nd and 4th alleles). Thus, this probability is equal to $p(1-p)^2 + (1-p)p^2$. The same quantity is found for the 3 other sampling probabilities, and moreover the probability of sharing either the 1st and 3rd or 1st and 4th or 2nd and 3rd or 2nd and 4th are all equal to each other, i.e., are equal to some constant, c. Therefore the total conditional probability is

$$\frac{4c\left[p(1-p)^2 + (1-p)p^2\right]}{4c} = p(1-p)^2 + (1-p)p^2,$$

as presented in the table.

If we know (from the pedigree relationship) the probabilities, z_0, z_1, and z_2, of sharing zero one or two alleles IBD, then multiplying the rightmost three columns of Table 2.2 by z_0, z_1, or z_2, respectively, and summing them together, we have the complete joint probability distribution of n_1 and n_2. Hence, we can compute the covariance of n_1 and n_2 as a simple weighted sum of the possible values of $[n_1 - E(n_1)][n_2 - E(n_2)] = (n_1 - 2p)(n_2 - 2p)$ with the weights given by the joint probability distribution for n_1 and n_2. A little bit of algebra shows that

$$\mathrm{Cov}(n_1, n_2) = (z_1 + 2z_2)p(1-p).$$

Since the variance of n_{jA} is equal to $2p(1-p)$ for both $j = 1$ and $j = 2$, we see that the correlation between the allele counts for the two individuals will be $\mathrm{Cor}(n_1, n_2) = (1/2)z_1 + z_2$ which is from above the expected fraction of shared alleles. From this we can write the $n \times n$ covariance matrix of a single SNP allele for all related subjects, as equal to

$$\mathrm{Var}(n_1, n_2, \ldots, n_N) = 2p(1-p)\mathbf{K}, \qquad (2.2)$$

where the matrix $\mathbf{K}$ has diagonal elements equal to 1 and off-diagonal elements equal to $k_{ij} = \langle (1/2)z_1 + z_2 \rangle_{ij}$ with z_1 and z_2 computed for each pair (i, j) of family members.

2.1.4 Coefficients of Kinship and of Inbreeding

Up until now the *relationship matrix* $\mathbf{K}$ has been a correlation matrix with diagonal elements all equal to 1. $\mathbf{K}$, however, does not have to be a correlation matrix and off-diagonal elements can in fact be greater than one. Note that $z_1 + 2z_2$ is the expected number of alleles shared identically by descent between two individuals. Now consider the following experiment: randomly sample two chromosomal segments, one from each individual, and then count the fraction of times that the two alleles are identical. It is easy to see that on average this fraction will (since there are four possible ways of sampling the two alleles) be equal to 1/4 times the expected number of shared alleles. It is this fraction, i.e., $(1/4)z_1 + (1/2)$ z_2 that is called the *coefficient of kinship*. Now think of a single individual and consider two independent draws from the same individual's chromosomes; if that individual's parents are unrelated, the two chromosomal segments of interest that comprise the two alleles are different, and the probability that the same one is sampled twice is 1/2. If however the parents are related with a coefficient of kinship equal to h, then the probability that the same chromosome is represented twice in that individual, rather than just once, will be equal to h. Thus when sampling two alleles at random with replacement from the same individual, the probability that the same allele is sampled twice is $(1/2) \times (1 - h) + 1 \times h$ or $(1/2)(1 + h)$. Moreover, it can readily be shown that the variance of the number of alleles carried by a single individual is $2p(1 - p)(1 + h)$. Here, h (i.e., the kinship between parents) is termed the *coefficient of inbreeding* and applies to individuals and identical twins. Thus for inbred populations, we continue to have the model for the variance-covariance matrix of a single marker measured for a total of N individuals equal to

$$2p(1 - p)\mathbf{K}, \tag{2.3}$$

but now with $\mathbf{K}$ being equal to twice the *kinship matrix* which we denote with the bold Greek lowercase letter kappa, $\boldsymbol{\kappa}$. The kinship matrix $\boldsymbol{\kappa} = (1/2)\mathbf{K}$ has off-diagonal terms equal to $\langle (1/4)z_1 + (1/2)z_2 \rangle_{ij}$ for $i \neq j$ and diagonal terms equal to $(1/2)(1 + h_i)$.

2.2   Relationship Between Identity by State and Identity by Descent for a Single Diallelic Marker

Identity by state (IBS) refers to the number of similar alleles shared (irrespective of descent) between two individuals at a particular locus. For example, if one subject has genotype aa and another subject genotype Aa, then one allele (the a) is said to be identical by state; if both subjects have genotypes equal to Aa and Aa, then two alleles are identical by state. From the joint distribution, in Table 2.2, of genotypes for two subjects given IBD status, we can easily compute the conditional probability distribution for sharing 0, 1, or 2 alleles by state, given the number of alleles that are identical by descent. This is shown in Table 2.3.

Table 2.3 The probability of allele sharing (IBS) given identity by descent (IBD) for a diallelic marker with allele frequency p

		Number of alleles shared IBD		
		0	1	2
Pr{IBS|IBD}	0	$2p^2(1-p)^2$	0	0
	1	$4p(1-p)^3 + 4p^3(1-p)$	$2p(1-p)^2 + 2p^2(1-p)$	0
	2	$4p^2(1-p)^2 + (1-p)^4 + p^4$	$(1-p)^3 + p(1-p)^2 + p^2(1-p) + p^3$	1

2.3 Estimating IBD Probabilities from Genotype Data

Table 2.3 motivates a simple method of moments estimate of IBD probabilities using a set of M markers, under the assumptions that subjects are drawn from a single population; improvements on this method to deal with finite sample sizes in estimation of allele frequency is given in [1] and maximum likelihood estimation is described in [2].

Changing notation to add an index ℓ distinguishing markers, we can estimate z_0 by counting the number of alleles ($\ell = 1, \ldots, M$) with IBS count equal to zero. Since from Table 2.3 the marginal probability, $\Pr(IBS(n_{i\ell}, n_{i'\ell}) = 0)$, of zero IBS sharing is equal to $z_0\{2p_\ell^2(1 - p_\ell)^2\}$ so that the expected number of alleles with IBS $= 0$ is $2z_0\sum_{\ell=1}^{M} p_\ell^2(1 - p_\ell)^2$. This suggests that we can estimate z_0 by equating the observed count, $\sum_{\ell=1}^{M} I\{IBS(n_{i\ell}, n_{i'\ell}) = 0\}$, of alleles with IBS $= 0$ with its expectation $2z_0\sum_{\ell=1}^{M} p_\ell^2(1 - p_\ell)^2$ and solve for z_0 as

$$\hat{z}_0 = \frac{\sum_{\ell=1}^{M} I\{IBS(n_{i\ell}, n_{i'\ell}) = 0\}}{2\sum_{\ell=1}^{M} p_\ell^2(1 - p_\ell)^2}. \tag{2.4}$$

Similarly, since the marginal probability that $IBS(n_{i\ell}, n_{i'\ell}) = 1$ is equal to $z_0\{4p_\ell(1 - p_\ell)^3 + 4p_\ell^3(1 - p_\ell)\} + z_1\{2p_\ell(1 - p_\ell)^2 + 2p_\ell^2(1 - p_\ell)\}$, we can estimate z_1 as

$$\hat{z}_1 = \frac{\sum_{\ell=1}^{M} I\{IBS(n_{i\ell}, n_{i'\ell}) = 1\} - \hat{z}_0\sum_{\ell=1}^{M} 4p_\ell(1 - p_\ell)^3 + 4p_\ell^3(1 - p_\ell)}{\sum_{\ell=1}^{M} 2p_\ell(1 - p_\ell)^2 + 2p_\ell^2(1 - p_\ell)} \tag{2.5}$$

and finally estimate z_2 as $\hat{z}_2 = 1 - \hat{z}_0 - \hat{z}_1$.

We must also estimate the allele frequencies, p_t as well generally using only unrelated subjects, and these frequencies are assumed known in the above. Note that the estimators for the IBD probabilities are only valid for members of homogeneous populations and do not apply when one or more non-mixing hidden strata exist. Applying these formulas to stratified samples overestimates z_2, the probability of sharing two alleles IBD, since a hallmark of population stratification is an overrepresentation of homozygotes (relative to that expected under HWE) for markers that are differentiated between two or more groups (see below).

2.4 The Covariance Matrix for a Single Allele in Nonrandomly Mixing Populations

We have just shown that when sampling related individuals, the covariance matrix for a single allele with frequency p is equal to $2p(1 - p)\mathbf{K}$ with the off-diagonal elements of $\mathbf{K}$ reflecting the relationships between subjects and the diagonals reflecting inbreeding. It turns out that for *structured populations*, i.e., ones where there are either hidden non-mixing populations and/or incomplete admixture between such groups, a similar model holds, except that in these cases the off-diagonal elements of $\mathbf{K}$ are not directly reflective of familial relationships between individuals but are rather influenced by the similarities or differences in genetic ancestry between individuals who would not normally be considered to be related (i.e., randomly selected members of a large racial/ethnic group) compared to other subjects (i.e., those from other such groups). The important thing (as shown for several examples below) is that in structured populations, the relationship matrix (or more properly *quasi-relationship* matrix since the elements of the matrix are not reflective of close familial relationships but rather of population history and ancestry) is the same for all variants (assuming neutral effects).

2.4.1 Hidden Structure and Correlation

Consider the between-person correlation in the allele counts for a given marker that is induced by the presence of hidden structure in a population. Intuitively it is clear that the individuals who are more alike (i.e., members of the same group) will have more similar values of a marker that has different allele frequencies in the different groups than do individuals who are in different groups. In order to quantify this and to make some general observations, we use a well-known model (the *Balding-Nichols* beta-binomial model) for the difference in allele frequencies in currently isolated groups which have originated from the same ancestral group, with the difference in allele frequencies being due to random drift in the frequencies through time. While a simplification of population genetics models for drift in allele frequencies [3], the model is used extensively [4].

The Balding-Nichols [5] beta-binomial model assumes that for any marker allele with frequency equal to p in the ancestral population, the allele frequency p_t in a modern population (here t indexes the different populations) will be distributed according to the beta distribution

$$p_t \sim B\left(\frac{1-F}{F}p, \frac{1-F}{F}(1-p)\right),\qquad(2.6)$$

so that p_t will have the same mean p as in the ancestral population and variance equal to $Fp(1-p)$. Here F is a parameter that is common for all SNPs and specifies the genetic distance, due to random drift in neutral allele frequency, between the modern day and ancestral populations. We assume that given the allele frequency, an individual's marker genotypes in the modern population (or populations) will then be distributed as draws from a binomial distribution—i.e., will satisfy Hardy–Weinberg equilibrium.

Now assume that a study sample is made up of subjects from total of T different subpopulations each with a genetic distance from the ancestral population equal to F_t and consider first single individuals and then pairs of subjects from the same or different populations. Again let n_i be the count of the number of copies of a given SNP for the person i in the sample, who happens to be in subpopulation t. We now compute the mean and variance of n_i unconditionally, i.e., incorporating the variability of the modern day allele frequency. The expected value of n_i can be computed as $E_{p_t}\left[E\left(n_i|p_t\right)\right] = E_{p_t}(2p_t) = 2p$, just as in the ancestral population. The variance of n_i is computed as

$$\mathrm{Var}(n_i) = E_{p_t}\left[\,\mathrm{Var}\left(n_i|p_t\right)\right] + \mathrm{Var}_{p_t}\left[E\left(n_i|p_t\right)\right].$$

With

$$E_{p_t}\left[\mathrm{Var}\left(n_i\mid p_t\right)\right] = E_{p_t}[2p_t(1-p_t)] = 2E_{p_t}(p_t) - 2E_{p_t}\left(p_t^2\right)$$
$$= 2p - 2\left(p^2 + F_t p(1-p)\right)$$

and

$$\mathrm{Var}_{p_t}\left[E\left(n_i|p_t\right)\right] = \mathrm{Var}_{p_t}(2p) = 4F_t p(1-p),$$

so that the unconditional variance of n_i equals $2p(1-p)(1+F_t)$. Notice that this is overdispersed relative to the binomial variance and implies that counts from a structured population will not follow the Hardy–Weinberg rule (and there will be an over abundance of homozygotes and a corresponding deficit in the number of heterozygotes compared to that expected under HWE). Of course if we knew which population individual i was sampled from, then we could compute the conditional variance, $2p_t(1-p_t)$ which does correspond to HWE, but here we are assuming that this is not possible.

Now suppose that two individuals i and j are sampled from the same subpopulations. Analogous to the rule for variances we have

$$\text{Cov}(n_i, n_j) = E_{p_t}\left[\text{Cov}(n_i, n_j | p_t)\right] + \text{Cov}_{p_t}\left[E(n_i | p_t), E(n_j | p_t)\right].$$

The first term is zero for all p_t (since we assume independence within each population). The second term is $\text{Cov}(2p_t, 2p_t)$, i.e., equals the variance of $2p_t$, which is $4F_t p(1 - p)$. Thus the covariance between the two genotypes is $4F_t p(1 - p)$ and the correlation between the two genotypes is $2\frac{F_t}{(1+F_t)}$. For individuals in different subpopulations, we easily see that the covariance and correlation between n_1 and n_2 is zero.

Note (Homework) that under this model the covariance matrix of the sum, s, of two independent alleles with ancestral allele frequency p_1 and p_2 is equal to $(2p_1(1 - p_1) + 2p_2(1 - p_2))\mathbf{K}$ and hence that the correlation of a sum of alleles between two individuals in the same population will also be equal to $2\frac{F_t}{(1+F_t)}$ just as for a single allele. This extends to *polygenes* composed of weighted sums of many different alleles.

2.4.1.1   Relationship Between Balding–Nichols' F Parameter and the Fixation Index F_{st}

Measures of the degree of population stratification in a given population include the fixation index F_{st} described initially by Sewall Wright [6] which quantifies degree of population separation by the difference in heterozygote frequency expected in stratified versus randomly mixing populations. This statistic can be written as $F_{st} = \frac{H_t - H_s}{H_t}$. Here H_t is the expected fraction of heterozygotes in the total stratified population if HWE could be assumed in that population, which we specify as $2\overline{p}(1 - \overline{p})$, and H_s is the average of the expected fraction of heterozygotes within each component of the stratified population, namely, $E(2p_t(1 - p_t))$. Now consider generating a SNP with ancestral frequency p for T equal-sized subpopulations using the beta-binomial model with all subpopulations sharing the same F. It is easy to see from the calculations immediately above that the expected number of heterozygotes in the full stratified population will be $E(2p_t(1 - p_t)) = 2p(1 - p)(1 - F)$. If we know the ancestral allele frequency, p, then we can say that the expected fraction of heterozygotes in the stratified population under HWE is $2p(1 - p)$, so that $F_{st} = F$. If we do not know the ancestral allele frequency, then we estimate $\overline{p}$ as $1/2$ the observed count of the generated allele over all populations. The expected value of $2\overline{p}(1 - \overline{p})$ (i.e., H_t) under the beta-binomial model can be shown to be equal to $H_t = 2p(1 - p)(1 - F/T)$ so that the calculated value of F_{st} is approximately $\frac{T-1}{T-F}F$ which converges to F as T (the number of populations) increases. See the simulation experiment in file BN_Fst.r. Note that we do not (in the simulation) calculate a separate F_{st} for each SNP and then average the F_{st}. Instead we calculate H_t and H_s for each SNP, then average these values over all the SNPs and form the ratio from the average values to estimate F_{st}.

2.4.2 Effects of Incomplete Admixture on the Covariance Matrix of a Single Variant

Population admixture occurs when individuals from two or more previously separated populations begin interbreeding. As mentioned earlier, even one generation of subsequent random mixing leads to alleles with a marginal distribution that are in Hardy–Weinberg equilibrium no matter how distinct the merging populations are. However, modern day admixture is more complicated than this, typical admixed populations show a greater than expected variation between members of the current population in the number of ancestors that derive from each of the mixing populations (compared to random mating after an initial mixing), and this between-person variation in ancestry is what leads to a failure of the Hardy–Weinberg rule to apply.

Consider two populations mixing, then as described by Chen et al. [7] the covariance matrix for a single SNP is of form $2p(1 - p)\mathbf{K}$ where the elements, k_{ij}, depend upon the fraction of ancestors α_i and α_j, that each subject has from one of the two mixing populations (with $1 - \alpha_i$ and $1 - \alpha_j$ from the other population). Here we are assuming that each sampled subject is unrelated to each other in the usual sense.

In this case the diagonal terms, k_{ii} of $\mathbf{K}$ will equal $1 + F_i$ with $F_i = F(1 + 2\alpha_i^2 - 2\alpha_i)$ and off-diagonal terms $F_{ij} = F(1 + 2\alpha_i\alpha_j - \alpha_i - \alpha_j)$. This reduces to the above model when $\alpha_i = 1$ and $\alpha_j = 0$ or vice versa. A subtlety noted by Chen et al. is that when all α_i are equal (i.e., there is complete mixing), the effects of admixture are no longer detectable, and replacing p from the ancestral population with the allele frequency in the completely admixed population (which is now $p_1\alpha + p_2(1 - \alpha)$ where p_1 and p_2 are the allele frequencies in the two mixing populations) allows one to drop the F_i and F_{ij} in the above calculations, i.e., the admixed population can be treated as any other homogeneous population when considered alone, at least in terms of the correlation of a single SNP.

2.5 Direct Estimation of Differentiation Parameter F from Genotype Data

We now consider the problem of using genotype data from two individuals to estimate a pair-specific differentiation parameter F. We concentrate here on the problem of there being hidden non-mixing populations, indexed by t. For simplicity we assume that all F_t are equal to a single value of F.

Using the index ℓ for distinguishing different markers from each other, note that the variances of the allele counts, $n_{i\ell}$, for each marker ℓ all have the same form, i.e., the variance is equal to $(1 + F)$ times the usual binomial variance $2p_\ell(1 - p_\ell)$ where p_ℓ is the allele frequency in the ancestral population. Similarly the covariance between variants for two individuals in population l is always equal to a constant, $2F$, multiplied by the usual binomial variance. While it is impossible to estimate the (unknown) differentiation parameter F between subjects based on just one marker observed in the two individuals, in a GWAS study we have hundreds of thousands of SNP markers available. Suppose for the time being that the ancestral allele frequency p_ℓ of marker ℓ is known. Then upon observing a total of M SNPs, we could form standardized alleles for each SNP and each individual, i, as

$$z_{i\ell} = \frac{n_{i\ell} - 2p_\ell}{\sqrt{2p_\ell(1 - p_\ell)}}. \tag{2.7}$$

Each of these has expected value 0 and variance $(1 + F)$. Moreover the covariance between two different standardized alleles, $z_{i\ell}$ and $z_{j\ell}$, for the same SNP but different individuals is equal to

$$\frac{\mathrm{Cov}\left(n_{i\ell}, n_{j\ell}\right)}{2p_\ell(1 - p_\ell)} = \frac{4Fp_\ell(1 - p_\ell)}{2p_\ell(1 - p_\ell)} = 2F.$$

This leads to the estimator of the covariance matrix of the counts of a given marker for individuals i and j as

$$2p_\ell(1 - p_\ell)\hat{\mathbf{K}}, \tag{2.8}$$

where $\hat{\mathbf{K}}$ is a 2×2 matrix with off-diagonal elements equal to

$$\frac{1}{M}\sum_{\ell=1}^{M} z_{i\ell}z_{j\ell} \tag{2.9}$$

and the ith diagonal element equal to

$$\frac{1}{M}\sum_{\ell=1}^{M} z_{i\ell}^2. \tag{2.10}$$

Extending this to consider all pairs of individuals, the resulting matrix is commonly used for describing the structure of a population sample and is the matrix computed, for example, in the principal components approach described by [4] and in the EIGENSTRAT program.

Although we have described it in terms of simple hidden structure problem (non-mixing hidden groups), this estimator is useful in many problems where we can model the covariance matrix for all SNPs as equal to a constant matrix $\mathbf{K}$ times a variance parameter unique to each SNP (here $2p_\ell(1 - p_\ell)$).

2.5.1   *Relatedness Revisited*

We have seen from our initial discussion of relatedness that the covariance matrix for the marker counts, $n_{i\ell}$ and $n_{j\ell}$, for two related subjects, i and j, coming from an otherwise unstratified population (i.e., randomly mixing) is equal to

$$2p_\ell(1 - p_\ell) \begin{pmatrix} 1 & \frac{1}{2}z_1 + z_2 \\ \frac{1}{2}z_1 + z_2 & 1 \end{pmatrix},$$

with z_0 and z_0 the IBD probabilities as defined above so that our estimate $\hat{\mathbf{K}}$ adapts to this setting as well.

If there is no hidden population structure, but we relax the assumption that all subjects are unrelated, then $\hat{\mathbf{K}}$ estimates the *relationship matrix* (i.e., twice the kinship matrix $\boldsymbol{\kappa}$ [8]) which has off-diagonal elements equal to $(1/2)z_1 + z_2$ and diagonal elements equal to $1 + h_i$ where h_i is the inbreeding coefficient for subject i, i.e., the kinship between subject i's parents. In the forgoing we refer to $\hat{\mathbf{K}}$ (computed now for all pairs of subject i and j) as the estimated relationship matrix, recognizing, however, that this name is only technically accurate in the absence of population stratification.

Note that if one was sure that the underlying population was not stratified, then we could also use (2.4) for $\hat{z}_0$ and (2.5) for $\hat{z}_2$ (and $\hat{z}_2 = 1 - \hat{z}_0 - \hat{z}_1$) to estimate $(1/2)$ $z_1 + z_2$, and this estimator may be better behaved when using markers with small allele frequencies p_k because division is delayed until after considerable simulation has taken place. Recently Yang et al. [9] have specifically noted that the diagonal estimate $\frac{1}{M} \sum_{\ell=1}^{M} z_{i\ell}^2$ is poorly behaved if many markers with small allele frequencies are used and have suggested the alternative

$$1 + \frac{1}{M} \sum_{\ell=1}^{M} \frac{n_{i\ell}^2 - (1 + 2p_\ell)n_{i\ell} + 2p_\ell^2}{2p_\ell(1 - p_\ell)},$$

which has the same expectation but a smaller sampling variance than does $\frac{1}{M} \sum_{\ell=1}^{M} z_{i\ell}^2$.

Even in situations where hidden stratification is present, it still is of interest to identify close relatives in a study especially in the process of performing data cleaning and outlier identification (see later chapters). One simple method of estimating IBD probabilities for close relationships that is not overly sensitive to population stratification is to simply exclude from the calculations of relatedness any markers that appear to be out of Hardy–Weinberg equilibrium. More complete estimation of z_1 and z_2 in a fashion that is relatively impervious to hidden structure is described in Purcell et al. [1] in their discussion of the GWAS analysis program, PLINK. The general approach is to bound the estimates of z_1 and z_2 so that they correspond to actual familial relationships. In almost all cases (except for identical twins, duplicated DNA samples, or extremely inbred population), the true probability of sharing two alleles IBD will be less than the probability of sharing one allele IBD, so that z_2 is generally much closer to zero than is z_1; in randomly mixing populations, z_2 can be no greater than the square of twice the kinship coefficient. Enforcing such constraints on z_2 helps to better estimate true close relationships in the presence of hidden structure.

As shown above for two individuals sampled from an admixed population derived from the (incomplete) mixing of two different ancestral populations, the covariance matrix for a given marker will again equal a constant matrix $\mathbf{K}$, with $\mathbf{K}$ not depending on which SNP is measured, multiplied by a variance parameter depending on SNP [7]. Even more general problems, such as admixture + relatedness or inbreeding within pedigree founders in a complex pedigree, can be modeled in this fashion [8, 10].

2.5.2   Estimation of Allele Frequencies

Next we need to point out that for our hidden subpopulation example that we have assumed that the ancestral population frequency is known when calculating the quasi-relationship matrix $\hat{\mathbf{K}}$. This is rarely if ever true in actual practice. What is done is to estimate p_ℓ as the frequency of marker ℓ within the sample that is available. In the hidden strata example, the overall sample allele frequency remains an unbiased estimator of p_ℓ, but it is not one with particularly good statistical properties. For example, it will not in general converge to the true ancestral p_ℓ as the number, N, of subjects in the study increases (only if the number of distinct hidden strata all derived from the same ancestral population increases with N would the sample allele frequency be expected to converge to p_ℓ). Rather than seeking to improve the estimate of p_ℓ, it makes better sense in most cases to simply accept the fact that $\hat{\mathbf{K}}$ measures the relative relatedness between subjects rather an absolute relatedness [10]. In fact if we use the sample estimated allele frequency in the calculations, then we will see that kinship estimates for certain pairs of subjects are negative reflecting that these pairs are more dissimilar to each other than are pairs from the same population. While some authors recommend setting negative off-diagonal elements to zero, this is not usually necessary for the kind of uses we make of this estimator [10] (as in Chap. 4).

2.6   Allele Frequency Distributions

2.6.1   Initial Mutations and Common Ancestors

One of the underlying principles of population genetics relevant to all association studies is that, at least in most cases, all carriers of a given genetic variant inherited that variant from a single most recent common ancestor (MRCA); i.e., we can trace back from generation to generation the variant allele to a single carrier chromosome or, more precisely, a single chromosomal segment, or *locus*, surrounding the variant allele. Indeed it is this "single origin" of a given variant that partly leads to the concept of association-based genetic studies, since the background pattern of other variants or genetic markers, and specifically SNPs, that were already present on the ancestral segment uniquely labels that given chromosome (distinguishing it from all other chromosomes with progeny in today's population). Searching for unique patterns of SNPs that are related to disease by association with causal alleles is at the core of what is meant by association studies.

This most recent common ancestral chromosome was not necessarily the earliest chromosome that ever carried that genetic variant, for at the time that the MCRA was extant, there may have been many other carriers of that same variant allele. Indeed the variant allele may already have been common in the population at that time. In essence, however, no other carrier of that allele at that time left progeny in today's population. As we see shortly, this is an overstatement, since a different genetic variant, for example, one on a different chromosome, will have a different most recent ancestral origin. It is not that the other carriers of the first allele have no progeny today; they just have no progeny today *at that locus*. It is through the process of recombination that different segments of the DNA have different origins.

This tracing back of carriers of a variant lying on a particular chromosomal locus or to its common origin can be modeled in terms of a tree-diagram called the coalescent. Coalescent theory has many important results, the simplest of which can be derived easily under restricted assumptions such as no recombination, no natural selection, random mating, and fixed population size, yielding essentially the Wright-Fisher model of neutral evolution [11].

Under the assumption of neutral evolution, if we consider a population of chromosomes which has been of constant size N over its history, we can construct a genealogy for that population by thinking of each offspring chromosome present at generation t as "randomly choosing" its parent chromosome from the population (also of size N) of chromosomes present at time $t - 1$, and from this we can derive the probability distribution of the time (counting backwards in generations) until any two chromosomal segments selected from among the current generation meet their MCRA or *coalesce*.

The probability that these two segments coalesce, i.e., choose the same parent, in the previous generation is $1/N$, while the probability that they do not coalesce is $1 - 1/N$. Repeating this process through earlier generations we see that the probability distribution of t the time (in generations counting backwards $t = 1, 2, \ldots$) until coalescent occurs is geometrically distributed with probability distribution function

$$P(t) = \left(1 - \frac{1}{N}\right)^{t-1} \frac{1}{N}.$$

The first term indicates the probability that the coalescence did not occur at times $t = 1, 2, \ldots, t - 1$, and the second term is the probability of a coalescence at time t. If N is large, this can be approximated as the exponential distribution

$$P(t) = \frac{1}{N} e^{-\frac{t}{N}},$$

which has mean N and variance equal to N^2.

More generally if we start with a sample of n chromosomal segments from among the population of size N, then we see that the time to the first coalescent (from among $_nC_2 = \begin{pmatrix} n \\ 2 \end{pmatrix}$ possible pairs) will be distributed as

$$P_n(t) = (1 - p_n)^{t-1} p_n,$$

where p_n is the probability of at least one coalescent occurring in one generation.

If N is large relative to n, then we can approximate p_n as

$$\frac{_nC_2}{N}$$

and also ignore the possibility that more one coalescent occurs in a single generation. Thus under the coalescent approximation, the number of distinct lineages decreases in steps of one back in time and the expected time from the kth coalescent until the $k + 1$st is equal to

$$\frac{N}{_{n-k}C_2}. \tag{2.11}$$

The expected time to the MCRA for the whole sample will be equal to the sum of the coalescent times or

$$N \sum_{k=0}^{n-2} 1 / _{n-k}C_2 = 2N(1 - 1/n). \tag{2.12}$$

We can also (for large N) approximate $P_{n-k}(t)$, the distribution of time between coalescent F and $k + 1$, as exponential with mean $\frac{N}{_{n-k}C_2}$.

This exponential approximation is heavily exploited for computer simulation of realistic genetic data [12]. For example, under the assumptions above, plus an assumption about the probability (per generation) of a new (neutral) mutation, we can take a population of chromosomal segments and simulate the occurrence of new genetic markers (such as SNPs or any other inheritable variant) on those segments by doing simulations backward in time, rather than forward. Moreover the program does not have to keep track of whether coalescences occur in each generation, instead it generates $N - 1$ independent exponential random numbers, with the appropriate mean, and independently of these a random bifurcating tree to construct the full genealogy describing the relatedness between all chromosomes in the current generation.

2.6.2   Mutations and the Coalescent

A basic simplifying assumption often useful in population genetics is that mutations only occur once at a given site with no possibility of backwards mutation or further changes at that site. This assumption is known as the infinite sites model, i.e., that there are an infinite number of mutation sites so that the chance of two mutations occurring at exactly the same site can be neglected. This model reflects the large number of base pairs in the genome as well as a very low per-base pair (10^{-8} or so) probability of change per generation or so in "higher organisms" [13]; the model appears to apply to SNPs considering, for example, the very small fraction of SNPs that have more than two alleles.

In coalescence models mutations are assigned along the branches of the tree, with exponential arrival times so that the number of new mutations along a particular path is distributed as a Poisson random variable with mean equal to the product of the mutation rate and the length of that path. To accommodate this notion in the simulation, each mutation is assigned not only a path position but also a unique chromosomal position.

Simulation programs based on the coalescent have wide usefulness in illuminating and comparing the properties of various statistical methods when they are to be applied to real data. Coalescent-based simulation programs, such as those given by Hudson [12] while based on this fundamental approach, can be modified to allow certain of the assumptions of the Wright-Fisher model to be relaxed, in particular population sizes can be allowed to change in time, and the migration of genes between populations can be accommodated.

See Fig. 2.1 for a depiction of a simulated coalescent tree.

2.6.3   Allelic Distribution of Genetic Variants

An important topic that impacts the design, analysis, and prospect for success of GWAS studies is the frequency distribution of variation in the genome and specifically of variation that is causative of disease or influences other phenotypes of interest. Much of the motivation for undertaking first candidate gene association studies and later GWAS studies was summarized in the *common disease-common variant* hypothesis, which argues that common, rather than rare, genetic variants underlay the heritability of common diseases. If this hypothesis is true then it has been shown [14] that genetic association studies will have more power than

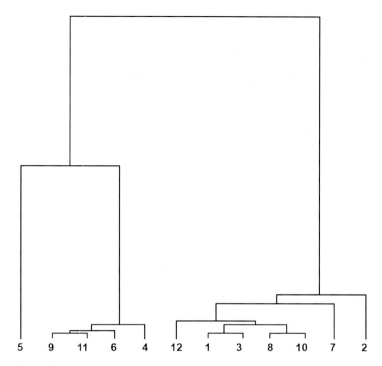

Fig. 2.1 Simulation of SNP data through the coalescent process

traditional pedigree-based linkage studies when it comes to finding the risk alleles. The arguments for the common disease-common variant hypothesis (c.f. [15–18]) include (1) weak or nonexistent selective pressure against variants involved in susceptibility for common diseases (especially late onset diseases which would tend not to affect reproductive success), (2) expansion of populations after passing through *bottlenecks* related to migration away from the earliest human groupings, and (3) a resulting distribution of alleles that involve susceptibility in which common variants predominate. The latter point follows from the first two; the distribution of frequencies of selectively neutral alleles in stable populations was described by Wright [19], further refined by Ewens [20], and has been updated to account for population growth and selection [17, 21].

An important implication of the neutral selection model is that, while there are many rare markers, if two individual chromosomes are compared to one another, most of the differences seen between the two chromosomes are due to common, rather than rare, alleles. Specifically, considering a specific site where the two genotypes differ, if we take a larger sample of individuals and examine the same site in each of the new individuals, in most cases many of them too will also be found to differ at this site as well. A heuristic argument for this can be made by considering the time to coalescence between the two individual chromosomes showing a different allele at a specific site. In order for the two sequences to differ

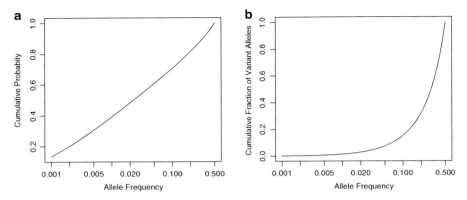

Fig. 2.2 (**a**) Expected cumulative distribution of allele frequencies of variants seen when genotyping a large number of sites in a sample population of size 500. (**b**) Expected cumulative distribution of total minor allele counts in same study

at a given site, the mutation at that site must have occurred after the time of coalescence for the two chromosomes (here we are focusing on segments short enough not to have been affected by recombination). The mean coalescent time is N generations in the past with an expected time of appearance of the mutation equal to $1/2N$ (assuming a constant rate of mutation over time). But this is early enough so that it would predate a very large number of coalescent events in the larger sample since the expected time to the MRCA for all the subjects in the sample is $2N(1 - 1/n)$ or roughly $2N$ for large n; in fact on average we would expect, from (2.11) and (2.12), that the last 3 coalescences take up time $3/2N$ so that all but these are (expected to be) yet to come by the (expected) time of the observed mutation. Thus a large fraction of the n members of the sample are likely to carry the mutation of interest. There is considerable variability in both the actual times of mutation and the number of coalescent events yet to take place at that time, but this argument can be fleshed out in further detail using coalescent theory.

For example, a formula for the expected number of sites, η_i, at which the less frequent base is present on i sequences out of a sample size of n sequences ($N = n/2$ individuals) is given by Wakeley [3] [(4.21), p. 105)] as

$$E(\eta_i) = \theta \frac{\frac{1}{i} + \frac{1}{n-i}}{1 + \delta_{i,n-1}} \quad 1 \le i \le [n/2], \tag{2.13}$$

where θ is the (scaled) mutation frequency, $[\cdot]$ is the largest integer (i.e., floor) function, and δ_{ij} is the Kronecker δ function equal to 1 if i and j are equal and equal to 0 otherwise. Figure 2.2a shows the expected cumulative frequency of minor allele frequencies for SNPs seen at least once in a sample of 1,000 chromosomes (500 diploid individuals) using this formula (by considering only SNPs seen at least once, we can drop the mutation frequency parameter from the calculations).

It is clear from Fig 2.2a that a large proportion of variants are expected to be "rare," with, for example, about 39 % of total alleles having allele frequency less than one percent while only about 20 % of variants will have frequency between 0.2 and 0.5. However, things look quite different when counting the total number of variant (e.g., minor) alleles seen, since each variant contributes an expected $2pN$ minor alleles; Fig 2.2b gives the expected cumulative contribution to the total number of minor alleles seen according to allele frequency. SNPs with frequency less than 1 % contribute hardly at all to the total variation, while common SNPs (frequency 0.2–0.5) contribute approximately two thirds.

This same argument applies to genetic variants (causal alleles) that increase susceptibility to diseases that have no relationship to reproductive success, either because they do not interfere with fitness or because they tend to be too late in onset to affect fertility. As will be shown in Chap. 7, common causal alleles are inherently more detectable than are rare alleles, all other things being equal, and would seem to contribute far more to risk of disease than rarer SNPs, unless there is a marked tendency for rarer variants to have higher risks associated with them.

2.6.4   Allele Distributions Under Population Increase and Selection

One factor in human population history that influences the number of rare variants (and potentially their contribution to risk) relative to the discussions above is the very large growth in human populations in the last 2–3 hundred years. This recent spectacular growth implies an excessive fraction of alleles are rare compared to the model given above. Recent large-scale sequencing in the *1000 Genomes Project* show that there is a surfeit of SNP alleles with frequency less than 0.5 % compared to that expected under the constant population size model [22].

An additional, and potentially more important factor influencing allele frequencies, is selection. Equation (2.13) is based on an assumption that all the alleles considered are neutral in the effects on reproductive success. A formula for allele frequency distributions in an infinite population that includes the effect of natural selection was given by Wright [23] who found that allele frequency p is distributed as

$$f(p) = kp^{(\beta_S-1)}(1-p)^{(\beta_N-1)}e^{\sigma(1-p)}, \tag{2.14}$$

with β_S as scaled mutation frequency (equivalent to θ above), β_N as scaled back-mutation (reversion) frequency, σ as the scaled selection rate, and k as a normalizing constant. Note that $f(p)$ in (2.14) is not really a probability distribution since its integral does not exist over the range (0–1) of interest. However, we can still use Wright's formula to evaluate questions involving the relative frequencies of ranges of alleles in an infinite population. The key parameter of interest to us here is the selection parameter σ; this is given in units of $4N_e s$ with N_e the effective sample size and s the reduction in reproductive success (expressed as the fractional reduction in

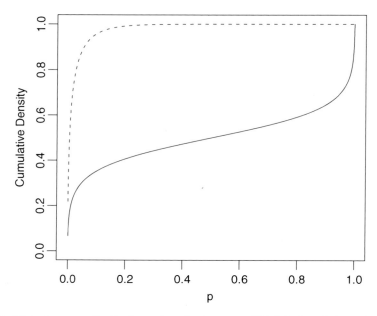

Fig. 2.3 Allele frequency distribution under selection or not. Wright's formula is used to depict the cumulative density of allele frequencies between frequency 0.001 and 0.999 under no selection (*solid line*) and selection with n_b (*dotted line*)

the number of offspring expected from carriers compared to noncarriers) associated with the allele of interest. Following Pritchard [24], we set σ to equal 12 to signify "weak selection" against the allele of interest and zero for no selection. Note that $\sigma = 12$ translates to a 0.03 % reduction in the probability of leaving offspring in each generation assuming a constant effective sample size of $N_e = 10,000$. Figure 2.3 plots the cumulative distribution of allele frequencies under this model. Even under this weak level of selection pressure, it is evident that there is a dramatic shift to rarer alleles compared to the neutral model. Does this mean that the *common disease-common variant* hypothesis that has underpinned GWAS studies to date is misconceived? This and related questions is taken up in Chap. 8.

2.7   Recombination and Linkage Disequilibrium

Note that in the coalescent depicted in Fig. 2.1 if two mutations (call them A and B) occur along a specific path segment between coalescences then in the resulting population all chromosomes that carry mutation A would also carry mutation B as well. This observation illustrates the first of two concepts (linkage disequilibrium) underlying the association-based approach to identifying risk alleles. The second is recombination.

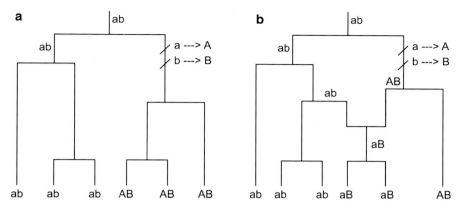

Fig. 2.4 Recombinations and the ancestral recombination graph. Two mutations are depicted as having occurred on the same branch. (**a**) No recombination. (**b**) Recombination that breaks the correlation between mutations A and B

Recombination is the exchange of genetic material during meiosis as two (homologous) chromosomes split at a certain point and reorganize after having traded the DNA sequence on one or the other side of the split with each other. Now markers A and B are no longer traveling together in the progeny issuing from that point forward thus altering (weakening) the pattern of correlation between these two markers. Approaching this backwards in time we note that when a recombination occurs, we can think of the child chromosome as having chosen two parents at that generation time, t, i.e., one for the position that A occupies and one for the position that B occupies. Figure 2.4 gives an illustration of such an ancestral recombination graph [25]. The ancestry of each position (one for A and one for B) marginally follows a coalescent. Ultimately even with recombination, there will be a single MCRA found from which both loci were inherited [25] and ultimately a single MCRA for all sites for the entire chromosome and genome, i.e., common ancestors for all living humans.

If the recombination occurs early in the coalescent process, the correlation between A and B will be weakened possibly considerably since a large number of both recombinant and nonrecombinant chromosomes may have progeny in the current generation. On the other hand, if the recombination event occurs much later down the tree than the initial occurrence of these two mutations, most, but not all, of the resulting (modern day) chromosomes that carry mutation A will also carry mutation B, i.e., the correlation between A and B will have been only partly diminished by the recombination. Here we have considered the impact of just one recombination event on the resulting correlations, but in fact if A and B are widely separated then many recombination events will generally have occurred, each one will tend to reduce the association between alleles like A and B.

The basic principles underlying association-based genetic studies is that markers are correlated with each other and with causal variants of any type which have

similar histories, for example, the allele A may be a variant that increases susceptibility to disease and B is a marker on the same chromosome that originated on the
same path segment (as in our simplified example) in Fig. 2.1. If there were no
recombination events anywhere on an entire chromosome, then marker B would not
be informative at all about the location of risk allele A; i.e., B could be placed
anywhere on the same chromosome and still be highly correlated with A, so that
B would appear to be associated with disease. However, when recombination does
occur, the correlations between markers are weakened. If the loci occupied by A and
B are distant from each other, then there will have been many recombinations taking
place over time so that the correlation between the marker B and the risk allele
A will be so low that B will no longer appear to be related to the disease of interest.[2]

The probability, in any generation, of a recombination occurring between the
loci that are occupied by A and B is termed the *genetic distance* between these two
sites. Genetic distance is an increasing function of the distance between sites, but
not uniformly so because recombination events do not occur at uniform rates at all
positions on a chromosome. There are certain regions where recombinations are
rare and certain regions where they are unusually common. These may be termed
recombination cold spots or hot spots, respectively [26–29]. Alleles between which
there have been low numbers of historical recombinations are said to be in linkage
disequilibrium (LD). The ongoing revolution in biotechnology has allowed the
inexpensive genotyping of hundreds of thousands of markers in large numbers of
people; the number of markers is so large that there is likely to be at least one
marker in high linkage disequilibrium with any given (common) variant affecting
risk of a disease or influencing some other phenotype that we are interested
in. Depending on the frequency of both the marker and the underlying causal
variant, this may result in a statistically detectable association between the disease
of interest and the marker. Once such an association has been detected, the
chromosomal region surrounding the marker becomes a candidate for a number
of additional analyses designed to first replicate the association, then further
localize and identify variants, and ultimately characterize the mechanism by
which a causal variant affects the disease or phenotype.

2.7.1 Quantification of Recombination

There are a number of standard statistics that are used to describe the pattern of
association between markers and to therefore characterize the extent of linkage
disequilibrium between markers. The two most important of these are Lewontin's

---

[2] Note that we are now talking about correlations between SNP allele counts of two different
markers at different locations, over a sample of individuals, $i = 1,\ldots,N$. In Sects. 2.1–2.5, our
focus was on the correlations (induced by structure or relatedness) of counts, n_A of a single marker
A for different individuals i and j.

Table 2.4 Haplotype probabilities for two loci

	b	B	
a	$(1-p)(1-q) + \delta$	$(1-p)q - \delta$	$1-p$
A	$p(1-q) - \delta$	$pq + \delta$	p
	$1-q$	q	1

[30] δ', while the second is the usual R^2 criterion applied to alleles at two loci. These two statistics are closely related; the first is designed to be a measure of linkage disequilibrium between the two independent of their allele frequencies, while the second depends on both the degree of linkage disequilibrium and the allele frequencies of the two markers. The R^2 statistic is most directly related to the performance of association-based genetic studies in the situation we described above, namely, when a nearby marker is measured as a surrogate for an unmeasured (and generally unknown) causal variant. Both δ' and R^2 can be initially considered in terms of a 2×2 table of two diallelic variants at two loci on a single chromosome. Each of the four possible combinations of the two alleles for the two variants is termed a *haplotype*. If we denote the two variants as having alleles a or A for the first variant and b or B for the second and if p is the probability of allele A (so that $1 - p$ is the probability of allele a) and q the probability of allele B, then the probabilities of the four haplotypes, $ab, aB, Ab,$ and AB, can be depicted as in Table 2.4.

Here δ is a disequilibrium parameter that measures the association between the two loci in the sense that if δ is zero, the two alleles are independent and otherwise are positively (for $\delta > 0$) or negatively ($\delta > 0$) associated. In fact, we see below that δ is the covariance in the population of haplotypes of the counts (0 or 1) of the number of alleles at each of the two loci. Because all haplotype probabilities must be nonnegative, we can immediately see that δ is bounded by $-\min((1 - p)(1 - q), pq)) \leq \delta \leq \min(p(1 - q), (1 - p)q)$. Since the labeling of the alleles (a vs. A or b vs. B) is completely arbitrary, yet affects the sign of δ, the interest is actually in $|\delta|$ which is bounded by

$$\delta_{max} = \begin{cases} \min\left[q(1-p), (1-q)p\right] & \text{if } \delta > 0 \\ \min\left[(1-p)(1-q), pq\right] & \text{if } \delta < 0 \end{cases}.$$

The scaled version of $|\delta|$ is defined as $\delta' = (|\delta|/\delta_{max})$ which takes values between zero and 1. Note that if δ' takes its maximum value of 1, then this means that at least one cell (i.e., haplotype) in Table 2.4 will have probability zero. Note that if all haplotypes have nonzero probability, then this constitutes proof (under the infinite sites model) that there has been a historical recombination between the two loci, i.e., the only way that all four haplotypes, $ab, aB, Ab,$ and AB could occur is if there was either (1) a second de novo occurrence of either A or B (assuming that ab is the ancestral allele), ruled out by the infinite sites model, or (2) that there was a recombination between the two loci to form, for example, AB from aB and Ab.

While a value of δ' close to one is evidence that there has been little or no recombination between the two loci δ' does not really measure the strength of the association between the two variant alleles in a way that is important for association testing. For example, if the allele frequencies p and q are very different (e.g., if p is close to 1/2 but q is much smaller), then the presence of only three haplotypes, for example, ab, aB, and Ab, means that while A always appears with b and never B, there are many instances of b not associated with A. When it comes to assessing the power of an association study that genotypes the loci occupied by B but not the loci occupied by A, the appropriate linkage disequilibrium criteria is simply the squared correlation R^2 between the count of the two alleles A and B.

Working within the haplotype framework, we introduce a slight variation on previous notation so that $n_A(h)$ counts the number of A alleles on haplotype h. Thus for haplotypes ab, aB, Ab, and AB, $n_A(h)$ takes values 0, 0, 1, and 1, respectively; similarly $n_B(h)$ counts the B allele.

From first principles $R^2 = \mathrm{Cov}[n_A(h), n_B(h)]^2 / \{\mathrm{Var}[n_A(h)]\mathrm{Var}[n_B(h)]\}$. The variance of the count, n_A, of the number of alleles of A (now a binary random variable since we are dealing with only one haplotype) is simply $p(1-p)$ and for n_B is $q(1-q)$, with the covariance between the two equal to $E[n_A(h)n_B(h))] - E[n_A(h)]$ $E[n_B(h)] = (pq + \delta) - pq = \delta$ so that $R^2 = \frac{\delta^2}{p(1-p)q(1-q)}$. It is worth noting first that R^2 does not depend upon which of the two alleles, a or A, is being counted, i.e., we could use n_A or n_a equivalently, and similarly for n_B or n_b.

2.7.2   Phased Versus Unphased Data and LD Estimation

While we have described R^2 as the squared correlation between binary variables (the n counters) in an experiment where we observe the haplotypes, ab, Ab, aB, and AB, directly, the same R^2 (or R for that matter) applies if we observe, rather than the haplotypes themselves, unphased genotypes for diploid chromosomes, so long as we assume that each haplotype is inherited independently; in this case n_A and n_B are correlated binomial random variables, which now take the values (0, 1, or 2), but with the same value of the correlation between them as if haplotypes were measured directly. Since we can certainly estimate the allele frequencies p and q as well from the unphased as from the haplotype data, a non-iterative estimate of δ based solely on the genotype data is simply $\hat{\delta} = \hat{R}\sqrt{\hat{p}(1-\hat{p})\hat{q}(1-\hat{q})}$. Here we have estimated R as the usual sample correlation estimate for n_A and n_B from genotypes obtained for a sample of individuals in the population. Other estimates of δ can be formed from genotype data, with the method of maximum likelihood easily implemented using an EM algorithm [31]. More about estimation of haplotypes based on genotype data is presented in Chaps. 5 and 6.

2.7.3   *Hidden Population Structure*

As we will see in Chap. 3, genetic association studies are based upon the assumption that because of recombination only markers that are in close proximity to a causal genetic variant that directly or indirectly influences disease risk or phenotype distribution should be statistically associated with that phenotype. However, there are a number of reasons why this may not be true. The most important of these is hidden population structure present in the study. When hidden population structure is present, LD appears to be of much greater extent than expected, and very large numbers of markers scattered over the entire genome may show unexpected levels of association with the phenotype of interest. At the root of this failure to localize associations is the extent of apparent LD that is brought about by the presence of such phenomenon as admixture, hidden stratification, and cryptic relatedness.

2.7.3.1   Stable Populations

Consider first a stable population of chromosomes that is isolated, in that there is no migration from the outside entering the region, and where there is random mixing between chromosomes (i.e., genetic variants are all assumed to be neutral in terms of reproductive fitness and unrelated to mating choice). In this case over time we will see two things: (1) an increase in the number of (neutral) mutations and (2) a loss of linkage disequilibrium between existing markers. For a given pair of markers t, it can be shown that the linkage disequilibrium parameter δ changes with generation, t, according to

$$\delta(t) = \delta_0(1 - \theta)^t, \tag{2.15}$$

where δ_0 is the initial value of δ and θ is the probability of a recombination between the two markers in one generation. Ultimately with enough time elapsed, recombination between markers would insure that only those markers that are extremely close to each other physically (i.e., with θ very close to zero) should be in LD with each other. As we will further illustrate later in this chapter, of the major continental populations (e.g., European, African, and Asian), it is the oldest continental population, i.e., people in or from Africa, that tends to show the lowest LD between markers and also the most common variants.

2.7.3.2   Out Migration and Population Expansion

Groups of Africans began to expand into Europe and Asia at the end of the last great ice age. Outmigration of a small number of founders and subsequent rapid population growth has profound effects upon linkage disequilibrium and frequency of markers. Since the founders may each have a great number of descendents, any mutation carried by a founder, no matter how rare in the ancestral population, will tend to be common in the descendant population. Moreover mutations that were in linkage equilibrium in the ancestral population, but which were both carried by a given founder chromosome, will be in linkage disequilibrium in the new population and remain in linkage disequilibrium until the force of recombination again weakens such disequilibrium. Thus recently founded isolated populations will tend to have higher levels of linkage disequilibrium than will older more stable populations.

For GWAS studies the extended linkage disequilibrium of recently derived isolated populations has sometimes been considered to be of benefit in that it would take fewer markers to find regions of the genome that were associated with disease- or phenotype-associated causal variants. Iceland, for example, has been described [32, 33] as an ideal setting for conducting GWAS studies because in this recently derived ethnically homogeneous island, LD patterns should be longer and coverage of causal variants with GWAS chips should therefore be more complete. In fact the GWAS studies in Iceland, conducted by deCode Genetics corporation, has had many important successes. It appears however that these successes had much more to do with the fact that DNA resources for a large fraction of the entire population of Iceland were available at an early stage, as well as the abilities of the deCode scientists, and less to do with better coverage of the genome, at least in comparison with other European populations. In particular, the discoveries in Iceland were very often reproduced by other similar sized GWAS studies of other less recent but still European-derived populations using similar genotyping technology.

A downside of using an isolated population in a GWAS is that not all alleles related to the phenotype of interest disease are likely to be present in that population (due to founder effects), and moreover extended linkage disequilibrium implies that localization of causal alleles underlying observed associations may be more difficult. Studies of disease and other phenotypes in populations of more ancient origins, notably African-derived groups, do require more SNPs to cover any one particular genetic region, or the genome as a whole, and this was one early impediment to progress in GWAS studies in such populations. The ability of commercial GWAS platforms to cover the variation in the African genome is gradually improving, and the shorter LD can be beneficial for the localization of the signal from GWAS findings, a crucial step in the ultimate identification of specific causal variants. The most crucial impediment now to GWAS studies in African populations is the less developed infrastructure of cohort and case–control studies with access to DNA samples in this (and other) non-European groups.

2.7.3.3   Population Admixture and Hidden Stratification

In the last few hundred years not only have population sizes grown immensely but also groups that had been relatively isolated for long periods are now in contact, because of migration patterns brought on by technological advances, the growth in trade and other economic relations between groups, and for less positive reasons including war, conquest, and slavery. Recent admixture between formerly isolated groups is an important feature of many of today's modern populations. Recent admixture introduces linkage disequilibrium between markers at two loci which have different allele frequencies in the original populations; this linkage disequilibrium is extensive and even affects markers that are on different chromosomes; if the resulting admixed population then mixes freely in subsequent generations, truly long-range linkage disequilibrium (between markers separated so that their recombination rate is near 1/2) will disappear rapidly , as indicated by formula (2.15), in subsequent generations. If mating practice is affected by admixture proportion (with mating more likely between similarly admixed than dissimilar subjects), then apparent linkage disequilibrium can remain high between markers throughout the genome for many generations. Admixture is an important aspect of such US populations as African Americans, Latinos, American Indians, and Native Hawaiians, and additional admixture among many populations may be expected to continue due to continued population movements and loosening of cultural prohibitions. As we will see in Chap. 4, it may be very important to control for admixture in an association study.

Hidden stratification occurs when an apparently homogeneous population contains unrecognized (or simply unmeasured in a given study) population structure, specifically the presence of subgroups within a larger population between which mixing is rare. Historically within the USA, we can think of many religious or ethnically based groups with prohibitions against marriage outside the group, but which may not be distinguished from each other in typical epidemiological studies. The distinction between hidden population stratification and admixture is not very clear in practice since in many cases traditional prohibitions are increasingly relaxed. The impact on LD structure of such stratification (while usually milder than the effect of recent admixture between continentally separated groups) can still be important in association studies especially in certain types of extreme studies, as we will see in later chapters.

2.7.3.4 Hidden Relatedness Between Subjects

Another potentially problematic issue for association studies is the presence of unexpected close relatives in studies. Many association studies that enroll a large number of participants from small populations are likely to encounter a fairly large number of quite closely related subjects, and even large-scale multisite studies occasionally find unexpected relatives (and even identical twins) when they look carefully at the genotypes that are generated. As we see in Chap. 4, *cryptic relatedness*, does, if many close relatives are genotyped in a study but the subjects were not recognized to be close relatives, have an important effect on the distribution of test statistics designed to detect associations between markers and phenotype.

While relatedness between individuals does not affect the marginal distribution of individual genotypes (here we are ignoring the possibility of inbreeding), it does affect the distribution of quantities such as the sum of two or more related individual's genotypes, for example, for two siblings (so that $z_0 = \frac{1}{4}$, $z_1 = \frac{1}{2}$, and $z_2 = \frac{1}{4}$) so that the correlation between n_1 and n_2 is equal to $1/2$ $z_1 + z_2 = 1/2$, then the sum, S, of $n_1 + n_2$ will have variance

$$\text{Var}(n_1) + \text{Var}(n_2) + 2\text{Cov}(n_1, n_2) = 6p(1-p)$$

compared to $4p(1-p)$ if the two counts were independent. This comparison is important because, as discussed in Chaps. 3 and 4, statistical tests that use inappropriate variance estimates are generally overdispersed under the null hypothesis, i.e., are prone to give inappropriate false-positive (type I) error rates.

2.7.4 Pseudo-LD Induced by Hidden Structure and Relatedness

For most of this chapter only one marker has been considered in the discussion of hidden structure and relatedness. Now consider an extension of the Balding-Nichols model to two markers, not in linkage disequilibrium in any individual population, sampled for a set of individuals ($i = 1, \ldots, N$) in a stratified population with substrata $l = 1, \ldots, L$. For the purpose of notational simplification, assume that both markers have the same frequency, p, in the ancestral population. The simulation process is as follows:

For the first marker, draw a set of subpopulation marker frequencies, p_{l1}, $l = 1, \ldots, L$ from the beta distribution with mean p.

For the first marker, draw a sample of marker values $n_{i,1}$, $i = 1, \ldots, N$ independently from the binomial distribution with index $= 2$ and frequency p_{l1}, where l corresponds to the substratum that individual i is assigned to.

Draw a set of marker frequencies, p_{2l}, $l = 1, \ldots, L$ from the same beta distribution for the second marker.

Draw sample of the second marker $n_{i,2}$, $i = 1, \ldots, N$ again stratified by subpopulation.

The following R code snippet illustrates the sampling procedure for $L = 2$ populations each of size 1,000 subjects:

```
> set.seed(10201) # to get the same results each time
> N<-1000 # number of subjects in each of L strata
> L<-2     # number of strata
> p=.3     # ancestral allele frequency for both markers
> F=.1     # differentiation between modern-day and ancestral populations
> n1<-rep(0,L*N) # holds values for first marker
> n2<-rep(0,L*N) # holds values for second marker
> p_l1=rbeta(L,p*(1-F)/F,(1-p)*(1-F)/F) # freqs of marker 1 in current populations
> p_l2=rbeta(L,p*(1-F)/F,(1-p)*(1-F)/F) # freqs of marker 2 in current populations
> for (l in 1:L){ # sample from appropriate binomial distribution
>        n1[((l-1)*N+1):(l*N)]<-rbinom(N,2,p_l1[l])
>        n2[((l-1)*N+1):(l*N)]<-rbinom(N,2,p_l2[l])
> }
```

Now consider testing for whether there is an association between markers 1 and 2. After running the above code, we type:

```
> summary(lm(n1~n2))
```

which gives results:

```
Call:
lm(formula = n1 ~ n2)
Coefficients:
             Estimate Std. Error t value Pr(>|t|)
(Intercept)   0.69113    0.02006  34.456  < 2e-16 ***
n2           -0.06808    0.02122  -3.208  0.00136 **

Signif. codes:  0 '***' 0.001 '**' 0.01 '*' 0.05 '.' 0.1 ' ' 1
```

Note that variables n_2 and n_1 appear to be associated despite being sampled independently, while the magnitude of the correlation is not very large (just $R = -0.07$), the p-value for testing association is equal to 0.00136 clearly something that is unlikely just by chance, in fact repeating this experiment many times gives a large number of quite small p-values.

The real source of this apparent association between independent markers is the failure to take account of the correlation structure of n_1 when we tested for association between n_1 and n_2.

The R function lm has underestimated the variance of the ordinary least squares estimate because it has assumed that the elements of n_1 are independent of each other, when instead the nonzero value of F used in the simulation has induced the between-marker correlation structure described above. When averaging over many runs, the correlation will be estimated to be equal to zero between the two markers; however, for any given run the usual tests for association are very likely to yield a very small p-value, i.e., a false-positive assessment of correlation, and this problem increases with sample size N.

A more detailed analysis (see Chap. 4) shows that the assumption that both n_1 and n_2 are differentiated according to population structure is required to produce this sort of induced correlation (this makes sense since we can always reverse the role of n_1 and n_2 in this problem). Note the use here of ordinary least squares (the R procedure lm) rather than glm to test for a relationship between two marker count variables; while this may seem nonstandard to many statisticians familiar with analysis of binomial data (e.g., using logistic regression), it is quick and gives very well-behaved tests of the null hypothesis of no association between the two markers for sample sizes as large (1,000 per strata) as used here (this can be observed in the behavior of the simulation program by setting F to zero and running the entire experiment again—only something very close to the expected number of small p-values will be observed), see Chap. 3 for more information.

Clearly the induced correlation described here behaves nothing like true linkage disequilibrium, which should die out as the genetic distance between the two markers increases; here we have simulated a situation that is analogous to markers lying on different chromosomes entirely. Interestingly as we will see in Chap. 4, even such weak apparent correlations (because they are spread over the entire genome) can have important consequences when it comes to distinguishing true marker/genotype associations between those induced by hidden structure or relatedness. This is most especially true for certain extreme analyses such as the case-only method for assessing gene x gene interactions [34] (see Chap. 7).

2.8   Covering the Genome for Common Alleles

As described above the common disease-common variant hypothesis is undoubtedly a simplification of a much more complex genetic architecture for many diseases, and while common disease-related alleles have been detected for many diseases, many questions remain about the relative role of common variants versus rare variants. Nevertheless the CDCV hypothesis motivates the use, in genetic association studies, of the technical breakthroughs that have led to the identification of millions of common SNPs, as well as cost-effective array-based large-scale genotyping of hundreds of thousands or even millions of SNPs.

A key issue then for GWAS studies is the "coverage" of common variants by the SNP arrays that are available commercially; coverage calculations are based on R^2 statistics between SNPs on the arrays and a target set of known variants. For each target variant, the goal is to have an SNP on the SNP array that is highly correlated with the target. Since these arrays are meant to be used generally, i.e., for all heritable phenotypes that could be of interest, target variants should not be simply be SNPs in candidate genes for one or more phenotypes but rather should as much as possible constitute a census of all common variation.

SNP array coverage statistics have been described for various populations by the companies that manufacture and sell the arrays, as well as by other investigators [35, 36]. However, at least three factors make the evaluation of coverage of the genome an ongoing project; first of all, the frequency domain of the target variants (which originally specified variants with minor allele frequencies at least 5 to 10 % frequency in one or more populations as common) is changing with rarer alleles increasingly being considered to be worthy targets; secondly the number of populations being assessed for genetic variation is increasing and this can lead to additional variants, common in specific populations being included in the target set; and finally techniques of SNP discovery are continuing to improve and to lead to increased discovery of variants not known to have existed. One additional factor that may also complicate the assessment of the coverage of common variation is inherent uncertainty in the measurement of some kinds of potential causal variants. Here I am referring to the possibility that haplotypes made up of SNPs or other variants could be causal variants (examples have been reported, e.g., [37]) rather than the SNPs: a "haplotype effect" means that a combination of SNPs falling on the same homologous chromosome could have a different effect than if the same SNPs were present, but on different homologs. Even if all the SNPs that constitute a SNP haplotype appear on the array, there still may be (depending on the degree of historical recombination between the SNPs making up that haplotype) considerable uncertainty in inferring the haplotype based upon the genotypes of those SNPs. We discuss haplotype uncertainty in more detail in Chap. 7. If we begin to consider not only all common SNPs and other sequence variants but also *all common haplotypes* of these SNPs as our target set of variants, then this greatly increases both the number of variants to be tested and also lowers overall coverage statistics due to haplotype uncertainty.

To date, the coverage target set of choice has been the SNPs (and other identified inherited variants) genotyped in the HapMap project (http://hapmap. ncbi.nlm.nih.gov/), specifically in phase 1 and phase 2 of this project [38]. As described below, phase 1 and phase 2 together genotyped over six million SNPs of which several millions were found to be common in at least one of four groups of samples. The DNA samples genotyped by the HapMap project originated from 270 people: 90 Africans (members of the Yoruba people, in Ibadan, Nigeria), 90 Americans of European descent from Utah, 45 Han Chinese from Beijing China, and 45 Japanese from Tokyo, Japan. The SNPs that were chosen to be genotyped in HapMap were those that had been previously reported to dbSNP (http://www.ncbi.nlm.nih.gov/snp/ [39]), an online repository of information about genetic variation contributed by scientists studying the human genome from around the world. In order to assess completeness of ascertainment of common SNPs by the HapMap, the HapMap project included within it an SNP discovery project focusing upon 10 different regions of the human genome, each of approximate length 500 kb, for which genetic sequencing was performed in 48 unrelated DNA samples (16 Yoruba, 8 Japanese, 8 Han Chinese, and 16 Europeans); all identified SNPs as well as all SNPs from dbGAP reported in these regions were genotyped in all the HapMap samples. Reports about the frequency and number of common variants in these regions as well as other statistics designed to use these regions to assess coverage over the full genome have been published [38].

More recently the 1000 Genomes Project [40] is in the process of using high-throughput sequencing methods to identify additional common sequence variants and also to begin to for the first time create a census of less common variants, specifically those within the range from 1 to 5 % frequency in at least one of the 14 populations considered. While these data are still (at the time of this writing) incomplete, there are already indications that not all common variants to be found in this project will have good surrogate SNPs either on the commercial arrays or indeed within the HapMap itself.

Table 2.5 shows the number of individual samples and type of sample (unrelated individuals or parent-offspring trios) for the HapMap phase 1 + 2 project, the HapMap phase 3 project, and the 1000 Genomes Project.

Table 2.5 Population description for HapMap and the 1000 Genomes Project (1KP)

Population designator	Population descriptor	HapMap 1 + 2	HapMap 3	1KG phase 1
ASW	African ancestry in southwest USA			
	N samples	0	90	61
	N founders	0	60	61
CEU	Utah residents with northern and western European ancestry			
	N samples	90	180	85
	N founders	60	121	85
CHB	Han Chinese in Beijing, China			
	N samples	45	90	97
	N founders	45	90	97
CHD	Chinese in Denver, Colorado			
	N samples	0	100	0
	N founders	0	100	0
CHS	Han Chinese, South			
	N samples	0	0	100
	N founders			100
CLM	Columbians in Medellin, Columbia			
	N samples	0	0	60
	N founders			60
FIN	Finnish in Finland			
	N samples	0	0	93
	N founders			93
GBR	British from England and Scotland			
	N samples	0	0	89
	N founders			89
GIH	Gujarati Indians in Houston, Texas			
	N samples	0	100	0
	N founders	0	100	0
IBS	Iberian populations in Spain			
	N samples	0	0	14
	N founders	0	0	14
JPT	Japanese in Tokyo, Japan			
	N samples	45	91	89
	N founders	45	91	89
LWK	Luhya in Webuye, Kenya			
	N samples	0	100	97
	N founders	0	100	97
MEX/MXL	Mexican ancestry in Los Angeles, CA			
	N samples	0	90	66
	N founders	0	60	66
MKK	Maasai in Kinyawa, Kenya			
	N samples	0	180	0
	N founders	0	150	0

(continued)

Table 2.5 (continued)

Population designator	Population descriptor	HapMap 1 + 2	HapMap 3	1KG phase 1
PUR	Puerto Ricans in Puerto Rico			
	N samples	0	0	55
	N founders	0	0	55
TSI	Tuscany in Italia			
	N samples	0	100	98
	N founders	0	100	98
YRI	Yoruba in Ibadan, Nigeria			
	N samples	90	180	88
	N founders	60	120	88

2.8.1 High-Throughput Sequencing

As of the time that this book is written, large-scale high-throughput sequencing [41] is beginning to be performed in association studies either focused on candidate regions, such as exons either of candidate genes, or for all known genes, regions containing GWAS hits; whole genome sequencing is beginning to be used despite the considerable expense and informatic burdens that large-scale sequencing involves. More on the rationale for collecting and approaches to the analysis of such data is given in Chap. 8.

2.9 Principal Components Analysis

One of the most useful methods for detecting and visualizing hidden structure and admixture is principal components analysis [42], and this technique has been widely advocated (and used) as an effective tool for addressing population structure in the analysis of data from association studies [4]. For the time being, we concentrate on principal components methods as a technique for display of sample or population features.

Reviewing very briefly, see Jolliffe [43], given samples of random vectors X with M components, the first principal component of X is a linear function $\alpha'_1 X$ of the elements of X which has maximum variance under the constraint that $\alpha'_1 \alpha_1$ equals 1. The second principal component is another linear function, $\alpha'_2 X$, which is uncorrelated with $\alpha'_1 X$ and again with maximum variance subject to $\alpha'_2 \alpha_2 = 1$. Proceeding in this fashion further up to M principal components can be found, but it is hoped that important characteristics of the variability of X will be captured by L principal components with L considerably less than M. These first L linear functions are called the *leading* principal components. They can be computed through a *spectral* or *eigenvector/eigenvalue* decomposition of the covariance matrix of X; specifically if $\boldsymbol{\Sigma}$ is the covariance matrix of X, then the *spectral decomposition* of $\boldsymbol{\Sigma}$ is

$$\boldsymbol{\Sigma} = \sum_{k=1}^{M} w_k \alpha_k \alpha_k^{\mathrm{T}},$$

where the w_k are each nonnegative scalars (the eigenvalues of $\boldsymbol{\Sigma}$), with $w_1 \geq w_2 \geq w_3 \ldots \geq w_M \geq 0$, and the α_k as the eigenvectors of $\boldsymbol{\Sigma}$ each having the property that $(\boldsymbol{\Sigma} - w_k \mathbf{I})\alpha_k = 0$. The fraction of total variance that is explained by the L principal components is computed as

$$\sum_{i=1}^{L} w_i \Big/ \left(\sum_{i=1}^{M} w_i \right). \tag{2.16}$$

Principal components analysis is used as a data summarization technique in a wide variety of data intensive fields and disciplines including bioinformatics for gene expression data, proteomics, and metabolomics [44, 45]. In nutritional epidemiology, there have been a number of papers relating risk of late onset disease (cardiovascular disease, cancer, etc.) to specific eating patterns captured by the first L (or leading) principal components of dietary data [46]. Many other uses of principal components analysis and its cousin, factor analysis, have been described in many different fields including bioinformatics, meteorology [47], and economics.

When variables are not all scaled similarly, it is customary to compute the principal components from the correlation matrix for the random vector X rather than from the covariance matrix. When dealing with massive amounts of SNP data (i.e., where M corresponding to the number of SNPs genotyped in a given study is very large), large-scale genetic association studies tend to approach principal components slightly differently than described above. For example, Price et al. [4] describes the extraction of the eigenvectors of the $N \times N$ kinship matrix $\mathbf{K}$, where N is the number of subjects, rather than starting with (as above) the eigenvectors of the $M \times M$ correlation or covariance matrix for the SNP data. The first L of these eigenvectors themselves (not their dot products with each individual's SNP data) are then termed "principal components" by Price et al., i.e., the ith element of the jth eigenvector is referred to as the value of the jth "principal component" for person i. While it is nonstandard terminology to call these the principal components, there is actually a close relationship between the classical principal components, calculated by decomposing the correlation matrix of the genotype data, to the eigenvectors of the relationship matrix (a matrix of dimension $N \times N$). While the relationship matrix is not a correlation matrix per se, note that we can compute the sample correlation matrix between the genotypes as

$$C = \frac{1}{(N-1)} X^T X, \tag{2.17}$$

where X is a $(N \times M)$ matrix with the (i, k) elements equal to the normalized values

$$x_{ik} = \frac{n_{ik} - \overline{n}_{.k}}{\sqrt{S_{.k}^2}}.$$

Here $\overline{n}_{.k}$ is the usual sample mean for SNP k and $S_{.k}^2$ is equal to the usual sample variance estimator $(1/N - 1) \sum_{i=1}^{N} (n_{ik} - \overline{n}_{.k})^2$. Note the similarity between this x_{ik} and z_{ik} in (2.7) which is used in the calculation of the estimated relationship matrix $\hat{K}$. In fact the estimate of the mean $\overline{n}_{.k}$ is exactly equal to $2\hat{p}_k$, and $\sqrt{2\hat{p}_k}(1 - \hat{p}_k)$ will be close (if HWE is not greatly violated) to $\sqrt{S_{.k}^2}$. This implies that the estimated relationship matrix (computed for all pairs of a total of N subjects) is "almost" equal to the $N \times N$ matrix $(1/M)XX^T$. Moreover it is easy to show that if α_l is the lth eigenvector of $(1/(N-1))X^TX$, the lth eigenvector of $(1/M)XX^T$ will be equal to a constant times $X\alpha_l$. Because of this, the eigenvectors of the relationship matrix while computed using the $z_{i,k}$ are generally almost proportional to the principal components computed using the eigenvectors of the correlation matrix computed from the $x_{i,k}$.

Note that if (as typical in a GWAS study) we have a larger number, M, of SNPs (several hundred thousand) genotyped than we have individuals, M (several thousand), then it may be much more computationally efficient to extract eigenvectors from the $N \times N$ relationship matrix than from the $M \times M$ correlation matrix. Given these considerations, it is reasonable to accept the slight abuse of terminology of Price et al. and refer to the eigenvectors of $\hat{K}$ as the principal components of the genotype data.

2.9.1   Display of Principal Components for the HapMap Phase 3 Samples

The HapMap project expanded the number of populations with genotypes available by (in phase 3) genotyping a total of 1,184 subjects from 11 different distinct population samples using a combination of the Affymetrix 6.0 and Illumina 1M SNP arrays, each of which genotyped about one million SNPs with approximately 400,000 SNPs genotyped using both arrays. We illustrate the power of principal components analysis to extract the main features of historical separation that arose between populations, as groups diverged from their ancestral origins, and more recently admixture between long-separated groups, by use of a sample of SNPs from these data. We illustrate the process here of using the HapMap website in order to read into R a sample of ~20,000 randomly chosen SNPs from each of the 11 HapMap phase 3 populations, perform the calculation of the relationship matrix and its principal components (e.g., eigenvectors), and then display simple plots of these data. Because we will only be using a small sample of the HapMap genotypes, we can do all of the statistical calculations and plotting reasonably quickly in R; for larger datasets, there are several other choices depending on the expertise of the statistician, for example, the stand-alone program EIGENSTRAT, introduced by Price et al. computes principal components, but then these must be read into other programs (such as R) for plotting, filtering of results, summarization, etc. The statistical package SAS and its principal components procedure PRINCOMP can also be used to compute and display eigenvectors of $\hat{\mathbf{K}}$. These programs are effective in computing eigenvectors for quite large matrices (~10,000 subjects or more) on a modern desktop computer with a large amount of main memory (8–16 Gb).

For the illustrative example here, the simplest way to retrieve data from the HapMap website is as a PLINK format file and to use PLINK (see Computer Appendix) to extract a random sample of SNPs. The following steps were followed:

Download HapMap phase 3 data set, *hapmap3_r1_b36_fwd.qc.poly.tar.bz2*, from the HapMap website ftp site *ftp://ftp.ncbi.nlm.nih.gov*. This file, which contains separate files for each of the 11 contributing population samples, can be decompressed using the linux command *bunzip* or the Windows program *winzip*. The 11 HapMap 3 populations each have files of type *.ped which contain genotypes and *.map files which contain SNP information.

Using PLINK, merge these 22 files together, make a random selection of approximately 20,000 SNPs to use in the PCA analysis, and perform the PCA analysis and plotting using R. To do so, we first run the following PLINK commands:

```
plink --file hapmap3_r2_b36_fwd.ASW.qc.poly --merge-list allfiles.txt --make-bed --out
hapmap3_allpops
plink --bfile hapmap3_allpops --recodeA --thin 0.02 -maf 0.05 --filter-founders --out
hapmap3_snp_sample
```

The first command refers to a list of all the files (*allfiles.txt*, created by the user) to be merged with the first file (ASW). The *allfiles.txt* file lists the remaining 10 genotype files to be merged starting with the first one as listed on the command line. It contains the list:

```
hapmap3_r2_b36_fwd.CEU.qc.poly.ped hapmap3_r2_b36_fwd.CEU.qc.poly.map
hapmap3_r2_b36_fwd.CHB.qc.poly.ped hapmap3_r2_b36_fwd.CHB.qc.poly.map
hapmap3_r2_b36_fwd.CHD.qc.poly.ped hapmap3_r2_b36_fwd.CHD.qc.poly.map
hapmap3_r2_b36_fwd.GIH.qc.poly.ped hapmap3_r2_b36_fwd.GIH.qc.poly.map
hapmap3_r2_b36_fwd.JPT.qc.poly.ped hapmap3_r2_b36_fwd.JPT.qc.poly.map
hapmap3_r2_b36_fwd.LWK.qc.poly.ped hapmap3_r2_b36_fwd.LWK.qc.poly.map
hapmap3_r2_b36_fwd.MEX.qc.poly.ped hapmap3_r2_b36_fwd.MEX.qc.poly.map
hapmap3_r2_b36_fwd.MKK.qc.poly.ped hapmap3_r2_b36_fwd.MKK.qc.poly.map
hapmap3_r2_b36_fwd.TSI.qc.poly.ped hapmap3_r2_b36_fwd.TSI.qc.poly.map
hapmap3_r2_b36_fwd.YRI.qc.poly.ped hapmap3_r2_b36_fwd.YRI.qc.poly.map
```

These files being merged are named according to the population descriptors for the 11 HapMap phase 3 groups: See Table 2.5.

The output of the second PLINK command is the file, hapmap3_snp_sample. raw, which is formatted in a way that the *R* command, *read.table*, can read directly. The *–recodeA* subcommand codes the SNP alleles as equal to 0, 1, or 2 copies of the minor allele with NA being the missing value indicator. The *–maf 0.05* command removes SNPs which have minor allele frequency less than 5 %, and the *–filter-founders* command indicates that only genotype data for the total of 988 founders (i.e., dropping offspring from any parent-offspring trios) is to be included.

With the addition of one other file (*IDgroup.txt* which contains the ID record for and group affiliation (ASW, CEU, etc. for each subject), we can now perform a simple PCA analysis in *R*.

Read data into *R* and compute the estimated relationship matrix for all *X* subjects:

```
>#  define function to calculate the Kinship matrix
>Calc_k<-function(x){
>        nsubj<-dim(x)[1]
>        nsnps<-dim(x)[2]
>        cfreq<-colMeans(x,na.rm=TRUE)/2
>        y<-t(t(x)-cfreq*2)
>        y<-ifelse(!is.na(y),y,0)
>        cv<-2*cfreq*(1-cfreq)
>        K<-t(t(y)/cv)%*%t(y)/nsnps
>        K
>}
>
>#  read the sample of ~20,000 SNPs
>pca_snps<-read.table("hapmap3_snp_sample.raw",header=T)
>
>#  read the group information for each sample
>IDgrp<-read.table(file="IDgrp.txt")
>grp<-as.character(IDgrp[,2])
>ID<-as.character(IDgrp[,1])
>
>#  compute the Kinship matrix K (a 988 by 988 matrix)
>ncols<-dim(pca_snps)[2]
>K<-Calc_k(pca_snps[1:nsubj,7:ncols]) #the first 6 columns do not contain genotypes
```

Next we compute eigenvectors and define and run a function *plotPC* used to display the results:

```
> # Compute the eigenvectors and eigenvalues
> e<-eigen(K)
>
> # Make plot distinguishing the different groups
> # make up a function to do this  ##### terrible code USE matplot instead
> #
> #
> plotPC<->function(e,GRP=c("ASW","CHB","CHD","GIH","JPT","LWK","MEX","MKK","TSI","YRI"),
>       COLOR=c("red","blue","green","yellow","orange","black","purple","pink","gray","violet"
>       ,"cyan>"),d1=1,d2=2,xl=c(-0.05,0.05),yl=c(-0.05,0.05),gp=grp)
>       {
>       matplot(rbind(e$vectors[gp=GRP[1],1]),e$vectors,xlim=xl,ylim=yl,col=COLOR,main="
>       ",xlab=paste("EV",d1,sep=""),ylab=paste("EV",d2,sep=""))
>          lr<-length(rest)
>          if (length(rest) >= 1) {
>                for (i in 2:length(rest))
>                   # add additional populatons
>                   lines(e$vectors[gp==rest[i-1],d1],e$vectors[gp==rest[i-1],d2],
>                   xlim=xl,ylim=yl,col=restc[i-1],type="p")
>          }
> }
> # run the plotting function
> plotPC(e)
```

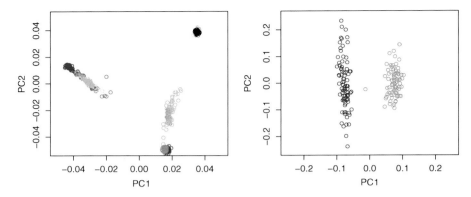

Fig. 2.5 Principal components plot for the HapMap phase 3 data. R code for this plot is given in the text. The *colors* correspond to group membership; see the *R* function plotPC, defined in the text, for color coding. The *left side plot* shows all 11 groups plotted, while the *right side plot* is only the Japanese and Chinese samples

The results of this first call to the function *plotPC* are given in Fig. 2.5a.

In Fig. 2.5a the main visible features are the clustering of the three continental groups (European, Asian, and African) as well as evidence of admixture for several groups including the African Americans (ASW) and the Mexican Americans (MEX). We can look in more detail at the two East Asian groups, Japanese from Tokyo (JPT) and Chinese from Beijing (CHB), by recomputing the K matrix that pertains to these two groups, recalculating the eigenvectors, and again calling the *plotPC* function:

```
>#  now look more closely at only the Japanese and Chinese groups
>grpJC<-(grp=="JPT")|(grp=="CHB")
>#  recalculate the Kinship matrix and eigenvectors
>KJC<-Calc_k(pca_snps[grpJC,7:ncols])
>ejc<-eigen(KJC)
>gJC<-grp[grpJC]
>#
>#Make a new plot just of the Japanese and Chinese samples
plotPC(ejc,gp=gJC,GRP="JPT",d1=1,d2=2,COLOR="orange",rest=c("CHB"),restc=("blue"),xl=c(-
>.25,.25),yl=c(-.25,.25))
>
```

The results are shown in Fig. 2.5b. Now the first eigenvector is sensitive to differences in SNP frequencies between the Japanese samples, compared to the Chinese samples. This plot shows that the principal components method can make more subtle distinctions than just the detection of large-scale continental variation. This Japanese group of samples appears to derive from China given the overall similarity of the two groups seen in Fig. 2.5a, but remains partly distinguishable as in Fig. 2.5b. The observed differences are probably related to founder effects and random genetic drift due to the relative isolation of Japan from the mainland of Asia over a number of generations [48].

Principal components analysis is of course interesting since it says much about historical relationships among population groups; it has also been stressed here

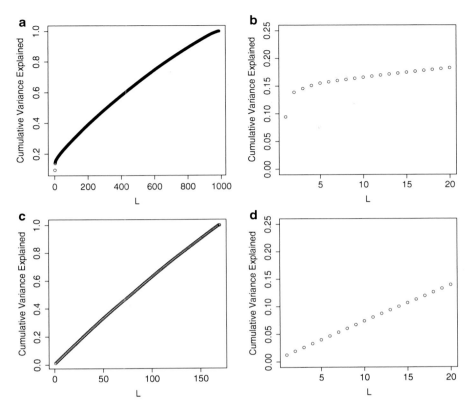

Fig. 2.6 Plots of the total variation explained by eigenvectors 1, ..., L for (**a**, **b**) the entire HapMap phase 3 dataset and (**c**, **d**) for the Japanese (JPT) and Chinese (CHB)

because of its utility as a tool in association studies as will be described in later chapters. Principal components can also be used as a QC tool in checking that batches of genotype data are not being disturbed by subtle factors (such as plate specific errors and DNA quality issues). Principal components are sensitive to each of population structure, relatedness between subjects, and to certain patterns of linkage disequilibrium, as well as such QC problems.

It is worth saying also that while principal components can distinguish groups that are quite closely related historically, the total amount of SNP variation that is explained by the first few leading principal components—i.e., the portion of SNP variation that can be directly related to racial/ethnic origins, is actually quite small. Figure 2.6 plots the cumulative percentage (2.16) of SNP variation explained by the first L eigenvectors for both the total HapMap phase 3 population and for the Japanese and Chinese separately. About 15 % of the total variation in the entire HapMap sample and much less (~2 %) of the variation of the SNP data for the Japanese and Chinese is explained by the two eigenvectors plotted in Fig 2.6a, b.

This illustrates the general concept that racial groups are ultimately much more similar than they are different, or more precisely that within-group genetic variation dwarfs between-group variation.

2.10   Chapter Summary

The chapter has presented a brief survey of topics related to population and quantitative genetics that are relevant to the motivation for and the design and analysis of large-scale genetic association studies. The concepts of linkage disequilibrium, population heterogeneity and relatedness, and the induced covariance between markers caused by population heterogeneity, as well as the techniques of principal component analysis, described here, are all followed up in the later chapters in this book.

Homework/Projects

1. If the vector of allele counts $\mathbf{n_1} = (n_{11}, n_{21}, \ldots, n_{N1})'$ for a given variant has covariance matrix $2p_1(1 - p_1)\mathbf{K}$ and that another variant with allele counts $\mathbf{n_2} = (n_{12}, n_{22}, \ldots, n_{N2})'$ independent of $\mathbf{n_1}$ which has covariance matrix $2p_2(1 - p_2)\mathbf{K}$:

   (a) Show that the sum of these two variants, $\mathbf{s} = \mathbf{n_1} + \mathbf{n_2}$, will have covariance matrix $(2p_1(1 - p_1) + 2p_2(1 - p_2))\mathbf{K}$.
   (b) Show that the correlation matrix of $\mathbf{s}$ is the same as the correlation matrix of $\mathbf{n_1}$ (or for that matter $\mathbf{n_2}$).
   (c) Define a *polygene*, $g_i = \displaystyle\sum_{j=1,\ldots,M} w_j n_{ij}$, as a weighted sum of M independent alleles each with the same covariance structure (covariance between subjects i and j) as above. Show that the covariance structure of the polygene is equal to $\gamma^2 \mathbf{K}$ with $\gamma^2 = \displaystyle\sum_{j=1,\ldots,M} w_j^2 2 p_j (1 - p_j)$

2. Give details of the calculations for several other probabilities in Table 2.2 following the method used for the (Aa, Aa) genotype.
3. For first cousins (where the grandparents are unrelated to each other):

   (a) Compute the probabilities z_0, z_1, and z_2 from first principles.
   (b) Suppose the first cousins marry and have two children, what is each offspring's inbreeding coefficient and the probabilities z_0, z_1, and z_2 between them?

4. Show using Table 2.2 that

$$\mathrm{Cov}(n_1, n_2) = (z_1 + 2z_2)p(1 - p).$$

5. Section 2.1.3: Suppose that DNA for a random sample of pairs of siblings is obtained and all DNA samples are genotyped for a polymorphism. How does

(2.1) need to be modified to give a confidence interval for the allele frequency of an allele A?

Hint: first find the variance of the allele frequency estimate for each sibling pair and then the average of this estimate over all pairs.

6. Section 2.1.4, inbreeding:

   (a) Show that if an individual's parents are related with coefficient of kinship equal to h then if n_A is the count of allele A for a given polymorphism $\{aA\}$ with frequency of A equal to p, the variance of n_A is $2p(1 - p)(1 + h)$.

   (b) Show also that the predicted fraction of heterozygotes equals $2p(1 - p)$ $(1 - h)$ in the same situation. This gives a definition of F_{st} for an inbred population, namely, as the average kinship between individuals in the population, which is estimated by the reduction of heterozygotes away from HWE.

   See Balding and Nichols' papers [49–51] for more details.

7. Section 2.5.1, relatedness: compute the variance of $\dfrac{1}{M} \displaystyle\sum_{\ell=1}^{M} z_{i\ell}^2$ under assumptions of (1) Hardy–Weinberg equilibrium for all SNPs (implying that this quantity has expected value equal to one), (2) that all variants are independent (not in LD) of each other, and (3) that all have the same allele frequency p. Compute the variance under the same conditions of the suggested estimator (Yang et al. [9])

$$1 + \frac{1}{M} \sum_{\ell=1}^{M} \frac{n_{i\ell}^2 - (1 + 2p_\ell)n_{i\ell} + 2p_\ell^2}{2p_\ell(1 - p_\ell)}.$$

   Hint: compute from first principals the mean and second moments of $z_{i\ell}^2$ under HWE by summation over its distribution, i.e., $z_{i\ell}^2$ takes value $(0 - 2p_\ell)^2/$ $(2p_\ell(1 - p_\ell))$ with probability $(1 - p_\ell)^2$, value $(1 - 2p_\ell)^2/(2p_\ell(1 - p_\ell))$ with probability $2p_\ell(1 - p_\ell)$, and $\frac{(2 - 2p_\ell)^2}{2p_\ell(1-p_\ell)}$ with probability p_ℓ^2.

8. Section 2.9, principal components. Why are the eigenvalues of a covariance matrix Σ considered to be equivalent to variances explained by eigenvectors, and why is (2.16) interpreted as the fraction of variance explained by the first L leading eigenvectors?

9. Section 2.7.4: Show that for a mixed population, Z, treated as a single population containing two subpopulations, X and Y, with proportion m and $(1 - m)$, respectively, that the disequilibrium between any two markers A and B in the mixed population is equal to

$$\delta_Z = m\delta_X + (1 - m)\delta_Y + m(1 - m)\left(p_{A,X} - p_{A,Y}\right)\left(p_{B,X} - p_{B,Y}\right),$$

with δ_X, δ_Y, and δ_Z as the disequilibrium parameters in populations, X, Y, and Z, respectively, and allele frequencies of markers A and B as $p_{A,X}, p_{B,X}, p_{A,Y}$, and

$p_{B,Y}$ in populations X and Y, respectively. Hint: see reference [52]. Note that this implies that markers which are unlinked in the originating populations ($\delta_X = 0$, and $\delta_Y = 0$) will be linked in a stratified populations only if the allele frequencies of both alleles are different.

10. Section 2.4.1.1: Based on the Balding–Nichols model used in that section give a formula for H_t and H_s and hence F_{st} when F remains the same for each population t, but the sample size in each population, N_t is different.

11. Section 2.6.3, selection and allele frequency distribution. Consider a cancer like breast cancer and assume that the only reduction in reproductive fitness related to occurrence of breast cancer is due to early mortality (e.g., mortality in the childbearing years from the cancer). We are interested in the following question: if a genetic variant of 10 % frequency increases relative risk of breast cancer mortality by 20 % per allele proportionately over a woman's lifetime, what value of σ in (2.14) would this correspond to, i.e., what reduction of fitness does this imply? What data would be needed in order to address this question?

12. Section 2.6.1, having two sexes raises an obvious question. Is there a most recent common female ancestor and a most recent common male ancestor? If so did they know each other? For a discussion, see http://scienceblogs.com/authority/2007/07/17/adam-eve-and-why-they-never-go/.

2.11 Data and Software Exercises

Here we assume that the JAPC and LAPC data mentioned in Chap. 1 are available to the student, either through a dbGaP request or otherwise. If other GWAS data are available to the student, these can in most cases be used instead.

1. Using available GWAS data (e.g., JAPC and LAPC) as well as the HapMap data described above, perform principal components analysis on the combined data. This consists of several steps:

    (a) Develop a list of SNPs that are genotyped in both the GWAS data and the HapMap data described above (hint: use the bim files to manipulate them in SAS or R) to form a list of the intersection of SNPs between all these files.
    (b) Sample perhaps 10,000 or so markers from the intersection above (SAS or R).
    (c) Pull out SNP data from each file (using PLINK commands). For HapMap do not use offspring who have parents with genotypes (PLINK command).
    (d) Merge the data for the 10,000 common markers into a single PLINK file (PLINK commands).
    (e) Recode this file to 0, 1, 2 coding (count of the number of minor alleles carried for each SNP) using PLINK commands.
    (f) Read this file into R and modify/run the R programs given above to extract principal components of the data and display these data as done above for the HapMap samples.

(g) Make a special run just on the JAPC data in combination with the JPT HapMap population. Describe the finer structure in the JAPC data; see [48] for a survey of population structure in Japan.

2. EIGENSTRAT for principal components estimation. We have shown a simple R program that can estimate the relationship matrix **K** using the formulae (2.8) and (2.9). This program will work reasonably well for a few thousand markers and few hundred subjects. A much more efficient program that can handle hundreds of thousands of markers and tens of thousands of subjects is EIGENSTRAT [53] available from http://genepath.med.harvard.edu/~reich/Software.htm. Review the use of this program.

3. STRUCTURE, Pritchard et al.[54]. This program is specifically designed to identify hidden structure in a population based upon SNP data and estimate population membership or admixture fraction for each individual in a study. The results of the STRUCTURE analysis (an individual's percent admixture from different populations) is often more interpretable than using principal components and has been used in many analyses. The program can be downloaded from URL http://pritch.bsd.uchicago.edu/structure.html.

(a) Try running this program on samples of the HapMap data described above. Estimate admixture fractions for individuals in the ASW group (African ancestry in Los Angeles CA).

(b) Using the JAPC data, does this program estimate the fine structure visible by contained in this population?

References

1. Purcell, S., Neale, B., Todd-Brown, K., Thomas, L., Ferreira, M. A., Bender, D., et al. (2007). PLINK: A tool set for whole-genome association and population-based linkage analyses. *American Journal of Human Genetics, 81*, 559–575.
2. Choi, Y., Wijsman, E. M., & Weir, B. S. (2009). Case-control association testing in the presence of unknown relationships. *Genetic Epidemiology, 33*, 668–678.
3. Wakeley, J. (2009). *Coalescent theory, an introduction.* Greenwood Village, CO: Roberts and Company.
4. Price, A. L., Patterson, N. J., Plenge, R. M., Weinblatt, M. E., Shadick, N. A., & Reich, D. (2006). Principal components analysis corrects for stratification in genome-wide association studies. *Nature Genetics, 38*, 904–909.
5. Balding, D., & Nichols, R. (1995). A method for quantifying differentiation between populations at multi-allelic locus and its implications for investigating identify and paternity. *Genetica, 3*, 3–12.
6. Wright, S. (1949). The genetical structure of populations. *Annals of Eugenics, 15*, 323–354.
7. Chen, G. K., Millikan, R. C., John, E. M., Ambrosone, C. B., Bernstein, L., Zheng, W., et al. (2010). The potential for enhancing the power of genetic association studies in African Americans through the reuse of existing genotype data. *PLoS Genetics, 6*, e101096.
8. Bourgain, C., Hoffjan, S., Nicolae, R., Newman, D., Steiner, L., Walker, K., et al. (2003). Novel case-control test in a founder population identifies P-selectin as an atopy-susceptibility locus. *American Journal of Human Genetics, 73*, 612–626.

9. Yang, J., Benyamin, B., McEvoy, B. P., Gordon, S., Henders, A. K., Nyholt, D. R., et al. (2010). Common SNPs explain a large proportion of the heritability for human height. *Nature Genetics, 42*, 565–569.

10. Astle, W., & Balding, D. J. (2009). Population structure and cryptic relatedness in genetic association studies. *Statistical Science, 24*, 451–471.

11. Nordborg, M. (2008). Coalescent theory. In D. J. Balding, M. Bishop, & C. Cannings (Eds.), *Handbook of statistical genetics* (3rd ed., pp. 843–877). New York: Wiley.

12. Hudson, R. R. (2002). Generating samples under a Wright-Fisher neutral model of genetic variation. *Bioinformatics, 18*, 337–338.

13. Haag-Liautard, C., Dorris, M., Maside, X., Macaskill, S., Halligan, D. L., Houle, D., et al. (2007). Direct estimation of per nucleotide and genomic deleterious mutation rates in Drosophila. *Nature, 445*, 82–85.

14. Risch, N., & Merikangas, K. (1996). The future of genetic studies of complex human diseases. *Science, 273*, 1516–1517.

15. Lander, E. S. (1996). The new genomics: Global views of biology. *Science, 274*, 536–539.

16. Chakravarti, A. (1999). Population genetics-making sense out of sequence. *Nature Genetics, 21*, 56–60.

17. Reich, D. E., & Lander, E. S. (2001). On the allelic spectrum of human disease. *Trends in Genetics, 17*, 502–510.

18. Pritchard, J. K., & Cox, N. J. (2002). The allelic architecture of human disease genes: Common disease-common variant...or not? *Human Molecular Genetics, 11*, 2417–2423.

19. Wright, S. (1938). The distribution of gene frequencies under irreversible mutation. *Proceedings of the National Academy of Sciences of the United States of America, 24*, 253–259.

20. Ewens, W. (1972). The sampling theory of selectively neutral alleles. *Theoretical Population Biology, 3*, 87–112.

21. Slatkin, M., & Rannala, B. (1997). The sampling distribution of disease-associated alleles. *Genetics, 147*, 1855–1861.

22. Abecasis, G. R., Auton, A., Brooks, L. D., DePristo, M. A., Durbin, R. M., Handsaker, R. E., et al. (2012). An integrated map of genetic variation from 1,092 human genomes. *Nature, 491*, 56–65.

23. Wright, S. (Ed.). (1949). *Adaptation and selection*. Princeton, NJ: Princeton University Press.

24. Pritchard, J. K. (2001). Are rare variants responsible for susceptibility to complex diseases? *American Journal of Human Genetics, 69*, 124–137.

25. Griffiths, R. C., & Marjoram, P. (1996). Ancestral inference from samples of DNA sequences with recombination. *Journal of Computational Biology, 3*, 479–502.

26. Myers, S., Bottolo, L., Freeman, C., McVean, G., & Donnelly, P. (2005). A fine-scale map of recombination rates and hotspots across the human genome. *Science, 310*, 321–324.

27. Wall, J. D., & Pritchard, J. K. (2003). Haplotype blocks and linkage disequilibrium in the human genome. *Nature Reviews Genetics, 4*, 587–597.

28. Reich, D. E., Cargill, M., Bolk, S., Ireland, J., Sabeti, P. C., Richter, D. J., et al. (2001). Linkage disequilibrium in the human genome. *Nature, 411*, 199–204.

29. McVean, G. A., Myers, S. R., Hunt, S., Deloukas, P., Bentley, D. R., & Donnelly, P. (2004). The fine-scale structure of recombination rate variation in the human genome. *Science, 304*, 581–584.

30. Lewontin, R. (1964). The interaction of selection and linkage. I.general considerations: Heterotic models. *Genetics, 49*, 49–67.

31. Thomas, D. C. (2004). *Statistical methods in genetic epidemiology*. Oxford: Oxford University Press.

32. Gulcher, J., & Stefansson, K. (1998). Population genomics: Laying the groundwork for genetic disease modeling and targeting. *Clinical Chemistry and Laboratory Medicine, 36*, 523–527.

33. Editorial Board. (1998). Genome vikings. *Nature Genetics, 20*, 99–101.

34. Bhattacharjee, S., Wang, Z., Ciampa, J., Kraft, P., Chanock, S., Yu, K., et al. (2010). Using principal components of genetic variation for robust and powerful detection of gene-gene

interactions in case-control and case-only studies. *American Journal of Human Genetics, 86*, 331–342.

35. Hao, K., Schadt, E. E., & Storey, J. D. (2008). Calibrating the performance of SNP arrays for whole-genome association studies. *PLoS Genetics, 4*, e1000109.

36. Barrett, J. C., & Cardon, L. R. (2006). Evaluating coverage of genome-wide association studies. *Nature Genetics, 38*, 659–662.

37. Nackley, A. G., Shabalina, S. A., Tchivileva, I. E., Satterfield, K., Korchynskyi, O., Makarov, S. S., et al. (2006). Human catechol-O-methyltransferase haplotypes modulate protein expression by altering mRNA secondary structure. *Science, 314*, 1930–1933.

38. Altshuler, D., Brooks, L. D., Chakravarti, A., Collins, F. S., Daly, M. J., & Donnelly, P. (2005). A haplotype map of the human genome. *Nature, 437*, 1299–1320.

39. Kitts, A., & Sherry, S. (2002). The single nucleotide polymorphism database (Dbsnp) of nucleotide sequence variation. In J. McEntyre & J. Ostell (Eds.), *The NCBI handbook [Internet]*. Bethesda, MD: National Center for Biotechnology Information.

40. 1000 Genomes Project Consortium. (2010). A map of human genome variation from population-scale sequencing. *Nature, 467*, 1061–1073.

41. Soon, W. W., Hariharan, M., & Snyder, M. P. (2013). High-throughput sequencing for biology and medicine. *Molecular Systems Biology, 9*, 640.

42. Cavalli-Sforza, L. L., & Feldman, M. W. (2003). The application of molecular genetic approaches to the study of human evolution. *Nature Genetics, 33*(Suppl), 266–275.

43. Jolliffe, I. T. (2002). *Principal component analysis* (2nd ed.). New York: Springer.

44. Yeung, K. Y., & Ruzzo, W. L. (2001). Principal component analysis for clustering gene expression data. *Bioinformatics, 17*, 763–774.

45. Rao, P. K., & Li, Q. (2009). Principal component analysis of proteome dynamics in iron-starved mycobacterium tuberculosis. *Journal of Proteomics and Bioinformatics, 2*, 19–31.

46. Chang, E. T., Lee, V. S., Canchola, A. J., Dalvi, T. B., Clarke, C. A., Reynolds, P., et al. (2008). Dietary patterns and risk of ovarian cancer in the California teachers study cohort. *Nutrition and Cancer, 60*, 285–291.

47. Preisendorfer, R. W. (1988). *Principal components analysis in meteorology and oceanography*. Amsterdam: Elsevier.

48. Yamaguchi-Kabata, Y., Nakazono, K., Takahashi, A., Saito, S., Hosono, N., Kubo, M., et al. (2008). Japanese population structure, based on SNP genotypes from 7003 individuals compared to other ethnic groups: Effects on population-based association studies. *American Journal of Human Genetics, 83*, 445–456.

49. Balding, D. J., & Nichols, R. A. (1994). DNA profile match probability calculation: How to allow for population stratification, relatedness, database selection and single bands. *Forensic Science International, 64*, 125–140.

50. Nichols, R. A., & Balding, D. J. (1991). Effects of population structure on DNA fingerprint analysis in forensic science. *Heredity Edinburgh, 66*(Pt 2), 297–302.

51. Balding, D. J., & Nichols, R. A. (1995). A method for quantifying differentiation between populations at multi-allelic loci and its implications for investigating identity and paternity. *Genetica, 96*, 3–12.

52. Chakraborty, R., & Smouse, P. E. (1988). Recombination of haplotypes leads to biased estimates of admixture proportions in human populations. *Proceedings of the National Academy of Sciences of the United States of America, 85*, 3071–3074.

53. Price, A. L., Zaitlen, N. A., Reich, D., & Patterson, N. (2010). New approaches to population stratification in genome-wide association studies. *Nature Reviews Genetics, 11*, 459–463.

54. Pritchard, J. K., Stephens, M., & Donnelly, P. (2000). Inference of population structure using multilocus genotype data. *Genetics, 155*, 945–959.

Chapter 3
An Introduction to Association Analysis

Abstract This chapter focuses on techniques commonly used in GWAS studies to estimate single SNP marker associations in samples of unrelated individuals; when the phenotype is discrete (disease/no disease) then case–control methods, *conditional* and *unconditional logistic regression*, are typically utilized. *Maximum likelihood estimation* for generalized linear models is reviewed, and the *score*, *Wald*, and *likelihood ratio* tests are defined and discussed. The analysis of data from nuclear family-based designs is also briefly introduced. Issues regarding confounding, measurement error, effect mediation, and interactions are described. Control for multiple comparisons is reviewed with an emphasis placed on the behavior of the *Bonferroni* criteria for multiple correlated tests. The effects on statistical estimation and inference of the loss of independence between outcomes are characterized for a specific model of loss of independence, which is relevant to the presence of *hidden population structure* or *relatedness*. These last results build on a basic theme described in Chap. 2 and are then carried forward in Chap. 4.

3.1 Single Marker Associations

As discussed in the previous chapter, an ideal SNP genotyping array for GWAS studies would provide surrogates for all of the variants in a comprehensive target set, with the target set guaranteed to represent, or even provide a census of, all common variations within the human genome. For any member of the target set there should be a predictor on the array which has a high value of R^2 with the target, so that testing for association between the phenotype of interest and the surrogate should be as nearly as possible equivalent to the testing of an association with the causal variant itself. The discussion for the time being is on single SNP analysis and is thus implicitly focused only on the targets (or causal variants) that are in high pairwise LD with at least one SNP on the array. As we discuss haplotype analysis we will see that there are difficulties in this one-marker per common causal variant

D.O. Stram, *Design, Analysis, and Interpretation of Genome-Wide Association Scans*,
Statistics for Biology and Health, DOI 10.1007/978-1-4614-9443-0_3,
© Springer Science+Business Media New York 2014

Table 3.1 Tabulation
of observed genotypes for
a single autosomal variant
for cases and controls

Disease status	aa	Aa	AA	
Controls	n_{00}	n_{01}	n_{02}	$n_{0.}$
Cases	n_{10}	n_{11}	n_{12}	$n_{1.}$
Total	$n_{.0}$	$n_{.1}$	$n_{.2}$	$n_{..}$

concept and haplotype analysis leads to an expansion of the number of tests, and the complexity of the type of tests, that are to be considered.

Consider a study in which the phenotype is disease or no disease and both cases with disease and controls without disease are genotyped and association of disease with a diallelic autosomal variant (taking values a and A) is to be tested. Table 3.1 gives a layout of a 3×2 table representing observed data.

3.1.1 Dominant, Recessive, and Co-dominant Effects

Here we consider a variety of tests for a relationship between disease status and genotype and then will relate these to tests that arise from logistic regression of disease status on individual genotypes. If we assume that both cases and controls come from the same randomly mixing population and are all unrelated to each other a number of tests immediately are suggested by the layout of Table 3.1. An omnibus Pearson test of no association between the rows and columns of Table 3.1 gives a chi-square test on two degrees of freedom, which can be computed as

$$\chi^2 = \sum_{i=0}^{1} \sum_{j=0}^{2} \frac{\left(n_{ij} - E_{ij}\right)^2}{E_{ij}}, \tag{3.1}$$

with $E_{ij} = n_{i.}n_{.j}/n_{..}^2$ being the expected value of n_{ij} conditional upon the row and column totals under independence. This test is sensitive to any association of genotype with disease probability; the statistic is distributed approximately as a chi-square for sample sizes that are large enough so that each expectation, E_{ij}, is reasonably large. The rule of thumb is that the chi-square approximation is reliable so long as each E_{ij} is at least equal to 5. This traditional standard is based upon analysis of the behavior in the tails of the two distributions at approximately the 95 percentile, i.e., for testing at the $a=.05$ level of significance, and needs modification since multiple testing requirements of GWAS studies require much smaller p-values to be computed accurately.

An allele that is more common in the cases than in the controls is said to be a *risk allele* while an allele that is more common in the controls than in the cases is said to be *protective*. A *dominant effect* of allele A on disease risk means that carrying either the aA or AA genotype has an equivalent association with risk compared to the homozogote aa. A *recessive effect* is when only the AA genotype and not the Aa genotype differs from aa in its association with risk. A one degree of freedom test for a dominant effect is therefore achieved by collapsing the 3rd and 4th columns of

Table 3.1 before computing the χ^2 statistic, with appropriate renumbering in (3.1), while a test for a recessive effect is achieved by collapsing columns 2 and 3. Note that if allele A is a risk allele with a dominant effect, then allele a shows a recessive protective effect and vice versa.

In many cases the association of the heterozygote genotype Aa with disease is somewhere midway between that of aa and aA. In classical genetics this is referred to as *incomplete dominance*. A one degree of freedom chi-square test for incomplete dominance can be constructed from the Cochran–Armitage [1] test:

$$
T^2 \equiv \frac{\left[\sum_{i=0}^{2} t_i\left(n_{1i}n_{0.} - n_{0i}n_{1.}\right)\right]^2}{\frac{n_1 n_0}{n_{..}} \sum_{i=0}^{2} t_i^2 n_{.i}(n_{..} - n_{.i}) - 2\sum_{i=0}^{1}\sum_{j=i+1}^{2} t_i t_j n_{.i} n_{.j}}.
\tag{3.2}
$$

```
# R-code for Armitage test
Armitage<-function(N,t){ # Cochran-Armitage test
        R<-rowSums(N)
        C<-colSums(N)
        NN<-sum(N)
        k<-dim(N)[2]
        if (!(dim(N)[1] == 2 )) {
                cat("error\n");0;   stop}
        top<-0
        for (i in 1:k)
        top<-top+t[i]*(N[1,i]*R[2]-N[2,i]*R[1])
        top<-top^2
        bot<-0
        for (i in 1:k)
        bot<-bot+t[i]^2*C[i]*(NN-C[i])
        for (i in 1:k) {
           j=i+1
           while(j<=k){
                   bot<-bot - 2*t[i]*t[j]*C[i]*C[j]

                   j=j+1
           }
        }
        bot<-bot*R[1]*R[2]/NN
        top/bot
}
```

In order to test for a linear trend (an approximation for incomplete dominance) in the association between the counts for $n(A)$ and disease the weights t_i take the values $t_0 = 0$, $t_1 = 1$, and $t_2 = 2$ (other values can be used to test other possible effects if desired). Note that if $t_0 = 0$ and if both $t_1 = 1$ and $t_2 = 1$, then the Armitage test agrees with the test of a dominant effect using (3.1) on the collapsed table. It is further worth noting that when $t_0 = 0$, $t_1 = 1$, and $t_2 = 2$ the trend test can be equivalently written in a rather different form from the raw data (rather than the table of cell counts) as $N\text{Cor}(n_{iA}, c_i)^2$ where N is the total number of observations (equivalent to $n_{..}$) and n_{iA} is the count of the number of A alleles carried by subject i and c_i is case–control status of subject i. The correlation coefficient Cor (n_{iA}, c_i) is computed in the usual way, i.e., as

$$\frac{\sum_{i=1}^{N}(n_{iA} - \overline{n}_A)(c_i - \overline{c})}{\sqrt{\sum_{i=1}^{N}(n_{iA} - \overline{n}_A)^2 \sum_{i=1}^{N}(c_i - \overline{c})^2}}.$$

As we will see shortly each of these tests is closely related or coincides with tests that stem naturally out of the tests of various hypotheses using either linear or logistic regression as described below.

3.2   Regression Analysis and Generalized Linear Models in Genetic Analysis

Univariate and multivariate regression analysis using *generalized linear models* provides a suitable framework for analysis of data from genetic association studies including both the testing of hypotheses and the estimation of parameters in models describing the relationship between measured genetic variants and the phenotypes of interest. This section gives a brief overview of using generalized linear models for regression analysis as will be used in the remainder of the book; it is based on the more extensive material from McCullagh and Nelder's book [2].

Generalized linear models begin with specifying that, conditional on all covariates of interest, the probability distribution, f, of the phenotype Y is known and is of exponential family form. The two exponential family probability distributions that this book will be considering are the normal distribution and the binomial distribution; other notable examples include the *Poisson*, gamma, and the inverse Gaussian distributions. Next a generalized linear model specifies that the mean $E(Y)$ of the phenotype Y is connected to one or more covariates X through a *link function* g. Link functions are invertible (smooth and monotonically increasing) scalar valued functions. The relationship between the mean and the covariates is written as

$$g[E(Y_i)] = \alpha_1 X_{i1} + \alpha_2 X_{i2} + \cdots + \alpha_r X_{ir}. \qquad (3.3)$$

Here the i indexes study participants, $i = 1, \ldots, n$, who will have observations of the outcome phenotype, Y_i, as well as covariate data $\mathbf{X_i} = (X_{i1}, X_{i2}, \ldots, X_{ir})^{\mathrm{T}}$. The parameters α are the regression parameters which are generally to be estimated in the course of the analysis and about which hypothesis tests, etc., are to be constructed. The right-hand side of (3.3) is known as the *linear predictor* for subject i and can be written as $X'_i \alpha$ with the un-subscripted α referring to the vector of parameters $(\alpha_1, \alpha_2, \ldots, \alpha_y)^T$. Defining the matrix $\mathbf{X}$ as the $n \times r$ matrix having rows X_i^T we can write the n-vector of linear predictors for all subjects simultaneously, $(\alpha^T X_2, \alpha^T X_2, \ldots, \alpha^T X_n)^T$, as $\mathbf{X}\alpha$.

For each probability function there is a so-called *canonical link function*, which plays a special role in the theory of the generalized linear model [2]. For the normal distribution the canonical link function is the identity link, i.e., $g(x) \rightarrow x$, for binary or binomial counts it is the logistic function $g(x) \rightarrow \log(x) - \log(1 - x)$, and for the Poisson the canonical link is the log function. Often but certainly not always the canonical link function is chosen as the link function g in the analysis. When, for example, the identity link function is used to analyze normally distributed data this yields *ordinary least squares* (OLS) regression.

In certain cases the canonical link function may not provide the simplest or best description of the data, however, and the flexibility of the general framework allows other choices. Note that model (3.3) can be written equivalently as

$$E(Y_i) = g^{-1}(\alpha_1 X_{i1} + \alpha_2 X_{i2} + \cdots + \alpha_r X_{ir}),$$

with g^{-1} being the inverse of the link function, for example, $g^{-1}(x) \rightarrow \exp(x)/(1 + \exp(x))$ for the logistic link function.

In case–control data, i.e., where Y_i is binary and where the sampling of study participants is conditional on the observed value (diseased or not diseased) of Y, the logistic link function plays a very special role. This is because most of the parameters, α, in the linear predictor for a typical *logistic regression* model (i.e., model (3.3) with logistic g and binary Y) are the log of *odds ratios*; A fundamental result about case–control studies (and also about their relationship to cohort studies) is that the interpretation of odds ratios, unlike other measures of risk, is not dependent on the sampling fraction of cases and controls.

When the Y_i are each independent of each other and the generalized linear model holds then maximum likelihood estimation of the parameters α is accomplished by use of an *iteratively reweighted least squares* algorithm, which is equivalent to OLS regression for the case of normal data with the identity link. For other GLMs (e.g., logistic regression) the iteratively reweighted least squares regression is equivalent to Fisher's scoring procedure (see Sect. 3.4 below). Hypothesis testing regarding the parameters α may be performed by several standard methods, such as likelihood ratio tests, score tests, or Wald tests which are based upon the asymptotic behavior (behavior as N gets large) of the likelihood function, its derivatives, and associated maximum likelihood estimates.

The choice of probability distribution f (e.g., normal, binomial, etc) also imposes a model for the variance of Y. For example, if the data can be interpreted as the number of successes from among m independent trials and therefore follow the binomial distribution then the generalized linear model for the *proportion of successes*, $Y = $ (number of successes/m) models the variance of Y as a function of the mean of Y_i, namely, $E(Y_i)(1 - E(Y_i))/m$. If the normal distribution is chosen the variance of Y is a constant value, σ^2, for all i, which is estimated along with the mean parameters α. For the Poisson distribution, the variance is also a known function of the mean, since $\text{Var}(Y_i) = E(Y_i)$ in this case. For other exponential family distributions also, such as the gamma and inverse Gaussian, where the variance is not a function of the mean, one additional (scale) parameter is estimated; the scale parameter for the normal distribution is σ^2.

It is possible also to alter the variance function of Y_i for the Poisson and for the binomial distribution with $m \geq 2$ in order to model *over-dispersed* count data, by introducing a pseudo-scale parameter into the fitting of these models as well. In this case the analog [3] to the iteratively reweighted least squares algorithm for fitting these models is a simple form of what more generally are known as *generalized estimating equations* [4].

3.3   Tests of Hypotheses for Genotype Data Using Generalized Linear Models

Consider a layout of phenotype and genotype as would be used in ordinary regression (either least squares or logistic regression); as above we use i to index each of the study participants from 1 to N and Y_i denotes the phenotype value (the dependent variable in the regression analysis) which can be either continuous or discrete; in case–control studies we may prefer to use D_i as a disease indicator taking the value 0 for controls and 1 for cases. For the time being we are considering only a single diallelic variant (e.g., an SNP), with alleles A and a, and a counter, n_{iA}, of the number of copies of allele A carried by subject i as an explanatory variable. Rather than putting the counts n_{iA} of this variant into the model directly, we expand this into three indicator variables for the specific genotypes: G_{i0} which is equal to 1 if and only if $n_{iA} = 0$ (i.e., if the genotype is *aa*); G_{i1}, an indicator for $n_{iA} = 1$; and G_{i2} indicating $n_{iA} = 2$. We will also consider the possible presence of additional covariates, X_{ij} with $j = 1, \ldots, r$, but for the time being we defer this aspect of the model. With slight change in notation from (3.3), we write

$$g[E(Y_i)] = \mu + \beta_0 G_{i0} + \beta_1 G_{i1} + \beta_2 G_{i2}. \qquad (3.4)$$

As written model (3.4) is over-parameterized, the constant μ is not separately estimable from the parameters β_0, β_1, and β_2, without placing constraints on the β parameters. The reason μ is introduced in the model is because we usually want to be able to interpret the β parameters as increments (in the log odds scale) of disease risk always compared to some baseline group parameterized by μ. This means that we will almost always impose constraints on the three β parameters. For example, to fit a model in which $g[E(Y)]$ is linear in genotype count n_A we constrain β_0 to equal zero and β_2 to equal twice β_1 which is equivalent to replacing $\beta_0 G_{i0} + \beta_1 G_{i1} + \beta_2 G_{i2}$ in model (3.4) with $\beta_1 n_{iA}$. In this case β_1 is interpreted as the additive increase (or decrease if β_1 is negative) of the log odds of disease (for logistic regression) or in the phenotype mean (for OLS regression) with each copy of the allele A compared to carriers of aa.

The constant μ can sometimes be taken as the population mean phenotype (transformed by g), or more often, if we constrain β_0 to equal zero, the (transformed) mean phenotype for subjects with genotype aa. As discussed above, in case–control studies, sampling is conditional on disease status and μ cannot be directly related to population disease prevalence. If there is no effect of genotype (all three β equal to zero) then μ is simply $g(S_y)$ where

$$S_y = \frac{\text{number of cases}}{\text{total cases} + \text{controls}}$$

is the sampling ratio.

3.3.1   Test of Hypothesis regarding Genotype Effects Testing Using Logistic Regression in Case–Control Analysis

All the hypothesis tests described in Sect. 3.1.1 (e.g., tests for additive, dominant, or recessive effects of genotype) can also be performed using GLMs. For example, a test of the null hypothesis of no effect of genotype on risk against the general two degrees of freedom test, i.e., the same hypothesis tested using the Pearson chi-square statistic given in expression (3.1), can be performed by setting β_0 to zero (i.e., removing G_{i0} from the model) and then fitting the remaining parameters in model (3.4) using the binomial distribution and the logistic link in order to estimate values for β_1 and β_2. The fit of this "full" model can be compared to the fit of the null model (estimated with all of $\beta_0 = \beta_1 = \beta_2 = 0$ so that only μ remains). For example, the likelihood ratio test (see below) compares the log likelihood of the null model with only μ in the linear predictor to the likelihood of the full model. Specifically twice the change in likelihood for the full compared to the null model is compared to a chi-square (with 2 degrees of freedom); see Sect. 3.4 below. For illustrative purposes we compute the likelihood ratio test, as well as the Pearson chi-square test for a simulated dataset representing a case–control study with 506 cases and 494 controls in which one SNP has been simulated. The data for case–control status and a simulated SNP, given as the count n_A of the allele A, are provided in "simul1.dat." The following R code reads the data, displays the first few lines of the raw data, and then summarizes the data using the R table command:

```
> x<-read.table("simul1.dat",header=T)
> names(x)
[1] "Y"      "n_A"
> x[1:10,]
    Y n_A
1   0   0
2   0   0
3   0   0
4   1   0
5   1   0
6   0   0
7   1   0
8   1   0
9   1   1
10  1   0
> Y<-x$Y
> n_A<-x$n_A
> TBL<-table(x)
> TBL

    n_A
Y     0   1   2
  0 418  71   5
  1 394 107   5
>
```

As we see in the box the data are organized in a way that is suitable for regression analysis, but then is summarized, using the *table* command, as in Table 3.1 above. We will use the generalized linear model (GLM) program in *R* (function *glm* in library *stats*) in order to compute the likelihood ratio test (see Sect. 3.4 for more information) of whether there is any association between case–control status and the genotypes. The *glm* function takes 2 primary arguments: a description of the outcome variable and linear predictor (separated by a ~) to form a *model formula*, and a specification of the probability model and link function. To organize the output of the *glm* function we use the generic *R* function *summary*. Specifically, we can run the code

```
> library(stats)
> M0<-summary(glm(Y~1,family=binomial(link="logit")))
> M1<-summary(glm(Y~factor(n_A),family=binomial(link="logit")))
> twice_change_loglikelihood<- M0$deviance - M1$deviance
> twice_change_loglikelihood
[1] 7.896825
pchisq(twice_change_loglikelihood,2,lower.tail=F)
[1] 0.01928529
```

to fit first the null model (M_0) with only μ in the linear predictor, using the model formula $Y \sim 1$ (see below), and then a model (M1) which estimates the three parameters μ, β_1, and β_2 to fit the model (3.4). The use of *factor(n_A)* in *R* on the right-hand side of the ~ in the model formula tells *R* to set up the dummy variables, G_0, G_1, and G_2, corresponding to the levels of n_{iA} by default *R* automatically drops G_0 in favor of estimating the constant μ. Here we display only the change in log likelihood for the two models.

The printed value 7.896825 is the value of the chi-square statistic, computed as the difference in *deviance* of the 2 models (in GLM notation this is twice the difference in the log likelihood) and the value 0.01928529 is the associated *p*-value for the test of the null hypothesis that both β_1 and β_2 are equal to zero, against the alternative than one or both are nonzero. To see that this test gives very similar results to the Pearson's chi-square test, we can use the built in R function chisq.test on the TBL object created earlier. We have

```
> chisq.test(TBL)

        Pearson's Chi-squared test

data:  TBL
X-squared = 7.8474, df = 2, p-value = 0.01977
```

We can test the fit of a dominant model to the data, compared to the fit of the null model similarly. To fit a dominant model using these data we impose the constraints that $\beta_0 = 0$ and that $\beta_1 = \beta_2$ so that the linear predictor in (3.4) is equal to

$$\mu + \beta_1(G_{i1} + G_{i2}).$$

This can be accomplished in R creating a new variable G_dom as (taking values 0 or 1) in

```
> G_dom<-as.numeric((n_A==1)+(n_A==2))
```

and then fitting and computing the p-value for the likelihood ratio test as

```
> M_dom<-summary(glm(Y~factor(G_dom),family=binomial(link="logit")))
>
> pchisq((M0$deviance-M_dom$deviance),1,lower.tail=F)
[1] 0.006163612
```

We can compare this to using the Pearson chi-square test on the collapsed (as described above) table.

```
> TBL_dom<-cbind(TBL[,1],TBL[,2]+TBL[,3])
> chisq.test(TBL_dom,correct=F) # no continuity correction

        Pearson's Chi-squared test

data:  TBL_dom
X-squared = 7.4601, df = 1, p-value = 0.006308
```

Again the resulting p-values are very similar. Fitting a model that is linear in n_A (by removing the call to *factor* in the model equation, see below for more information about R model formula) gives a likelihood ratio test (p-value $= 0.0116$) that is very close to the that of the Armitage test (p-value $= 0.0119$) computed for these data (The R code for the Armitage test in R is given in the sidebar above)

```
> M_lin<-summary(glm(Y~n_A,family=binomial(link="logit")))
> pchisq((M0$deviance-M_lin$deviance),1,lower.tail=F)
[1] 0.01160770
>
> pchisq(Armitage(TBL,c(0,1,2)),1,lower.tail=F)
          1
0.01191033
```

3.3.2 Interpreting Regression Equation Coefficients

So far we have not seen any really good reason to prefer the GLM approach to these data compared to the use of either the Armitage test or Pearson's chi-square test. That is partly because up to now we have been "hiding" the regression output, other than to compute the likelihood ratio tests from the change in model deviances that were calculated using the *glm* function. We now examine the results of fitting models M_1 and M_lin. For clarity's sake we recompute model M1 and print the resulting summary object

```
> M1<-summary(glm(Y~factor(n_A),family=binomial()))
> M1
Call:
glm(formula = Y ~ factor(n_A), family = binomial())

Deviance Residuals:
    Min      1Q   Median      3Q      Max
 -1.356  -1.152    1.009   1.203    1.203
Coefficients:
             Estimate Std. Error z value Pr(>|z|)
(Intercept)  -0.05913    0.07022  -0.842  0.39973
factor(n_A)1  0.46928    0.16841   2.787  0.00533 **
factor(n_A)2  0.05913    0.63634   0.093  0.92597
---
Signif. codes:  0 '***' 0.001 '**' 0.01 '*' 0.05 '.' 0.1 ' ' 1

(Dispersion parameter for binomial family taken to be 1)

    Null deviance: 1386.2  on 999  degrees of freedom
Residual deviance: 1378.3  on 997  degrees of freedom
AIC: 1384.3

Number of Fisher Scoring iterations: 4
```

To reiterate we are estimating the model,

$$g[E(Y_i)] = \mu + \beta_1 G_{i1} + \beta_2 G_{i2}, \tag{3.5}$$

using the (default for the binomial family) logistic link function. We focus on the *coefficients* portion of the *R* output. As mentioned before the intercept parameter estimate is not very meaningful for case–control data. If sampling had been random with respect to case–control status then the intercept parameter in this output could be interpreted as an estimate of the log odds of disease in homozygotes (individuals carrying *aa*) for the *a* allele, i.e.,

$$\log \frac{P(Y = 1 | n_{iA} = 0)}{P(Y = 0 | n_{iA} = 0)}.$$

Here that estimate of the *odds* as $(\exp(-0.05913) = 0.9426))$ reflects mainly the close to 1:1 matching of cases to controls in this "study." The next two estimates are more meaningful; the *glm* output for the second coefficient is the estimate of the log odds ratio of disease in the heterozygote carriers compared to the homozygote carriers of *aa*. To be more specific what we have estimated is

$$\beta_1 = \log \frac{P(Y = 1 | n_{iA} = 1)/P(Y = 0 | n_{iA} = 1)}{P(Y = 1 | n_{iA} = 0)/P(Y = 0 | n_{iA} = 0)}.$$

The exponent of the estimate exp(0.46928) = 1.598842 indicates that the odds of disease in carriers of heterozygote, *aA*, are estimated to be approximately 60 % greater than in homozygotes. The odds of disease for carriers of the homozygote *AA* are estimated to be exp(0.05913) = 1.060913 or only 6 % greater than for homozygotes *aa*. The number of subjects (10 total) with this genotype is small however. When we display the fit of the linear logistic model M_lin we see that the per allele increase in the odds ratio is estimated to be exp(0.38139) = 1.464319 or about a 46 % increase per copy. Compared to model M1 the slope is much closer to the estimate of the heterozygote odds ratio than the homozygote reflecting the paucity of subjects with an *AA* genotype. The deviance of the two models M1 and M_lin (which can be displayed as M1$deviance and M_lin$deviance) is very close (1378.234 and 1379.781, respectively) so that there is little evidence that the log linear model, M_lin, is inferior to M1.

```
> M_lin<-summary(glm(Y~n_A,family=binomial()))
> M_lin

Call:
glm(formula = Y ~ n_A, family = binomial())

Deviance Residuals:
   Min      1Q   Median      3Q     Max
-1.491  -1.156   1.041   1.199   1.199

Coefficients:
            Estimate Std. Error z value Pr(>|z|)
(Intercept) -0.05071    0.06989  -0.725   0.4681
n_A          0.38139    0.15255   2.500   0.0124 *
---
Signif. codes:  0 '***' 0.001 '**' 0.01 '*' 0.05 '.' 0.1 ' ' 1

(Dispersion parameter for binomial family taken to be 1)

    Null deviance: 1386.2  on 999  degrees of freedom
Residual deviance: 1379.8  on 998  degrees of freedom
AIC: 1383.8

Number of Fisher Scoring iterations: 4
```

Note that we could have fit model M1 using the identity link function, i.e., specify *family* = *binomial(link* = *"identity"*), in place of the logistic, and achieved an identical fit to the data (as measured by the log likelihood of the model). This is because in estimating each $E(Y_i)$ M1 has used all 3 available degrees of freedom (one for each of μ, β_1, and β_2) in modeling the relationship between the genotype (taking 3 levels) and case–control status. The fit of model M1 is therefore equivalent to the fit of any other binomial model with three degrees of freedom in the linear predictor. While the fit of the identity link function would have been identical, the parameter estimates would not be.

The logistic link function is usually preferred when analyzing case–control data because the interpretation of odds ratios is not dependent on the case–control sampling ratio and hence is applicable to the population sampled in the study. The numerical values of the parameters being estimated when using an identity link function, for example, would depend on the case–control sampling ratio.

The fit (as measured by the log likelihood) of the linear model M_lin (i.e., with n_A treated as a continuous trend variable rather than a categorical factor, i.e., $g(E(Y_i)) = \alpha + \beta n_{iA}$) would, on the other hand, be different if the identity link is used as g compared to using the logistic link function, since with the logistic link function the log odds ratios, rather than the case–control probabilities, are being modeled as linear in the genotype count.

3.4   Summary of Maximum Likelihood Estimation, Wald Tests, Likelihood Ratio Tests, Score Tests, and Sufficient Statistics

Here we provide some general information about likelihood-based inference based closely upon the classic discussion of these methods provided in McCullaugh and Nelder [2].

Let $f(Y;\theta)$ be the probability mass or density function of the random variable, Y, which depends upon the parameter vector θ (for generalized linear models θ includes the regression parameters, $\alpha_1 \ldots \alpha_y$, in model (3.3) as well as the scale or variance parameter if needed). Then the likelihood function $L(\theta;Y)$ is identical to $f(Y;\theta)$ but treated as a function of θ with Y fixed.

Specific Examples

1. Normal distribution for scalar Y with $E(Y) = \mu$ and $\mathrm{Var}(Y) = \sigma^2$:

$$L(\theta; y) = \frac{1}{\sqrt{2\pi\sigma^2}} \exp\left\{\frac{-1}{2\sigma^2}(y - \mu)^2\right\}.$$

2. Binomial distribution with index (number of independent trials) m (integer >0), with number of successes Y and probability of success equal to π:

$$L(\pi; Y) = \binom{m}{Y}\pi^Y(1 - \pi)^{(m-Y)}.$$

Note that if Y is defined to be equal to the proportion of successes, i.e., (number of successes)/m, rather than the number itself the binomial likelihood is rewritten as

$$L(\pi; Y) = \binom{m}{mY} \pi^{mY} (1 - \pi)^{(m-mY)}.$$

3. Normal distribution for n independent normal random variables, $Y_1, Y_2, \ldots, Y_n$ with mean $E(Y_i) = \alpha_0 + \alpha_1 X_i$ and variance σ^2:

$$L(\theta; Y_1, Y_2, \ldots, Y_n) = \prod_{i=1}^{n} L(\alpha_0, \alpha_1, \sigma^2; Y_i),$$

$$\prod_{i=1}^{N} \frac{1}{\sqrt{2\pi\sigma^2}} \exp\left\{ -\frac{1}{2\sigma^2} (Y_i - \alpha_0 - \alpha_1 X_i)^2 \right\}. \qquad (3.6)$$

4. Binomial distribution for the proportion of successes Y_i, for n independent binomial observations, with binomial index m_i with mean

$$E(Y_i) = \frac{\exp(\alpha_0 + \alpha_1 X_i)}{1 + \exp(\alpha_0 + \alpha_1 X_i)},$$

$$L(\theta; Y_1, Y_2, \ldots, Y_n) = \prod_{i=1}^{n} L(\alpha_0, \alpha_1; Y_i),$$

$$= \prod_{i=1}^{n} \binom{m_i}{m_i Y_i} \left(\frac{\exp(\alpha_0 + \alpha_1 X_i)}{1 + \exp(\alpha_0 + \alpha_1 X_i)} \right)^{m_i Y_i} \left(1 - \frac{\exp(\alpha_0 + \alpha_1 X_i)}{1 + \exp(\alpha_0 + \alpha_1 X_i)} \right)^{(m_i - m_i Y_i)}.$$

This is the likelihood for the logistic regression model for binomial data with a single explanatory variable. For binary case–control data this likelihood with all $m_i = 1$ is used; the constant parameter α_0 here is equivalent to μ above.

3.4.1   Properties of Log Likelihood Functions

For the vector, Y, of independent observations, $Y_1, \ldots, Y_n$, define the log likelihood, $\ell(\theta; Y)$, as the natural log of the likelihood function $L(\theta; Y_1, \ldots, Y_n) = \prod_{i=1}^{n} L(\theta; Y_i)$, so that we have

$$\ell(\theta; \mathbf{Y}) = \sum_{i=1}^{n} \log\{L(\theta; Y_i)\}.$$

Now consider the derivatives of the log likelihood function. If θ is a scalar then we find that

$$E\left\{\frac{\mathrm{d}}{\mathrm{d}\theta}\ell(\theta; Y)\right\} = 0 \tag{3.7}$$

and

$$\mathrm{Var}\left\{\frac{\mathrm{d}}{\mathrm{d}\theta}\ell(\theta; Y)\right\} = -E\left\{\frac{\mathrm{d}^2}{\mathrm{d}\theta^2}\ell(\theta; Y)\right\}. \tag{3.8}$$

For example, to show that (3.7) holds we simply differentiate the identity (applying to any probability distributions or density functions) that

$$\int f(Y; \theta)\mathrm{d}Y = 1,$$

with respect to θ. This gives

$$0 = \frac{\mathrm{d}}{\mathrm{d}\theta}\int (Y; \theta)\mathrm{d}Y = \int \frac{\mathrm{d}}{\mathrm{d}\theta}f(Y; \theta)\mathrm{d}Y.$$

By dividing and multiplying the integrand above by $f(Y;\theta)$, we have

$$\int \frac{\frac{d}{d\theta}f(Y; \theta)}{f(Y; \theta)}f(Y; \theta)dY = 0.$$

Equation (3.7) follows because

$$\frac{\mathrm{d}}{\mathrm{d}\theta}\log\left(f(\theta; Y)\right) = \frac{\frac{\mathrm{d}}{\mathrm{d}\theta}f(Y; \theta)}{f(Y; \theta)}.$$

Similar techniques are used to prove (3.8).

Note that (3.7) and (3.8) appear to be suitable for forming hypothesis tests about the parameter θ. To test a null hypothesis that $\theta = \theta_0$ we compute the observed value of the derivative of the log likelihood evaluated at θ_0, and compare it to its standard deviation, also computed at θ_0, to see if the derivative is close to zero. If the derivative is small compared to its standard deviation then we would accept the null hypothesis; otherwise we would reject it. This argument forms the basis of the *score test* described below. Equation (3.8) says that we can compute this standard deviation as the square root of the expected value of minus the second derivative of the log likelihood.

When θ denotes a vector of 2 or more parameters (3.7) holds for all partial derivatives and (3.8) generalizes to

$$\text{Cov}\left\{\frac{\partial}{\partial\theta_i}\ell(\theta;Y),\frac{\partial}{\partial\theta_j}\ell(\theta;Y)\right\} = -E\left\{\frac{\partial^2}{\partial\theta_i\partial\theta_i}\ell(\theta;Y)\right\} \quad \text{for } i,j$$

$$= 1,\ldots,r. \tag{3.9}$$

The resulting variance matrix (of size $r \times r$) is fundamental in making likelihood-based inference about the parameters as described below.

3.4.2   Score Tests

The derivative of the log likelihood, $U(\theta,Y) = \frac{\partial}{\partial\theta}\ell(\theta;Y)$, is called the *score statistic* and its variance matrix is the *expected information*, also known as the *Fisher's information*, denoted herein as $i(\theta)$. Several important large sample results apply to $U(\theta,Y)$ and $i(\theta)$. For example, under suitable regularity conditions the growth of the information matrix $i(\theta)$ with n we have

$$U(\theta,Y)'i(\theta)^{-1}U(\theta,Y),$$

as asymptotically distributed as a chi-square random variable with r degrees of freedom. This forms the basis of the score test for θ which is a generalization of the method of inference discussed briefly above. Specifically, a test of the hypothesis that $\theta = \theta_0$ is constructed by comparing the observed value of

$$U(\theta_0,Y)'i(\theta_0)^{-1}U(\theta_0,Y) \tag{3.10}$$

to critical values of the cumulative distribution function for a chi-square random variable, χ_r^2, with r degrees of freedom. Speaking somewhat crudely, for large samples, (3.10) follows a central chi-square distribution because $U(\theta_0,Y)$ converges to a multivariate normal random variable (with mean 0 and variance $i(\theta)$) under the null hypothesis; this follows because it is a sum of independent random variables each with mean zero and variance $i_i(\theta_0)$ which is the contribution of the ith individual to $i(\theta_0)$. If the observed value of expression (3.10) is larger than the critical value then the hypothesis is rejected at the chosen level of significance.

If the main interest is only in certain of the components of the parameter vector θ then θ can be partitioned into sub-vectors (γ,λ), with γ regarded as the parameter or parameters of interest and λ as the nuisance parameters. Here the vector of nuisance parameters, λ, is of length q and γ of length $r - q$.

Then the information matrix is partitioned as

$$i(\theta) = \begin{bmatrix} i_{\gamma\gamma} & i_{\gamma\lambda} \\ i_{\lambda\gamma} & i_{\lambda\lambda} \end{bmatrix},$$

with inverse

$$i^{-1}(\theta) = \begin{bmatrix} i^{\gamma\gamma} & i^{\gamma\lambda} \\ i^{\lambda\gamma} & i^{\lambda\lambda} \end{bmatrix},$$

and from the formula for a partitioned inverse $i^{\gamma\gamma} = (i_{\gamma\gamma} - i_{\gamma\lambda}i_{\lambda\lambda}^{-1}i_{\lambda\gamma})^{-1}$. A score test of the hypothesis $\gamma = \gamma_0$ with the nuisance parameters λ unspecified is formed as

$$U(\gamma_0, \hat{\lambda}, Y)^T i^{\gamma\gamma} U(\gamma_0, \hat{\lambda}, Y). \tag{3.11}$$

Here $U(\gamma_0, \hat{\lambda}, Y)$ are the elements of $U(\theta, Y)$ corresponding to γ and $\hat{\lambda}$ is chosen so that the remaining q components of the score are equal to zero.

Upon calculation of the value (3.11) it is compared to the critical values for the $\chi^2_{\gamma-q}$ distribution, rejecting the hypothesis that $\gamma = \gamma_0$ for larger observed values.

3.4.3 Likelihood Ratio Tests

The value, $\hat{\theta}_{\text{MLE}}$, of θ that maximizes the log likelihood is known as the maximum likelihood estimate (MLE). For large samples (and under regularity conditions) we have the approximation that

$$2\ell(\hat{\theta}_{\text{MLE}}, Y) - 2\ell(\theta, Y) \to \chi^2_\gamma.$$

This yields the *likelihood ratio test*. We can test the hypothesis that $\theta = \theta_0$ by computing

$$2\ell(\hat{\theta}_{\text{MLE}}, Y) - 2\ell(\theta_0, Y)$$

and comparing this value to the critical value for a chi-square statistic, χ^2_γ. Note that in the terminology for generalized linear models adopted by the R package -2ℓ (θ, Y) is termed the model deviance and increases in (twice) the likelihood are computed as declines in model deviance.

If there are nuisance parameters, λ, in the model and we are interested in testing the null hypothesis that $\gamma = \gamma_0$ with λ unrestricted, we do this in two steps. First we form the profile maximum likelihood estimate, $\hat{\lambda}_{\gamma_0}$, which maximizes $2\ell(\gamma_0, \lambda; Y)$ with respect to λ with γ fixed at γ_0. Next we calculate

$$2\ell(\hat{\gamma}_{\text{MLE}}, \hat{\lambda}_{\text{MLE}}, Y) - 2\ell(\gamma, \hat{\lambda}_{\gamma_0}, Y)$$

where $\hat{\gamma}_{\text{MLE}}$ and $\hat{\lambda}_{\text{MLE}}$ are the unconstrained maximum likelihood estimates of θ under the null hypothesis. This value is then compared to the critical values of a $\chi^2_{\gamma-q}$ random variable and the null hypothesis is rejected for larger observed values.

3.4.4   Wald Tests

Wald tests use an asymptotic approximation of the behavior of the MLE estimate itself for inference; specifically it is assumed that for large N that the MLE $\hat{\theta}_{\text{MLE}}$ is normally distributed with mean equal to the true value of the parameters θ and with variance matrix equal to $i(\theta)^{-1}$. A Wald test of $\theta = \theta_0$ is constructed as

$$\left(\hat{\theta}_{\text{MLE}} - \theta_0\right)' i\left(\hat{\theta}_{\text{MLE}}\right)\left(\hat{\theta}_{\text{MLE}} - \theta_0\right)$$

and the observed value of this statistic is compared to the critical values for a χ^2_γ random variable. In the nuisance parameter case

$$(\hat{\gamma}_{\text{MLE}} - \gamma_0)^{\text{T}}(i^{\gamma\gamma})^{-1}(\hat{\gamma}_{\text{MLE}} - \gamma_0)$$

is compared to the critical values of a χ^2_{r-q}. When hypotheses for a single parameter are of interest, i.e., when the dimension of γ is 1, Wald tests are often reported as $Z = (\hat{\gamma}_{\text{MLE}} - \gamma_0)/\sqrt{i^{\gamma\gamma}}$ and referred to the standard normal distribution; here $\sqrt{i^{\gamma\gamma}}$ is the standard error of the estimate $\hat{\gamma}_{\text{MLE}}$.

3.4.5   Fisher's Scoring Procedure for Finding the MLE

Fisher's scoring procedure provides updated values θ_1 of initial values θ_0 of the parameter vector according to

$$\theta_1 = \theta_0 + i^{-1}(\theta_0)U(\theta_0; Y) \tag{3.12}$$

with the calculations repeated until convergence. For generalized linear models the Fishers' scoring procedure for estimating the regression parameters α is equivalent to the *iteratively reweighted least squares algorithm* (IRWLS) of McCullagh and Nelder which has the added value of providing useful initial values for the regression parameters α_0 as a part of the algorithm. For generalized linear models the Fisher's scoring procedure will usually converge in a few iterations to the maximum provided that the parameters are identifiable, which requires for example that the $n \times r$ matrix $\mathbf{X}$ having rows $\mathbf{X}$ be of full column rank. In some cases, generally involving small sample sizes, or nearly singular $\mathbf{X}$, Fisher's scoring may diverge or reach a local rather than a global maximum of the likelihood. Some further discussion of this behavior is provided when discussing the analysis of rare variants in Chap. 8.

Equation (3.12) is also important because we can often approximate the behavior of the MLE θ compared to the true value θ by substituting true θ for θ_0 and $\hat{\theta}$ for θ_1 so that

$$\hat{\theta} - \theta \cong i^{-1}(\theta)U(\theta; Y). \tag{3.13}$$

Since $U(\theta, Y)$ is the sum of independent elements each with mean zero, i.e., $U(\theta, Y) = \sum_{i=1}^{n} U_i(\theta; Y)$, then in most cases we can appeal to the (multivariate) central limit theorem to argue that $\hat{\theta}$ will converge in distribution to a normal random variable with mean θ and variance–covariance matrix $i^{-1}(\theta)\text{Var}(U(\theta;Y))$ $i^{-1}(\theta)$ which equals $i^{-1}(\theta)$, thereby justifying the Wald test. The likelihood ratio test can be motivated in a similar way. Specifically the change $\ell(\hat{\theta}; Y) - \ell(\theta; Y)$ can be approximated around θ as $U(\theta; Y)(\hat{\theta} - \theta) + \frac{1}{2}(\hat{\theta} - \theta)'i(\theta)(\hat{\theta} - \theta)$. Since the expectation of $U(\theta;Y)$ is zero at the true parameter value we can ignore the first term leaving $2\ell(\hat{\theta}; Y) - 2\ell(\theta; Y) \approx (\hat{\theta} - \theta)'i(\theta)(\hat{\theta} - \theta)$ which can be assumed to converge to a χ_r^2 random variable.

3.4.6   Scores and Information for Normal and Binary Regression

Starting from expression (3.3) for the relationship between $E(Y_i)$ and covariates this section gives some specifics for the two most relevant GLMs: those using the normal distribution with identity link functions (i.e., OLS regression) and the binary distribution with logistic link (logistic regression). Expression (3.6) for simple OLS regression generalizes to

$$\ell(\alpha, \sigma^2; Y) = -\frac{n}{2}\log(2) - \frac{n}{2}\log(\pi\sigma^2) - \sum_{i=1}^{n} \frac{1}{2\sigma^2}\left(Y_i - X_i'\alpha\right)^2,$$

so that the score for the regression parameters α is simply

$$U(\alpha, \sigma^2; Y) = \frac{1}{\sigma^2}\sum_{i=1}^{n}\left(Y_i - X_i'\alpha\right)X_i, \tag{3.14}$$

and the information matrix $i(\theta)$ is simply

$$\frac{1}{\sigma^2}\sum_{i=1}^{n} X_i X_i'. \tag{3.15}$$

For logistic regression the log likelihood is

$$\ell(\alpha; Y) = \sum_{i=1}^{n} Y_i \log\left(\frac{\exp(X_i'\alpha)}{1 + \exp(X_i'\alpha)}\right) + (1 - Y_i)\log\left(1 - \frac{\exp(X_i'\alpha)}{1 + \exp(X_i'\alpha)}\right),$$

with score equal to

$$U(\alpha; Y) = \sum_{i=1}^{n}\left(Y_i - \frac{\exp(X_i'\alpha)}{1 + \exp(X_i'\alpha)}\right)X_i \qquad (3.16)$$

and information

$$i(\alpha) = \sum_{i=1}^{n}\left(\frac{\exp(X_i'\alpha)}{(1 + \exp(X_i'\alpha))^2}\right)X_iX_i'. \qquad (3.17)$$

For binary logistic regression there is no scale or variance parameter to be estimated since the variance of any binary random variable Y_i is strictly a function of the mean, i.e., equal to $E(Y_i)(1 - E(Y_i))$. For normal regression the variance parameter σ^2 is estimated as $1/(n - r)$ times the sum of squares of the residuals, $Y_i - X_i\hat{\alpha}$.

For binary regression we can reexpress (3.17) as

$$i(\alpha) = \sum_{i=1}^{n} v_i X_i X_i',$$

with $v_i = \mu_i(1 - \mu_i)$ with $\mu_i = (\exp(X_i'\alpha))/(\exp(1 + X_i'\alpha))$. Note that μ_i and v_i is the mean and variance respectively of binary Y_i under the logistic model.

For normal linear regression the three testing procedures (score, likelihood ratio, and Wald) described above are equivalent—i.e., they produce the same value of the criteria (see Homework). However none of these tests are equal to the standard F and t-tests for parameters as described in linear models theory, which are based upon exact rather than approximate inference for the normal distribution. This is very easily remedied, however, since dividing the chi-square statistic obtained by a likelihood ratio test first by the number of degrees of freedom, $r - q$, and then by $\hat{\sigma}^2$ yields the usual F statistics with $r - q$ and $n - r$ degrees of freedom for the numerator and denominator, respectively. Similar comments of course apply to Wald and score tests since they are equivalent in this setting.

For logistic regression the three tests (score, likelihood ratio, and Wald) can give different results and it is natural to ask which of the tests is more reliable when they do differ. An interesting point about the Wald test for logistic regression is that it has unexpected poor behavior when effects are very strong, for example (see Chap. 8), when a very rare SNP has large effects it is possible that the only observed minor alleles will be among the cases. In this setting the logistic regression estimate of the effect of that SNP will diverge to infinity during Fisher's scoring, but so will its variance estimate (at an even faster rate) so that a Wald test computed at the end of each iteration converges to zero as the iterations proceed.

It is for this sort of behavior, see Hauck 1977 [5] for further discussion, that, when the tests differ, it is the Wald test that is generally considered to be the least reliable.

One reason to prefer the likelihood ratio test to the other two is to note that it is invariant to parameter transformation, whereas neither the score nor the Wald test is invariant; if there exists a re-parameterization of the problem that produces very nicely normally distributed estimates, then this parameterization should be used over some other parameterization when constructing the Wald test. For example, in a logistic regression involving a parameter β_1 we can directly estimate the odds ratio $OR = \exp(\beta_1)$ rather than the log odds ratio β_1 and then compute a Wald test for $OR = 1$ as $(\hat{O}R - 1)/\sqrt{\text{Var}(\hat{O}R)}$ this test will in general give different values of the chi-square statistic than the usual Wald test that $\beta_1 = 0$ computed as $\hat{\beta}_1/\sqrt{\text{Var}(\hat{\beta}_1)}$ even though they are testing exactly the same hypothesis. Furthermore if on the original scale β_1 is close to being normally distributed (so that the Wald test is very accurate) on the exponential scale $\hat{O}R$, equal to $\exp(\hat{\beta}_1)$, would tend to be distributed as a log normal random variable. This could reduce the accuracy of the Wald test, since a log normal random variable divided by the square root of its variance may be far from normally distributed. The likelihood ratio tests of either $OR = 1$ or $\beta_1 = 0$ on the other hand will be identical.

Note however that these concerns go away as the sample size gets larger and larger and both β_1 and $\exp(\hat{\beta}_1)$ are asymptotically normally distributed except in pathological cases.

3.4.7   Score Tests of $\beta = 0$ for Linear and Logistic Models

Note that the score (i.e., the first derivative of the log likelihood) for both linear and logistic regression takes the form

$$U(\theta; Y) \propto \sum_{i=1}^{n} (Y_i - \mu_i)X_i,$$

where μ_i is the mean of Y_i; see (3.14) and (3.16). Intuitively it makes sense that U here is measuring the covariance between the variables X and Y. We make this clear below for logistic regression by considering the score test in the simplest case when only a slope and an intercept are being fit. In this case each regression vector $\mathbf{X_i}$ has two elements, a 1 (for the intercept) and the variable of interest X_i so that $\mu_i = g^{-1}(a + bX_i)$. The score vector for logistic regression evaluates to

$$
\begin{bmatrix}
\sum_{i=1}^{n} Y_i - \mu_i \\
\sum_{i=1}^{n} (Y_i - \mu_i)X_i
\end{bmatrix}
$$

and the information is

$$
\frac{\exp(a)}{(1 + \exp(a))^2}
\begin{bmatrix}
n & n\overline{X} \\
n\overline{X} & \sum X_i^2
\end{bmatrix}.
$$

The information has matrix inverse equal to

$$
\frac{(1 + \exp(a))^2}{\exp(a)} \frac{1}{n\sum X_i^2 - n^2\overline{X}^2}
\begin{bmatrix}
\sum X_i^2 & -n\overline{X} \\
-n\overline{X} & n
\end{bmatrix}.
$$

Therefore the score statistic for testing that the slope $b = 0$ is equal to zero is

$$
\left(\sum_{i=1}^{n} X_i Y_i - \frac{\exp(\hat{a})}{1 + \exp(\hat{a})} \sum_{i=1}^{n} X_i \right)^2 \frac{(1 + \exp(\hat{a}))^2}{\exp(\hat{a})n\mathrm{Var}(X)},
$$

with $n\mathrm{Var}(X)$ equal to the sum of squares of X or $\left(\sum X_i^2 - n\overline{X}^2\right)$. Here the estimate $\hat{a}$ of a is to be its MLE under the null hypothesis which is $\hat{a} = \log(\overline{Y}) - \log(1 - \overline{Y})$. After this substitution the score test for $b = 0$ simplifies to

$$
\frac{\left(\sum_{i=1}^{n} X_i Y_i - n\overline{Y}\,\overline{X} \right)^2}{n\mathrm{Var}(X)\overline{Y}(1 - \overline{Y})}.
$$

Because the numerator is equal to the square of the sample covariance of X and Y multiplied by n and because $\overline{Y}(1 - \overline{Y})$ is the estimate of the variance for a binary random variable it follows that this equals $n\mathrm{Cor}(X,Y)^2$ as mentioned above.

Note that for univariate linear regression the usual F or t^2 test for a slope b can be written as $(n - 2)R^2/(1 - R^2)$ which is similar to the score test for logistic regression if n is large and if R^2 is small. When there are other adjustment variables to be used in the model the test for linear regression is $(n - p - 1)R^2_{\text{partial}}/(1 - R^2_{\text{partial}})$ where p is the number of adjustment variables (including the intercept as an adjustment variable) and where R^2_{partial} is the squared partial correlation between X and Y after adjustment. The extent to which score tests from multivariate logistic regression can be approximated using R^2_{partial} is the subject of homework exercises.

3.4.8   Matrix Formulae for Estimators in OLS Regression

For ordinary least squares regression, i.e., when using model (3.3) with g equal to the identity, it is very helpful to be familiar with matrix expressions for the estimators of both the regression parameters and for the variance σ^2. Here these results are briefly introduced. First we define the vector of outcomes, Y, as $(Y_1, Y_2, \ldots, Y_N)'$ and the matrix of covariate values as

$$\mathbf{X} = \begin{pmatrix} 1 & X_{11} & X_{12} & \cdots & X_{1,r-1} \\ 1 & X_{21} & X_{22} & \cdots & X_{2,r-1} \\ \vdots & \vdots & \vdots & & \vdots \\ 1 & X_{N1} & X_{N2} & \cdots & X_{N,r-1} \end{pmatrix}.$$

Further we define the vector of parameters to be estimated as $\beta = (\mu, \beta_1, \beta_2, \ldots, \beta_{r-1})'$. Here we assume that the matrix $\mathbf{X}$ is of full rank r (so that linearly dependent parameters have already been removed). Furthermore we assume that (conditional on the covariates $\mathbf{X}$) that the elements of Y are uncorrelated and each has variance parameter σ^2 so that we can write the variance–covariance matrix $\sum$ of Y as $\sigma^2 \mathbf{I}$ where $\mathbf{I}$ is the $N \times N$ identity matrix.

In this case then it is easy to show that the maximum likelihood estimate, $\hat{\beta}$, of the regression parameter β is equal to

$$\hat{\beta} = \left(\mathbf{X}'\mathbf{X}\right)^{-1}\mathbf{X}'Y. \tag{3.18}$$

The usual estimate of σ^2 can be written in matrix form as

$$\hat{\sigma}^2 = \frac{1}{N-r}Y'\left(\mathbf{I} - \mathbf{X}(\mathbf{X}'\mathbf{X})^{-1}\mathbf{X}'\right)Y. \tag{3.19}$$

We can show that both β and $\hat{\sigma}^2$ are unbiased (i.e., have expectation β and σ^2, respectively) by understanding several properties of matrix manipulation of random vectors (and matrices) the first is that for any fixed matrix $\mathbf{A}$ and random vector V that are conformable, i.e., $\mathbf{A}$ has the same number of columns as V has elements then $E(\mathbf{A}V) = \mathbf{A}E(V)$ where $E(V)$ is the vector containing the expected values of the elements of the random V. (This rule also holds when V is replaced with **V** a matrix of random variables conformable with **A**.) Furthermore the variance-- covariance matrix for **A**V is equal to **A** Var(V)**A**$'$ where Var(V) is the variance-- covariance matrix of V.

Using the rule for expectations we can see that

$$E(\hat{\beta}) = E\left(\mathbf{X'X}\right)^{-1}\mathbf{X'}Y = \left(\mathbf{X'X}\right)^{-1}\mathbf{X'}E(Y) = \left(\mathbf{X'X}\right)^{-1}\mathbf{X'X}\beta = \beta,$$

so that $\hat{\beta}$ is unbiased. Using the rule for variances if follows that that

$$\text{Var}(\hat{\beta}) = \left(\mathbf{X'X}\right)^{-1}\mathbf{X'}(\sigma^2\mathbf{I})\mathbf{X}\left(\mathbf{X'X}\right)^{-1} = \sigma^2\left(\mathbf{X'X}\right)^{-1}.$$

In order to show that $\hat{\sigma}^2$ is unbiased it is helpful to invoke some additional matrix properties, specifically rules about the trace function defined as the sum of diagonal elements and denoted tr(**X**) for a square matrix **X**. Specifically suppose that **A** and **B** are matrices where **A** has the same number of columns as **B** has rows and in addition **B** has the same number of columns as **A** has rows (so that both products **AB** and **BA** are defined and square) In this case it is easy to show that tr(AB) = tr (BA). Furthermore it can be easily shown that if **V** is a random matrix then E(tr $(V)) = \text{tr}E(V)$

A somewhat more complicated but very useful result [6] concerns the trace of the matrix $X(X'X)^{-1}X'$ in expression (3.19) for $\hat{\sigma}^2$. The general rule is that for any *idempotent* matrix **P** (so that $PP = P$) then tr(P) = rank(P) implying that tr(X $(X'X)^{-1}X'$) = rank(X) = r. Note also that $\mathbf{I} - X(X'X)^{-1}X'$ is idempotent with rank equal to N–r.

Application of these rules shows that

$$E(\hat{\sigma}^2) = E\left[\frac{1}{N-r}\text{tr}\left\{Y'\left(\mathbf{I} - \mathbf{X}(\mathbf{X'X})^{-1}\mathbf{X'}\right)Y\right\}\right]$$

$$= \frac{1}{N-r}\text{tr}\left\{\left(\mathbf{I} - \mathbf{X}(\mathbf{X'X})^{-1}\mathbf{X'}\right)E(YY')\right\}$$

$$= \frac{1}{N-r}\text{tr}\left\{\left[\mathbf{I} - \mathbf{X}(\mathbf{X'X})^{-1}\mathbf{X'}\right]\left[E(Y)E(Y)' + \sigma^2\mathbf{I}\right]\right\}.$$

$$= \frac{1}{N-r}\text{tr}\left\{\left[\mathbf{I} - \mathbf{X}(\mathbf{X'X})^{-1}\mathbf{X'}\right]\left[\mathbf{X}\beta\beta'\mathbf{X'} + \sigma^2\mathbf{I}\right]\right\}$$

$$= \frac{\sigma^2}{N-r}\text{tr}\left\{\left[\mathbf{I} - \mathbf{X}(\mathbf{X'X})^{-1}\mathbf{X'}\right]\right\}$$

$$= \sigma^2$$

We use calculations like these in several other places in this book, particularly as we explore the results of population structure on OLS estimation of linear models (and by implication upon the estimation of other general linear models).

When Y_i are not independent and the covariance matrix $\boldsymbol{\Sigma}$ of the vector Y is known, then the *best linear unbiased estimate* (BLUE) of the parameters β in the mean model $E(\mathbf{Y}) = \mathbf{X}\beta$ is

$$\hat{\beta} = \left(\mathbf{X}'\boldsymbol{\Sigma}^{-1}\mathbf{X}\right)^{-1}\mathbf{X}'\boldsymbol{\Sigma}^{-1}Y \tag{3.20}$$

and the variance of $\hat{\beta}$ is equal to $(\mathbf{X}'\boldsymbol{\Sigma}^{-1}\mathbf{X})^{-1}$. If in addition Y is multivariate normal then $\hat{\beta}$ is the maximum likelihood estimate. In this case when there are parameters in $\boldsymbol{\Sigma}$ that are unknown and must be estimated then $\hat{\beta}$ with $\boldsymbol{\Sigma}$ replaced by an estimate $\hat{\boldsymbol{\Sigma}}$ remains the maximum likelihood estimate.

3.5 Covariates, Interactions, and Confounding

The importance of generalized linear models has a great deal to do with the simplicity in which the model can be extended to incorporate covariates, by adding these to the linear predictor. Control for additional variables, beyond the ones of direct interest, is often useful simply in order to sharpen inference; for example, if the phenotype of interest in a study of smokers is blood or urine levels of a nicotine metabolite then controlling for reported tobacco use (e.g., number of cigarettes consumed per day) will reduce the inherent variability of the phenotype and allow the effects, presumably more subtle, of a particular genetic variant of interest to be more readily detected. In addition it may be that we are interested in interaction effects; i.e., does the effect of an SNP allele increase or decrease with increasing exposure? In the nicotine example it may be that the SNP is most related to levels of the metabolite when smoking is at a low or intermediate level, with the SNP effect being swamped by the exposure at higher levels of smoking; adding an interaction term between smoking and the coded SNP genotype to the genetic model allows us to improve the quantification of the SNP effect. If such effects are assumed to exist a priori then we may even be able to improve the detection of SNP effects in a scan by simultaneously testing for the existence of either a genetic "main effect" or a gene × smoking interaction or both [7].

Often the most important covariates to consider including in the association modeling are potential *confounders* of the genetic variants. Confounding variables are variables that are themselves associated both with the study phenotype and with the explanatory variable of real interest to the investigator. For example, obesity is related to diabetes risk in nearly all populations [8], and therefore SNPs that affect obesity levels may appear to be risk factors for diabetes even if they are really only related to risk of obesity. An SNP in the FTO gene has been found to be associated with both obesity [9] and diabetes [10] as well as with diabetes-related phenotypes [11] including fasting insulin and glucose levels. However in the regression analysis of Freathy et al. [11] a very strong significant relationship between the FTO SNP and fasting insulin or glucose disappeared after including *body mass index* (BMI, **weight/height**^{2}) in the model; the effect of the SNP allele was no longer statistically significant in the regression models. It therefore appears that the variant in the FTO gene may not be related directly to diabetes risk but rather the increase in obesity caused by this variant is the *mediator* of the increase in diabetes risk seen in carriers.

Mediation of effects may or may not be regarded as confounding; this depends on the purpose of the analysis; if we are interested in innate disease susceptibility, not due to already known risk factors, then obesity is certainly a potential confounder; however, if estimation of the overall genetic component of diabetes risk is the primary focus then SNPs in FTO clearly remain important. For individual prediction, however, appropriate measurement of obesity itself may trump the FTO SNPs as predictors.

In other analyses, which have been called *Mendelian randomization* [12], testing for the marginal effect on disease risk of an SNP which is known to be related to a potential (but unproven) risk factor for a disease may help show that the unproven risk factor is indeed important as a causal factor for disease and is not for example a simple byproduct of disease. To give a recent example, the protein MSP is abundantly secreted by the prostate and has been recently suggested as a biomarker for prostate cancer risk [13]; it has also been shown [14] that an SNP allele in the MSMB gene (which encodes MSP) strongly predicts circulating levels of this protein. The fact that this SNP is both a predictor of MSMB levels and a known prostate cancer risk factor [15] helps to alleviate concerns about whether MSP levels are a by-product of cancer occurrence, rather than a predictor of cancer risk, since an SNP for which the only known effects are to alter MSP levels is predictive of prostate cancer risk.

Again taking smoking as an example, there are SNPs [16, 17] in a region of chromosome 15 that contains nicotinic acetylcholine receptor genes that have strongly and reproducibly been associated with risk of lung cancer. Since nicotine itself is not a suspected lung carcinogen it is very likely that these SNPs, and the underlying causal variants, are actually associated with smoking carcinogen exposure level, rather than innate susceptibility to lung cancer; i.e., they affect personal smoking behavior rather than individual sensitivity to the effects of smoking. If we can condition on true exposure to lung carcinogens then these SNPs may not appear to be predictive. However the situation here may be even more complicated than described above in the FTO/obesity/diabetes example. This is because smoking behavior may not be well characterized by the available information about cigarette consumption available in these studies; counting the number of cigarettes smoked per day does not capture individual differences in number of puffs taken per cigarette or in depth of inhalation. Simply including cigarettes per day in a model for lung cancer may not fully capture the variation in smoking behavior so that disease susceptibility will still appear to depend upon the SNPs in chromosome 15 because they "pick up additional information" about carcinogen exposure. This problem of incomplete control for confounders is also known in the epidemiologic literature as *residual confounding* [18].

We have already begun our discussion of population stratification in the previous chapter, and for genetic studies that involve participants from multiple racial/ethnic groups control for ethnicity is of great importance; self-reported racial/ethnic group membership can either be controlled for as a confounder or in case–control studies, treated as a matching factor when the study is designed (see discussion below on stratification). However self-reported ethnicity may provide insufficient control for population stratification in many cases (with particularly acute problems in admixed groups) and SNPs or other variants that are predictive of racial/ethnic origins may appear to be predictive for many phenotypes even after controlling for self-reported ancestry. This issue is discussed at length below, but many of the basic issues are the same as dealing with other confounders. In order to be a confounder individual racial/ethnic background must not only vary from person to person within a study but must also be related to the disease or phenotype distribution. For such phenotypes *residual confounding* occurs when available information concerning ancestral background is insufficiently informative, and all SNPs or other variants that are related to ancestral origin will appear to remain related to disease.

3.6   Conditional Logistic Regression

Matching of cases and controls at the design stage of a case–control study is an attempt to reduce the chance that heterogeneity due to either known or unknown factors will influence results. In genetics studies the use of sibling case–control pairs ensures that both the cases and the controls have the same ancestral background, thus eliminating concern about the effects of population stratification, admixture, etc., on results. The standard approach to the analysis of such data is conditional logistic regression. Conditional logistic regression constructs a different probability model than the usual (unconditional) model. For one-to-one matching the likelihood of the data from each matched pair is computed as the probability that the observed case had the disease conditional on the fact that exactly one of the two members of the pair had disease. Thus if the unconditional probability of the event follows a logistic regression model with the linear predictor for the case equal to $\alpha' \mathbf{X_1}$ and for the control $\alpha' \mathbf{X_0}$ then from first principles this conditional probability is written as

$$\frac{\text{logit}^{-1}(\alpha'\mathbf{X_1})\left(1 - \text{logit}^{-1}(\alpha'\mathbf{X_0})\right)}{\text{logit}^{-1}(\alpha'\mathbf{X_1})\left(1 - \text{logit}^{-1}(\alpha'\mathbf{X_0})\right) + \text{logit}^{-1}(\alpha'\mathbf{X_0})\left(1 - \text{logit}^{-1}(\alpha'\mathbf{X_1})\right)}.$$

This reduces immediately to

$$\frac{\exp(\alpha' \mathbf{X_1})}{\exp(\alpha' \mathbf{X_1}) + \exp(\alpha' \mathbf{X_0})}. \tag{3.21}$$

Note also that any terms in $\alpha^T X_i$ that are common to the case and the control (including the intercept parameter) will cancel out of the likelihood (and we assume that these have all been removed). The contribution of each pair to the kth element of the score vector and the k, k' element of the information matrix will be equal to

$$\frac{\exp(\alpha' \mathbf{X_1})}{\exp(\alpha' \mathbf{X_0}) + \exp(\alpha' \mathbf{X_1})} (X_{1k} - X_{0k})$$

for $k = 1, \ldots, r$ and

$$\frac{\exp(\alpha' \mathbf{X_1})}{[\exp(\alpha' \mathbf{X_0}) + \exp(\alpha' \mathbf{X_1})]^2} (X_{1k} - X_{0k})(X_{1k'} - X_{0k'})$$

for $k, k' = 1, \ldots, r$, respectively. These contributions are summed over all pairs to compute the full score and information. If there is only one parameter of interest, then the score test for the null hypothesis that this parameter is zero is easily seen to be equal to

$$\frac{\left(\sum_i (X_{i1} - X_{i0}) \right)^2}{\sum_i (X_{i1} - X_{i0})^2}, \tag{3.22}$$

which is essentially a test that the mean value of X for the cases differs from the mean value of X for the controls.

For more complicated matching, the conditional likelihood, i.e., the probability that the particular observed combination of cases and controls was observed given that there were N cases from among the $N + M$ subjects, involves complicated summations. However the best of today's modern software (e.g., PROC LOGISTIC in SAS) implements very fast and effective means to perform or approximate these computations.

3.6.1   Breaking the Matching in Logistic Regression of Matched Data

Even for data that has been collected using a matched design it is often desirable to break the matching, i.e., to use an unconditional logistic model for analysis of the study. Notice that for a 1:1 matched design that if either a case or a control is missing a covariate value then both the case and control in that stratum are no longer available for a given analysis; the situation is even worse for 1:M design if a case is missing data since then M + 1 subjects will no longer be available for analysis. This means that a matched design will often lose somewhat more cases and controls to missing data than would an equivalent unmatched design. Another common rationale for breaking the matching of a 1–1 study is to investigate subtypes of disease, restricting attention, for example, to ER- or ER + cancers rather than all disease in a breast cancer GWAS. By breaking the matching many more controls remain available than if the matching is retained. When faced with missing data or for subset analyses epidemiologists will generally break the matching and use unconditional logistic regression when they can.

Breaking the matching produces reliable results so long as the influence of the matching variables can be parsimoniously modeled using known covariates; here parsimoniously means "without introducing too many new parameters in the model." When breaking the matching it is important to use the original matching variables as adjustment variables in the unconditional analysis. To give an extreme example suppose that cases and controls were matched by race/ethnicity and some other variables but with the complexity that for one ethnicity a 1:1 matching of controls to cases is performed, but for another group a 1:2 matching was used. If the matching is broken then any variables (such as SNP counts n_A) that have different distributions in the two subgroups will appear to be strongly related to disease unless ethnicity is included in the unconditional (matches broken) model.

More generally whenever the variable of interest is itself associated with one or more of the variables used in the matching it is important to include the matching variables as adjustment variables in unconditional analysis: In particular when both the matching variables and the variables of interest are strongly associated with risk and are themselves correlated, then leaving out the matching variables from the unconditional analysis will lead to low powered analysis compared to the conditional matched logistic regression. Figure 3.1 shows the results (obtained by running "break_matching.r") of five different tests for the effect of a single SNP for data where (1) age is a very important predictor of disease and (2) the study is designed to be either individually matched on age or is unmatched (with equal numbers of cases and controls). Shown are box plots of the Z-statistics (estimate/ standard error) for the following tests of a nonzero SNP effect (see the R program for details of the model).

1. Conditional logistic regression analysis using the individual matching.
2. Breaking the matching (and using unconditional logistic regression) with no adjustment for age.
3. Breaking the matching with adjustment for age as a continuous variable.
4. Breaking the matching with adjustment for age as a categorical variable (5-year age groups).
5. Analysis of an unmatched case–control sample drawn from the same population, with adjustment for age.

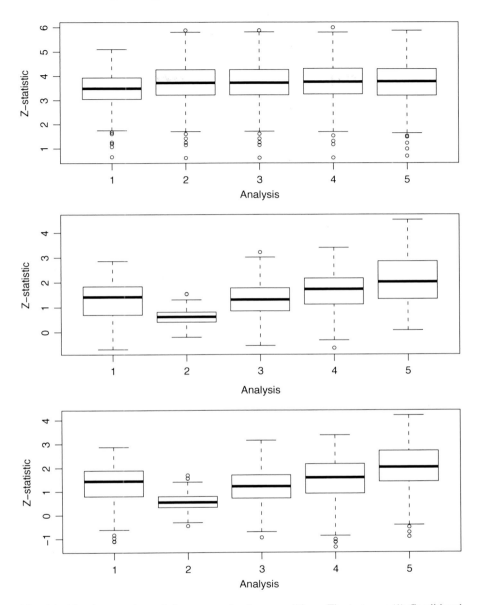

Fig. 3.1 Visual comparison of five tests under three conditions. The tests are (1) Conditional logistic regression analysis for individually matched data; (2) breaking the matching (and using unconditional logistic regression) with no adjustment for age; (3) breaking the matching with adjustment for age as a continuous variable; (4) breaking the matching with adjustment for age as a categorical variable (5 year age groups); (5) analysis of unmatched case control sample drawn from the same population. The *upper panel* gives the results of these tests when the variable of interest (snp count) is uncorrelated with age and the middle panel when the snp1 count is strongly correlated with age (correlation approximately equal to 0.85). This illustrates the importance of

We see from the top two panels of Fig. 3.1 that all analyses seem to have similar power when age and the SNP are not highly correlated with each other; i.e., the Z-statistics computed in each of analyses (1–5) are similarly distributed. However for the middle panel, where age and SNP count are highly correlated then analysis 2 is very underpowered. Adjusting for age seems to make up this power loss quite nicely (in analyses 3 and 4) even though by design the distribution of age is the same in the cases as in the controls. This can be understood because conditional on a given value of SNP count the age distribution of the cases will now be different than the age distribution of controls, because of the strong correlations between both age and outcome, and between age and SNP, even though averaging over the SNP counts there is no such correlation. Modeling the association of SNP and outcome given age (by including age as an adjustment variable) then improves the power of the analysis. In this setting analysis 5 (actually a different design than analyses 1–4, since the data are collected unconditionally) has similar power to that of analyses 1, 3, and 4.

While we did not see much difference between the power of unmatched (analysis 5) and matched studies(analysis 1) in the top 2 panels of Fig. 3.1, it is important to realize when an unmatched study might be a better design than a matched study. From a study design perspective matching has a price to pay compared to the unmatched analysis whenever (1) the variables being matched on are not strongly related to disease, but (2) the variables being matched on are related to the variable (here SNP) of interest; this is often called *overmatching* since we are matching (for no good reason) on a non-influential variable that is correlated with the exposure of interest. In this setting the comparison of the 5 analyses considered above is different (see Fig. 3.1 lower panel) in particular the unmatched design; i.e., scenario (5) above provides the most powerful analysis. Note also that analysis (2), breaking the matching with no adjustment for age, is again the least powerful analysis, emphasizing again that matching variables should be included as adjustment variables in the unconditional analysis of matched data.

Note (Homework) that in a matched analysis that if the matching variable is correlated with the variable of interest (here the SNP count) with correlation R then the correlation between the exposure of interest seen when comparing the values of the cases and controls will be equal to R^2. This observation allows us to now consider *sibling matched designs* where a case is matched to his or her unaffected sibling. Prior to the advent of large-scale genotyping studies, where principal components and other analyses are possible, the matching factors (basically the complete ancestry of the parents) could not be summarized parsimoniously so that if we break the family matching we could only do an analysis equivalent to analysis (2).

Fig. 3.1 (continued) control for age after breaking the matching since analysis (2) is much inferior to the remainder of the analyses when there is a strong correlation between the matching factor (here age) and the variable of interest (here a snp count). In the lower panel we are assume that age is not a predictor of the effect but that there is still a strong correlation (0.85) between SNP count and age. In this case it is clear that the best analysis is the unmatched design (adjusting for age) whereas all the other analyses (of matched data) are inferior

It was shown in the previous chapter that the correlation between SNP counts for siblings is equal to 1/2. From the comment above this is equivalent to assuming that the correlation between SNP count and matching factor (which would be a hypothetical parsimonious representation of the ancestry of each sibling pair) must be the square root of (1/2) or roughly 0.71. Thus the results from the middle and lower panel of Fig. 3.1 (where a similar high correlation was assumed between the variable of interest and the matching variable) would seem to apply to the sibling matched design. In this case, analysis (2), breaking the matching and ignoring the matching variable (which we must then do since we can't measure the hypothetical parsimonious representation of ancestry), has much poorer power than keeping the matching, so therefore we would always choose to keep the matching in the analysis of such a study. However, when considering whether to design such a study, we should realize that there is a considerable loss of power in choosing a sibling matched case–control design over an unmatched design unless some unmeasured characteristics varying among families[1] are strongly predictive of outcome. If all the families have the same disease risk (i.e., matching on family is unneeded) matching on family is equivalent to choosing design (1) over design (5) for the bottom panel of Fig. 3.1; i.e., there is severe loss of power. In the past the problem with choosing the unmatched design was that there was no way to adjust for the influence of hidden population structure, admixture, etc. Modern large-scale genotyping studies can make up for this deficit.

3.6.2 Parent Affected-Offspring Design

Another family-based design specifically the *parent affected-offspring design* [19, 20] also provides protection against population stratification. Here outcome data (disease of interest) are only collected for an affected offspring, but genotypes are available for both the *affected offspring* and the parents. Analysis of these data can be presented in a variety of ways including as a conditional logistic regression problem [20], although that is not our emphasis here. Consider the triplet ($n_{f,A}$ $n_{m,A}$ $n_{o,A}$) of allele counts for father, mother, and offspring for a given variant of interest (with alleles a and A). Conditional on the genotypes for the father and mother, the distribution of the number of copies can be readily computed under Mendel's law. Moreover the mean and variance of the offspring allele counts can be computed as well, as given in Table 3.2 below.

Table 3.2 is computed under the null hypothesis. If however the SNP is linked to a disease variant then the affected offspring will tend to have more copies of the risk allele than expected given their parental genotypes (under an additive model for the effect of having 0, 1, or 2 copies of allele A). Given data for family $i = 1, \ldots, N_{trios}$

---

[1] Hidden stratification or admixture + either cultural practices affecting disease risk varying by ethnicity and/or the presence of an unmeasured polygene are obvious candidates.

Table 3.2 Conditional distribution of offspring allele count, n_{oA}, of allele A given parental allele counts n_{mA} and n_{fA}

Parental genotype (n_{fA}, n_{mA})	Pr(n_{oA})			$E(n_o|n_f, n_m)$	Var$(n_o|n_f, n_m)$
	0	1	2		
(0, 0)	1	0	0	0	0
(0, 1)	1/2	1/2	0	1/2	1/4
(0, 2)	0	1	0	1	0
(1, 0)	1/2	1/2	0	1/2	1/4
(1, 1)	1/4	1/2	1/4	1	1/2
(1, 2)	0	1/2	1/2	3/2	1/4
(2, 0)	0	1	0	1	0
(2, 1)	0	1/2	1/2	3/2	1/4
(2, 2)	0	0	1	2	0

a test of the null hypothesis of no effect of A on risk against an additive alternative can be computed as

$$
T^2 = \frac{\left(\sum_{i=1,N_{\text{trios}}} n_{ioA} - E\left(n_{ioA} \big| n_{ifA}, n_{imA} \right) \right)^2}{\sum_{i=1,N_{\text{trios}}} \text{Var}\left(n_{ioA} \big| n_{ifA}, n_{imA} \right)}.
\tag{3.23}
$$

With T^2 distributed as approximately χ_1^2 under the null hypothesis. A more general test would be to construct a multi-degree of freedom test for any distortion in Mendelian segregation among the affected offspring. Note that many of the parental genotypes are non-informative (no variability in the offspring genotype given the parental genotypes). These can of course be eliminated from the calculations. The test statistic, T^2, in (3.23) can be shown to be equivalent to the *transmission-disequilibrium TDT* test [19] (see Homework) and to the score test for the conditional logistic regression discussed by [20].

Case–parent trios allow for the investigation of a number of unique effects that cannot be addressed in only unrelated individuals. For example, parental origin of an allele may be important because of imprinting (see Chap. 1); that is, an allele could have a different effect on risk of disease depending upon whether it was transmitted from the mother versus the father. Since parental origin of each allele can be inferred for 14 of the 15 nonzero cells in Table 3.2 (the exception is when each of the parents and the offspring are heterozygous) it is possible to make appropriate comparisons that include not only the observed genotype for the affected offspring, but also the parental origin of that genotype. For example, if we saw similar numbers of parent affected-offspring trios falling into the $(n_{fA}, n_{mA}, n_{oA}) = (1,0,1)$ cell compared to the $(1,0,0)$ cell of Table 3.2 but saw more trios falling into the $(0,1,1)$ cell than in the $(0,1,0)$ cell this might be evidence that an A allele is only related to risk if it was transmitted from the mother. See Weinberg [21] for a careful discussion.

3.7   Case-Only Analyses

3.7.1   Case-Only Analyses of Disease Subtype

Consider first case-only analysis in the context of distinguishing between risk factors for one form or type or grade of disease from another such form of disease (say low stage versus high stage disease, nonaggressive versus aggressive disease, biomarker positive versus biomarker negative, etc.). For example, many cancers of the prostate and thyroid are low grade at diagnosis and may remain indolent for many years. In a GWAS devoted to such an outcome a natural question is whether it is possible to find risk genetic variants that predict susceptibility to high stage or aggressive disease but not (or to a lesser degree) low state disease. A simple but effective approach for analysis of such data is simply to redefine the case status variable so that high-grade cases are defined as $D = 1$, the remaining cases as $D = 0$, and the controls are dropped from this portion of the analysis. With this redefinition standard logistic regression analyses are utilized. When associations between markers and this new case status variable are detected, these can be interpreted as interactions between genes and grade of disease. For example, in breast cancer research most associations found in the first few GWAS studies appeared to be restricted to increasing the risk of ER + breast cancer and not the risk of ER disease. Testing and affirming the significance of such an apparent interaction using case-only analysis add credibility to the assertion that these two forms of the disease have distinct etiology as well as being of prognostic importance.

3.7.2   Case-Only Analysis of Gene × Environment and Gene × Gene Interactions

Consider fitting a model

$$\text{logit}(\Pr(D_i = 1)) = \mu + \beta_1 n_{iA} + \beta_2 E_i + \beta_3 (E_i \times n_{iA}), \tag{3.24}$$

where the primary interest is in the parameter β_3, i.e., in the interaction between the count, n_{iA}, of allele A and the additional (environmental) variable E_i. If we knew that in the population sampled that E_i and n_{iA} are independent of each other then in certain situations it is possible to exploit this independence in order to test for multiplicative interactions between E_i and n_{iA} affecting the mean, $\Pr(D_i = 1)$, of D_i. A classic paper by Piegorsch et al. [22] pointed out that under this assumption interactions can be tested for by testing explicitly for an association between E_i and n_{iA} among the cases in the study. When disease is rare so that all terms in the model can be approximated to be multiplicative, then Piegorsch et al. show that this test is more powerful than the usual test for $G \times E$ interaction using both cases and controls. To give intuition to the results of Piegorsch et al., the R program *case-*

only.r in the online materials illustrates what is going on. First it is helpful to understand that testing for a $G \times E$ interaction using model (3.24) is nearly equivalent to testing whether the association between the G and E variables differs by case–control status. For example, in the R program mentioned above two models are fit in each simulation:

1. glm(E[case] ~ G[case],family = binomial)
2. glm(E[control] ~ G[control] ,family = binomial)

   Then the coefficients for the slope parameter (called e_1 for cases e_0 for controls in the program) as well as their variances (v_1 for cases and v_0 for controls) are extracted from the summary of these models and a simple test for equality of independent estimates is performed as $(e_1 - e_0)^2/(v_1 + v_2)$, which is compared to a chi-square statistic with 1 degree of freedom to assess significance. In addition the usual case–control main effect + interaction model is fit

3. glm(Y ~ G + E + G*E,family = binomial)

   and the Wald test for the $G*E$ interaction (also of 1 degree of freedom) is performed. Finally the case-only test that $e_1 = 0$ is computed from the fit of the first glm model (as e_1^2/v_1). Figure 3.2 shows the results of 50 such analyses using simulated data with parameters chosen for illustrative purposes. The figure suggests the near equivalence of the standard $G \times E$ test (*x*-axis) with the test that compares the association between E and G between cases and controls, as well as the striking increase in power seen in the case-only analysis relative to the usual test. It should be noted here that the model being fit is nearly multiplicative because for rare diseases and modest effects (of E, G, and $G*E$) the logistic function behaves similarly to the logarithmic function. The logistic function is $\log(x) - \log(1 - x)$ so that if the operand x is close to zero (as in a rare disease) the second term is also close to zero.

   In many cases it seems very reasonable to assume independence between genetic and environmental variables (i.e., here between E_i and n_{iA}). The best case would be as in a clinical trial if treatment is assigned randomly to individuals. However most randomized trials are studies of common, rather than rare, events (e.g., relapse after treatment for an initial cancer). When the event probability is close to 1/2 in the population of interest the usual test for interaction is more powerful than the case-only analysis. This is reasonable because of the relative efficiencies between the test that (using the above terminology) $e_1 = e_2$ and the case–control test. If the disease is common (close to 50 % probability) then the controls are under as much (or more) selection than are the cases, and it is the selection that causes e_1 to be nonzero. For example, in the above simulation the expected values of e_2 would no longer be close to zero (and would be opposite in direction than e_1) and so the test that $e_1 = e_2$ (~equivalent to the case–control test for interaction) becomes more powerful than the test using only the cases that $e_1 = 0$. Of course for very common outcomes a "control-only" analysis would become an attractive alternative.

   In epidemiologic studies without the benefit of randomization the assumption of G and E independence may still be plausible, and even if a few genes are not

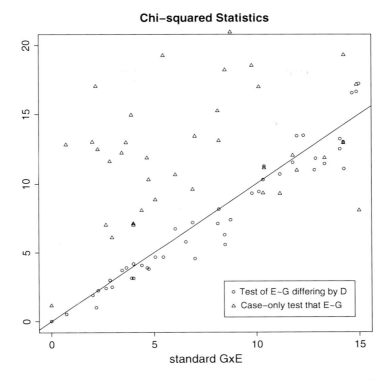

Fig. 3.2 Plot of chi-squared statistics for two alternative tests plotted against the chi-squared statistic for the standard G × E test using case control data. The first alternative is a test that the association between *E* and *G* differs between the cases and controls (*circles*), the second is for the case-only test (*triangles*). This figure suggests the near-equivalence of the standard *G* × *E* test with the comparison between cases and controls of association between *E* and *G* as well as the striking increase in power in the case-only analysis, when, as here, it is appropriate

independent of exposure this may not matter on the larger scale. For example, alcohol intake is related to ability to metabolize alcohol and it is well known that certain SNPs in the alcohol dehydrogenase gene are related to alcohol intake and these could be ignored in the results of a *G* × alcohol genome-wide survey.

A number of authors [7, 23–25] have sought to find some way of combining the case–control and case-only analyses in ways that can provide protection against a failure of assumption of independence between *E* and *G*. One of the most interesting proposals is by Murcray et al. [26] who suggest first testing for association between *E* and *G* for all individuals (cases and controls) and then moving associations that pass a certain threshold of significance into traditional case–control analysis. Murcray et al. show that the two tests are formally independent of each other; i.e., for a given association the outcome of the case–control analysis will not depend upon that of the initial screen. Moreover by fine-tuning the thresholds for significance in this "two-stage" testing, both for the initial case-only analysis and the follow-up case–control analysis, Murcray et al. are able to preserve power and control for multiple testing [27]. Intuitively, however, the Murcray et al.'s approach still rests upon the rare-disease assumption, since if both cases and controls are common in the population then the initial screen will have diminished power since the sample roughly speaking reflects the full population, and so no association will be detected between G and E when the independence assumption is true.

Case-only analyses are susceptible to population stratification; i.e., in structured populations it could well be that exposures are related to culture or ethnicity; thus careful control for population stratification can be important. This is especially true when case-only analysis is performed to test for gene by gene ($G \times G$) interactions. Associations between unlinked SNPs, e.g., SNPs very far away from each other on the same chromosome or on different chromosomes must be analyzed carefully before they can be considered to be evidence of interactions (when observed among cases), since as seen below, correlations between unlinked SNPs are a hallmark of hidden population structure [28].

3.8 Non-independent Phenotypes

So far in this chapter it has been assumed that each of the outcomes Y_i is independent of each other so that likelihoods can be multiplied (and log likelihoods summed) over the independent observations. It is worthwhile to consider situations where phenotypes Y_i and Y_j ($i \neq j$) might NOT be independent of each other and what the effects of such lack of independence will be.

Consider the effects of unexpected relatedness between subjects. Suppose that the mean of Y_i and Y_j depended not only on the measured genotypes $n_i(A)$ and $n_j(A)$ but also on an unmeasured variant with allele counts $n_i(U)$ and $n_j(U)$. If $n_i(U)$ and $n_j(U)$ are independent of each other we could still regard Y_i as being independent of Y_j given only the known genotypes for the first variant. However if $n_i(U)$ and $n_j(U)$ are dependent then Y_i and Y_j will also be dependent; for example, for linear models (i.e., g is the identity function) that are linear in $n(U)$ (with parameter β_u) the covariance between Y_i and Y_j is equal to $\beta_u Cov[n_i(U), n_j(U)]$, where this covariance is calculated conditionally on the values of the measured variables and $n_i(A)$ and $n_j(A)$.

3.8.1 OLS Estimation When Phenotypes Are Correlated

Here we expand our discussion in Sect. 3.4.8 of the mean and variance of β to the case when phenotypes are correlated according to a special structure; namely, we assume that the model for the expectation of phenotype vector Y remains

$$E(Y) = \mathbf{X}\beta$$

and assume that Y has variance–covariance matrix equal to $\sum = \sigma^2\mathbf{I} + \gamma^2\mathbf{K}$. We will see that this model is highly relevant to the issues of relatedness and hidden structure described in Chaps. 2 and 4. For this model we can show (from the rules used in Sect. 3.4.7) that the ordinary least squares estimate $\hat{\beta}$ of (3.18) has expectation β, i.e., is unbiased, but it now has variance equal to

$$\mathrm{Var}(\hat{\beta}) = \left(\mathbf{X}'\mathbf{X}\right)^{-1}\mathbf{X}'\Sigma\mathbf{X}\left(\mathbf{X}'\mathbf{X}\right)^{-1}$$

$$= \sigma^2\left(\mathbf{X}'\mathbf{X}\right)^{-1} + \gamma^2\left(\mathbf{X}'\mathbf{X}\right)^{-1}\mathbf{X}'\mathbf{K}\mathbf{X}\left(\mathbf{X}'\mathbf{X}\right)^{-1}. \qquad (3.25)$$

Further we can show that under this model the estimate of σ^2 in (3.19) is no longer unbiased; in fact with a little algebra similar to that used in Sect. 3.4.7 the usual estimate, $\hat{\sigma}^2$, can be shown to have expectation equal to (for Proof see Appendix below)

$$\sigma^2 + \gamma^2 \frac{\left[\mathrm{tr}\{\mathbf{K}\} - \mathrm{tr}\left\{(\mathbf{X}'\mathbf{X})^{-1}\mathbf{X}'\mathbf{K}\mathbf{X}\right\}\right]}{N - r}. \qquad (3.26)$$

Notice that since the variance of any given observation, Y_i, conditional on covariate data $\mathbf{X}$ is under this model equal to $\sigma^2 + \gamma^2 K_{ii}$ $\hat{\sigma}^2$ underestimates the variability of Y_i if $\frac{\left[\mathrm{tr}\{\mathbf{K}\} - \mathrm{tr}\left\{(\mathbf{X}'\mathbf{X})^{-1}\mathbf{X}'\mathbf{K}\mathbf{X}\right\}\right]}{N-r}$ is less than K_{ii}. When $\mathbf{tr}\{(\mathbf{X}'\mathbf{X})^{-1}(\mathbf{X}'\mathbf{K}\mathbf{X})\}$ is large then the true variability will be most underestimated. It turns out that the problem of finding a maximum value of $\mathbf{tr}\{(\mathbf{X}'\mathbf{X})^{-1}(\mathbf{X}'\mathbf{K}\mathbf{X})\}$ is similar to the eigenvector/eigenvalue problem. In particular when columns of $\mathbf{X}$ load on the largest eigenvectors of $\mathbf{K}$, then both the variance of observations Y_i and therefore the variance of $\hat{\beta}$ will be underestimated. More on these effects is described in the following chapter when correction for population stratification and relatedness is discussed.

3.9 Needs of a GWAS Analysis

In GWAS studies several hundred thousand to more than one million SNP markers are genotyped often in thousands of study participants. One of the most obvious differences between GWAS studies and traditional epidemiological studies is the sheer number of models fit and effects tested. This has an impact both on the software that we choose to analyze the data (to complete the analyses in a reasonable length of time) as well as upon the sample sizes that are needed to keep control of type I error rates in a major study. Single SNP analyses with no or only few covariate variables included in the model are very simple to fit computationally but nonetheless represent a serious burden for most software: the data are very voluminous, and the computer software must be able to rapidly access the data for each SNP in turn during the course of the analyses. Simple naïve use of the usual statistical packages familiar to most statisticians, including R, will not work on datasets this large, unless special methods are adopted. In R perhaps the most important problem to deal with is speeding up access to the data from disk to memory, which is far slower using standard R methods, such as the read.table command illustrated above, than can be regarded as acceptable for large-scale studies.

3.9.1　Hardware Requirements for GWAS

A typical GWAS dataset may involve manipulating many gigabytes of data for a single study. For most but not all analyses, stand-alone machines costing in the rough range of 5–10 thousand dollars including access to several terabytes of disk space and 16 gigabytes memory or more are adequate with most analyses running in a few hours. One exception to this, often regarded as an essential part of quality control, is to estimate IBD probabilities for all pairs of subjects in a study in order to identify unexpected close relatives or unknown duplicates, often with the intention being to remove one member of each such pairs from analysis (or both if sample mix-ups are suspected as a cause). For these and some other (multivariate) analyses, for example, involving scans of the entire genome for haplotype effects using sliding windows, as described in Chap. 6, it is extremely helpful if not essential to have access to a reasonably large cluster of interconnected computers. Calculation of principal components may require specialty software; i.e., general purpose programs such as SAS PROC PRINCOMP may be inadequate for larger problems, while programs like EIGENSTRAT (see Chap. 2) remain feasible to run on single user systems (although EIGENSTRAT only runs on Linux or UNIX systems).

3.9.2　Software Solutions

A basic dilemma arises when considering the choice of software, i.e., whether to abandon, in favor of specialty software, tried and true statistical packages, which while not optimized for the GWAS setting, but which provide extremely flexible model fitting, and also allow for a great deal of automation, either through macrogeneration (e.g., in SAS) or through user-defined functions (in R).

　　There are some very impressive stand-alone programs available for analysis of GWAS data that are optimized for dealing with hundreds of thousands or even millions of SNPs. The best of them, such as the PLINK program [29], provide capabilities for both processing large files containing SNP data and for dealing with special problems that such data pose. These include providing procedures to deal with quality control for these data such as computing genotype completion rates, performing Hardy–Weinberg tests, and checking for Mendel errors for family data, providing help with strand issues when two or more sources of genetic data are to be merged or compared, as well as performing specialized analyses, such as relatedness checking, etc. Such packages, however, are not optimized for data display or more generally for post-analysis manipulation of results. A compromise procedure is often adopted; i.e., a familiar statistical package is used for initial data manipulation of the raw data coming from genotype calling software for the purpose of the setup of files for analysis in PLINK or other external software, which may include genotype files, subject description files, SNP information files, additional covariate information, etc. When the external program finishes, the results of the external program are again manipulated with a highly flexible package such as *R* or SAS. By using the ability of the statistical package (such as the *R system* command or SAS *X* command) to call external programs, and then to read and manipulate the results files for data display or other post processing, much of the pre- and post-analysis data manipulation process can be automated by a statistical programmer working within a statistical package such as SAS or in the *R* language. Writing, documenting, and saving a program script that orchestrates as much of the analyses as is possible are an essential part of ensuring that results obtained can ultimately be traced back to the original data and samples, even if the same analysis is not expected to be repeated many times.

   It is possible to run large-scale GWAS problems in *SAS*, and this allows for use of the large range of features available in *PROC LOGISTIC* (use of offsets, conditional logistic regression, calculation of score and likelihood ratio tests, etc.). The main issue in SAS is to reduce the number of calls to PROC LOGISTIC from one per variable, to one call per large number of variables, using a BY statement in SAS to break up SNPs. For example, if there are 10,000 SNPs being run for 5,000 individuals in single SNP analyses, a file can be created with only a few columns, one of them named SNP, and an additional column, labeled SNPNAME, e.g.,

```
Proc Logistic data=long_skinny;
class age sex;
model D=age sex SNP; by SNPNAME;
```

the data file *long_skinny* is the concatenation of files needed to run a single SNP, i.e., there may be only 5 columns in *long_skinny*, i.e., those needed to contain D, age, sex, SNP, and SNPNAME, but there are 10,000 × 5,000 rows; since each of the 10,000 SNPs being analyzed (all named SNP) needs the covariate data for all 5,000 individuals, SNPNAME contains the SNP identifier distinguishing the SNPs.

   For larger numbers of SNPs many *long_skinny* files may need to be created in sequence (and discarded after processing, to save space), but surprisingly the whole procedure can be implemented in SAS macros and run in times that are highly competitive with stand-alone programs such as PLINK, while keeping the greater flexibility of the SAS regression programs.

3.10   The Multiple Comparisons Problem

A GWAS study is *designed* to provide an *unbiased* search for regions of the genome that contain variants that are related to risk of disease. As such GWAS studies are inherently exploratory, and hundreds of thousands to millions of often correlated tests are produced. For a given disease or other phenotype of interest the ultimate *goals* of the scientific enterprise that GWAS studies play a part in are to understand at a fundamental level the genetic portion of individual variability of that phenotype. Because of the work involved in following up GWAS results for the identification of causal variants and (ultimately) their mechanistic relationship to phenotypic variability it is necessary to carefully control the rate of false-positive reports coming out of GWAS studies.

Currently the de facto standard that in order to be accepted as a true association by the community of interested scientists (and accepted for publication in a good journal) a novel finding (generally an SNP/phenotype association not previously known or suspected) should be

1. *Globally significant* in the original GWAS—which may have been performed in several stages, so that not all subjects need to have been genotyped for all SNPs (see discussion of the design of two-stage studies, Chap. 7).
2. Be replicated in at least one other study that is completely independent of the original discovery sample.

For the present attention is focused here on issue (1). By *globally significant* it is meant that starting with an initial set of SNPs (i.e., those present on the genotype array), the *sequence of analyses* that was followed in the GWAS study in order to declare a novel finding significant would have produced no false-positive results in the vast majority of all such investigations (i.e., if the entire study was somehow able to be repeated again a large number of times). Thus the phrase *global significance* means controlling the overall *experiment-wise* type I error rate, α, typically at the generally accepted *5 % level*. From a practical stand point, since the details of the sequence of analysis followed by a specific study may be obscure, a standard for *nominal significance* that is generally accepted as implying global significance, at least for a single SNP association, is that the p-value for the observed association is less than 5×10^{-8}. This standard for nominal significance to equal global significance fluctuates a bit depending upon circumstances since LD patterns vary by race/ancestry and by the frequency spectrum of the alleles that are to be interrogated. The justification of the use of this (or other similar p-values) is not so much based upon a Bonferroni test (i.e., dividing 0.05 by the total number of SNPs that are genotyped), but rather upon considerations involving a hypothetical *effective number* of independent single marker associations that could be tested if we were to capture, through linkage disequilibrium with the set of genotyped markers, all common variations in the human genome. This criterion for nominal significance is designed to allow for the use of a particular type of multi-SNP analysis, namely, predicting (and testing for association) ungenotyped SNPs or other known common variants, using disequilibrium patterns. For a number of years the set of common variants that have been targeted in such analyses were the common SNPs genotyped in the Phase 2 HapMap data [30, 31]. Such analyses typically include examination of the ENCODE regions that have been more extensively sequenced for discovery purposes, in order to estimate the "capture" rates for common variants that have been achieved by the Phase 2 HapMap itself. It is very possible that these criteria will need to be changed with the more extensive discovery of both common and rarer variation provided by the ongoing 1000 Genomes Project.

3.11 Behavior of the Bonferroni Correction with Non-Independent Tests

The Bonferroni correction for multiple comparisons is based upon a very simple concept; for any set of random events (whether independent or non-independent) the probability that at least one of the events occurs is less than or equal to the sum of the marginal probabilities of the events. In the hypothesis testing framework if we perform N tests of hypotheses, each one with type I error rate α/N, the probability, if all the null hypotheses are true, that we will falsely reject one or more of them is less than or equal to α. Use of the Bonferroni criteria is an effort to control the overall type I error rate α of the experiment, under the *global null* hypothesis that all of the individual null hypotheses are true.

Bonferroni correction works very well in controlling the false-positive rate for large numbers of independent or nearly independent tests. For example, if the test statistics are all independent, then under the global null hypothesis the probability that one or more tests is rejected is calculated as $1 - (1 - \alpha/N)^N$ which as N increases converges rapidly to $1 - \exp(-\alpha)$. At $\alpha = .05$ using the Bonferroni calculation will be slightly over-conservative since $1 - \exp(-0.05) = 0.04877$ rather than the desired α of 0.05.

For non-independent tests, where the rejection of one hypothesis means that another hypothesis is more likely to be rejected as well, the Bonferroni correction worsens as an approximation to the true experiment-wise type I error rate; it is conservative in the sense that the probability of a false-positive experiment is smaller than the nominal significance level α. When testing massive amounts of SNP data, each SNP one at a time, association tests of nearby SNPs are non-independent because the SNPs are in linkage disequilibrium with their neighbors.

In the model

$$E(Y_i) = \mu + \beta_1 n_i(A),$$

if we reject the hypothesis that $\beta_1 = 0$, in favor of a two-sided alternative, then if B is another nearby SNP allele with high correlation to A, i.e., high R^2 between $n(A)$

and $n(B)$, we are also likely to reject the hypothesis $\beta_1 = 0$ when testing SNP allele B (i.e., replacing $n_i(A)$ with $n_i(B)$ above).

In special cases it is possible to quantify the loss of accuracy of the Bonferroni correction due to such correlation. For example, consider a study in which evenly spaced markers are each tested, to form the z-scores, Z_i and Z_j, from Wald or other tests of $\beta_1 = 0$ at the two marker positions, i and j. Now assume that short-range linkage disequilibrium decays so that for two test statistics at marker positions i and j, we have $Cor(Z_i, Z_j) = \exp(-\lambda\Delta)$ with Δ being the distance between markers and λ a positive rate of decay parameter. This model for decay in the correlation between test statistics with distance, Δ, has some theoretical justification when recombination events are regarded as occurring independently with a rate constant over the genome. Such a sequence of correlated normal random variables is called an Ornstein–Uhlenbeck process after the physicists who first studied it (see Siegmund and Yanik's book [32] Sect. 3.3 for additional discussion of this process and its relevance to genetic studies and including R code to perform the computations).

For this process the probability that the maximum z-score is larger in absolute value than the positive number z can be well approximated as

$$\Pr\left(\max_i |Z_i| \geq z\right) \approx 1 - \exp\left\{-2C[1 - \Phi(z)] - 2\lambda Lz\phi(z)v\left(z\{2\lambda\Delta\}^{1/2}\right)\right\}, \quad (3.27)$$

with $\Phi(z)$ and $\phi(z)$ being the probability distribution and density functions, respectively, of the standard normal distribution, where L is the total genetic length, and C the number of chromosomes, being considered in the scan. The third function, $v(\cdot)$, can be approximated as

$$v(y) = \frac{(2/y)(\Phi(y/2) - 0.05)}{(y/2)\Phi(y/2) + \phi(y/2)}.$$

Equation (3.27) can be used to study the behavior of an approximation to the true experiment-wise rate, when using the Bonferroni criteria to control that rate, but when the marker z-scores for pairs of adjacent markers are correlated with correlation equal to the value $R > 0$. For example, in a study with one million markers assumed to be evenly spaced over 3 billion base pairs (a spacing of one SNP every 3 kb) over 23 chromosomes, we can calculate the Ornstein–Uhlenbeck approximation (3.27) using values $C = 23$, $L = 3 \times 10^9$, $\Delta = 3,000$, $\lambda = -(1/3,000)$ $\log(R)$, and $z = 5.45$. Here, $z = 5.45$ defines the critical value for significance required by the Bonferroni test, i.e., $Pr(|Z| > 5.45131) = 5 \times 10^{-8}$, and λ is chosen so that the correlation between nearby z-scores, $\exp(-\lambda\Delta)$, is equal to R. Figure 3.3 gives values of the Ornstein–Uhlenbeck approximation for R ranging from 0.01 to 0.99. From Fig. 3.3 the simple Bonferroni correction appears to perform very reasonably until correlations between neighboring tests become rather large. Only with $R > 0.88$ does the Ornstein–Uhlenbeck approximation to the true experimental-wise type one error rate decrease below 0.04.

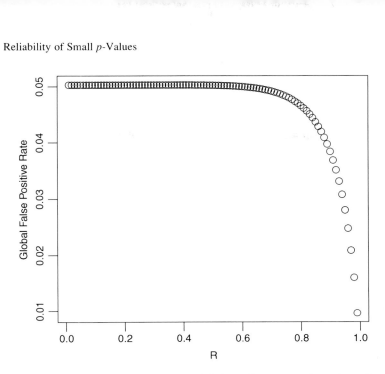

Fig. 3.3 Ornstein–Uhlenbeck approximation to global type I error rate when using a Bonferroni approximation for one million evenly spaced correlated markers. Correlations, R, between z-scores for single marker tests range from 0.01 to 0.99

The implication of Fig. 3.3 is that for simple one-marker tests it is quite "hard to beat" the Bonferroni approximation so long as marker correlations die out within a few score kilo basepairs. For other types of tests, such as the sliding window haplotype approach described in Chap. 7, the correlations between tests can get very large however, and for these types of approaches it may be very important to consider alternative methods to estimating the global significance of any apparent associations found [33].

3.12   Reliability of Small *p*-Values

One practical consideration that merits addressing is the validity of the asymptotic approximations used to approximate the distribution of the score tests and likelihood ratio tests when very small *p*-values for significance are required (as when applying a Bonferroni criteria in genome-wide analyses). While little has been published on this subject concerns have often been raised that "rule of thumb" criteria developed for the reliability of *p*-values close to 0.05, e.g., that the expected counts for each cell of a table (say of genotype by case–control status) must be equal to 5 or so before a chi-square approximation to the distribution of a test of independence of genotype by status can be relied upon, may be completely inappropriate for p-values in the range of 5×10^{-8}. We contrast two very simple tests, one where such a "rule of thumb" is very bad and another where it appears to be quite good.

3.12.1   Test of a Single Binomial Proportion

Consider a one-sample test of binomial proportion, adapted to testing for allele frequencies for an autosomal SNP (under Hardy–Weinberg equilibrium). The standard test that the true value of the allele frequency $\hat{p}$ is equal to p is

$$T^2 = 2N \frac{(\hat{p} - p_0)^2}{\hat{p}(1 - \hat{p})}.$$

The "standard" rule would be that this can be treated as chi-squared (1df) random variable for values of $2Np \geq 5$. The following simulation in R examines this for a given value of N and p. Figure 3.4 shows the resulting Quantile–Quantile (QQ) plot of the p-value from the statistic assuming that this is a chi-square with 1 degree of freedom, for two choices of p (large and small) and N (small and large, respectively) with $2Np = 10$

```
>  nsim=100000;
>  p=.5;n=10  # 2*n*p = 10
>  yhat=rep(0,nsim)
>  vyhat=rep(0,nsim)
>  t2<-rep(0,nsim)
>  for (i in 1:nsim) { # simulation loop
>            y<-rbinom(1,n*2,p)/(2*n)  #  each element of y has mean p and
>                                      #  variance p*(1-p)/(2 *n)
>            yhat[i]=y
>            v=y*(1-y)
>            vyhat[i]<-v
>            t2[i]<-2*n*(y-p)^2/v
>  }
>  x=seq(1/nsim,1,1/nsim)
>  pval=sort(pf(t2,1,Inf,lower.tail=F))
>  plot(-log10(x),-log10(pval),main="N=10, p=.5",xlab="-log10(expected)", ylab="-log10(p)")
>  abline(0,1)
```

It is clear from the Fig. 3.4a, b that this approximation is very bad for p-values less than 10^{-3} or so, much less 10^{-8}. In fact (personal communication Kenneth Rice, University of Washington) a much better approximation is to treat T^2 not as a chi-square random variable, but rather as an F with 1 and Np degrees of freedom. This is shown in Fig. 3.4c for the case of small p and large N.

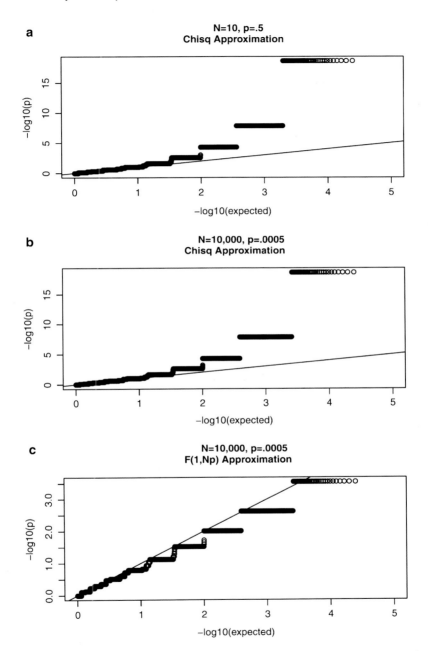

Fig. 3.4 QQ plot showing the distribution of the test statistic for one sample test of proportions

Fig. 3.5 Quantile–Quantile plot for the null distribution of the test of two binomial proportions, small p, large N, expected number of alleles in each group equal to $2Np = 10$

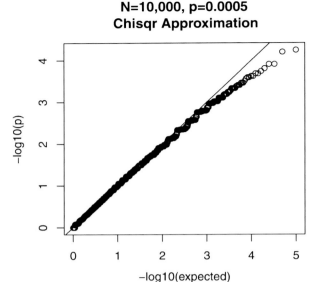

3.12.2   Test of a Difference in Binomial Proportions

Interestingly the usual chi-square approximation is more acceptable for testing for a difference in binomial proportions even when the total number of allele counts for each cell is quite small. The R code to run a similar example to the above is provided below, which produces Fig. 3.5.

```
>  nsim=100000;
>  p=.0005;n=10000 # 2n*p=10
>  t2diff<-rep(0,nsim)
>  for (i in 1:nsim) { # simulation loop
>  y1<-rbinom(1,n*2,p)/(2*n)
>  #  each element of y has mean p and variance p*(1-p)/(2*n)
>          y2<-rbinom(1,n*2,p)/(2*n)
>  #  each element of y has mean p and variance p*(1-p)/(2*n)
>          v=(y1*(1-y1)+y2*(1-y2))/(2*n)
>          t2diff[i]<-(y1-y2)^2/v
>  }
>  x=seq(0,1/nsim,1/nsim)
>  # make plot to examine the test for differences
>  pval=sort(pf(t2diff,1,Inf,lower.tail=F))
>  plot(-log10(x),-log10(pval))
>  abline(0,1)
```

For very low expected counts ($2Np = 10$ here) the chi-square approximation has slightly smaller variance compared to the simulated distribution; however, as $2Np$ increases this tail behavior improves rapidly (not shown). We should note that the test a difference in binomial frequencies used here is sensitive to failures of HWE and so it is generally better to use an Armitage test instead (Homework).

3.13   Chapter Summary

This chapter has described several of the main techniques used as well as issues relating to testing individual markers for association with risk. The theory of maximum likelihood estimation for the generalized linear model has been reviewed, general issues regarding confounding are introduced, the behavior of regression tests when outcomes are not independent was briefly touched on, and the problem of multiple comparisons was described. In addition some comments on hardware and software requirements have been discussed. Each of these topics will be taken up again in later chapters.

Homework

1. Show that if random variable X is correlated with variable W with correlation coefficient equal to R, and if Y is correlated with W with correlation coefficient R as well, and finally that X and Y are independent given W that X and Y are correlated with correlation coefficient R^2. See last paragraph of Sect. 3.6.1.
2. Consider a model for Poisson regression in which the log link function is used and a slope and intercept term fit. What is the score vector and information matrix for the two parameters?

    Suppose that instead of a log link function for Poisson data, the identity function is used. Then what is the score and information?
3. What is the score and Fisher's information for the variance parameter σ^2 in a OLS regression model with

    (a) Only an intercept, μ, in the model
    (b) An intercept and slope model, $\mu + \beta X$
    (c) What is the covariance between the score for σ^2 and those for μ and β?

4. Prove expression (3.8)

    (a) when the parameter θ is a scalar
    (b) for multivariate θ.

5. The layout of the conditional distribution of offspring genotypes given parental genotypes in Table 3.2 can be used to motivate several different multi-degree of freedom tests. Suppose that we tabulate affected-offspring data according to parental genotypes for a total of 645 trios as below:

	Offspring genotypes	Maternal genotypes								
		aa			aA			AA		
		aa	aA	AA	aa	aA	AA	aa	aA	AA
Parental	aa	394	0	0	68	44	0	0	4	0
genotypes	aA	46	51	0	5	16	3	0	0	1
	AA	0	10	0	0	1	2	0	0	0

(a) Compute the expected number of offspring counts conditional on the parental counts for each cell of the above layout.

(b) Compute the statistic T^2 in (3.23) for these data.

(c) Compute a statistic for an overall failure of Mendelian segregation in these data and relate that to the appropriate χ^2 distribution. How many degrees of freedom should be used? If we explicitly assume that there is no "parental origin effect" can this table be further collapsed?

6. Consider the first entry for the table above; there are 394 offspring homozygous for aa for whom both parents were *aa*. Thus each of the fathers has one *a* allele transmitted and one *a* allele not transmitted similarly for the mother. If we create a table of transmitted and untransmitted alleles then we have 394.

		Transmitted		
		A	a	Total
Not transmitted	A	0(a)	68(b)	
	a	0(c)	394 + 394 + 68(d)	
	Total			

fathers with genotype *aa* who transmitted one *a* and did not transmit one *a* allele which adds 394 to cell (d) of the table and similarly for the mothers. For the next nonzero cell in the same row there were 68 offspring with genotype *aa* whose father's genotype was *aa* and mother's genotype was *Aa*. This means the fathers each transmitted one *a* allele and failed to transmit the other *a* allele, adding 68 to the (d) cell of the table, whereas the mothers each transmitted one *a* allele and failed to transmit one *A* allele adding 68 to the (b) cell of the Table. Finish the calculation of this transmission table.

		Transmitted		
		A	a	Total
Not Transmitted	A	(a)	(b)	
	a	(c)	(d)	
	Total			

(a) What is the resulting Table?

(b) Perform McNamar's test (search web if necessary) of whether the A allele is more or less often transmitted than untransmitted. Compare the chi-square with that seen in problem 4. What conclusion would you make if one allele is transmitted to the affected offspring significantly more often than the other allele?

7. Simulation experiment: simulate data from model logit $E(Y_i) = \mu + \alpha_1 n_{i,A} + \alpha_2 X_i$ where X_i is either a weak or strong predictor of Y_i. Compare the power and type one error of the score test, or likelihood ratio test, of $\alpha_1 = 0$ to a test based on the partial correlations between Y and n_A adjusting for X. Do this for the following situations: (1) Y is a rare disease (frequency ~ 1 %) and X is a weak predictor, (2) Y is rare and X is a strong predictor, (3) Y is common and X is a weak predictor, and (4) Y is common and X is a strong predictor.

8. Modify the code *case-only.r* to change the prevalence of disease in the population (by modifying the intercept parameter in the model used to generate the data). How prevalent does the disease have to be (in the simulation given) before the power of the case–control test of interaction becomes equal to or greater than the power of the case-only test?

9. One problem with the test of binomial proportions given in Sect. 3.12.2 is that it is dependent upon HWE holding in each population. The Armitage trend test (which can be computed as $N\mathrm{Cor}(c,n)^2$) is more robust to deviations from HWE. Redo the simulations and QQ plot shown in Fig. 5.3 by modifying the R code in Sect. 3.12.2 to use this test.

10. Show that the score test for ordinary least squares linear regression (assuming normal errors and a linear link function) that all slope parameters $(\alpha_1, \alpha_2, \ldots, \alpha_p)$ are equal to a known value $\boldsymbol{\alpha}_0$ is equal to the Wald test of the same hypothesis. It is OK to assume that the variance parameter σ^2 is known.

    Hint, start with the score statistic expressed in matrix form as $U = (1/\sigma^2) \mathbf{X}' (\mathbf{Y} - \mathbf{X}\boldsymbol{\alpha}_0)$ and the information matrix expressed as $\imath = (1/\sigma^2)\mathbf{X}' \mathbf{X}$ and multiply out terms in $U' \imath^{-1} U$ to show that these become equal to the Wald test expressed as $(1/\sigma^2)(\hat{\boldsymbol{\alpha}} - \boldsymbol{\alpha}_0)'\mathbf{X}'\mathbf{X}(\hat{\boldsymbol{\alpha}} - \boldsymbol{\alpha}_0)$

12. The best linear unbiased estimate BLUE is the estimate, linear in outcomes $\mathbf{Y}$, that has the smallest variance among all linear unbiased estimates.

    (a) Find a proof (web search OK but pick one that you understand) that when $E(\mathbf{Y}) = \mathbf{X}\beta$ and the covariance matrix is $\boldsymbol{\Sigma}$ (assume known), $\hat{\beta} = \left(\mathbf{X}'\boldsymbol{\Sigma}^{-1}\mathbf{X}\right)^{-1}\mathbf{X}'\boldsymbol{\Sigma}^{-1}\mathbf{Y}$ is the BLUE estimate of β. Note that this does not require normality of the outcome vector $\mathbf{Y}$.

    (b) Is $\hat{\beta}$ still the BLUE estimate if $\boldsymbol{\Sigma}$ is not known but must be estimated?

Data and Software Exercises

1. Use PLINK to estimate associations in the JAPC data. In order to make sure the programs are running correctly (and to save wasted time and electricity if they are not) first randomly select 1 % of the SNPs (using the "–thin" command) and use these SNPs to test the programs before running the entire dataset.

Perform two tests, those using "–assoc" and "–logistic," and compare the results. Does adjustment for age or principal components (in the logistic regression) affect the distribution of resulting p-values? For computation of principal components, see *Data and Software Exercises* for Chap. 2.

2. For a small number of SNPs use the –recodeA command to create a file that can be read into R or SAS and merged with the covariates used. Check that you can reproduce the tests performed by PLINK. What test is being performed with the "–assoc" command?

3. A score test of a single variable in SAS PROC LOGISTIC can be performed using the following code. Here we assume that SNP is the variable of interest and that we are adjusting for AGE and principal components PC1–PC10

```
PROC LOGISTIC data=x;
        class AGE;
        model status=AGE PC1-PC10 SNP/ selection=forward include=11 details slentry=0;
run;
```

Compare the score test to the Wald test and likelihood ratio test for the SNPs in problem

4. Write code to do the score test for logistic regression in R. Hint: you have to roll your own; the standard *glm* procedure in R will not compute it without additional help.

   (a) Here a brute force example downloaded from https://stat.ethz.ch/pipermail/r-help/2009-March/190406.html which can get you started. (Included in *Score_Test_in_R.r*):

```
> # If the response y is given as a binary 0,1 variable,
> #and y, p, x, and z are vectors of length M, and the model is logit(p) =
> #b0 + b1*z + b2*x then for the score test for the null hypothesis b2=0 use
> des<-matrix(c(rep(1,M),z,x),M,3) # the design matrix with columns (1|z|x)
> m0<-glm(y~z,family=binomial()) # fit the model with z but without x
> f<-fitted(m0)        # save the fitted values -- estimate of the mean for each
>                 #observation
> efscor<-rep(0,3) # computes the score stat
> for (i in 1:3)
> {
> efscor[i]<-sum((y-f)* des[,i])
> }
> fim<-matrix(0,3,3)
> for (i in 1:3) # computes the Fisher's information
> {
> for (j in 1:3)
> {
> fim[i,j]<-sum(des[,i]*des[,j] *f*(1-f))
> }
> }
> ifim<-solve(fim) # invert the information
> scoretest<- t(efscor)%*%ifim%*%efscor # calculates the scoretest
> scoretest
```

   (b) Note here that only the 3rd element of *efscor* is numerically nonzero (explain why) so that this implies that the test is equal to

```
scortest<-efscor[3]^2%*%ifim[3,3]
```

(c) Generalize this code to allow for expansion of the model (to allow for more than one nuisance variable *z* and more than one variable of interest to be used in the score test). Allow for both single and multivariate score tests.

5. This score test can also be done using one additional step of Fisher's scoring after having fit the null model (here *m0*).

   In the above example we can use the following *R* code to perform the same test by adding the following code:

```
> m1<-glm(y~z+x,family=binomial(),start=c(m0$coefficients,0),maxit=1)
> summary(m1)
```

The *start* parameter uses the initial model results (without *x* in it) as the starting values for a model that includes the variable *x* (with a starting value of zero). Then the *maxit* = *1* parameter is used to make the program stop after just one iteration of the Fisher's scoring estimation procedure mentioned above. Notice then that the usual Wald test for the effect of variable *x* (the square of the reported *z value* for this variable) gives the same numerical result as the score test in 4 above.

(a) Prove based on the discussion of Fisher's scoring algorithm above that computing the usual Wald test (estimate/std error)^2 after allowing only Fisher's scoring 1 iteration away from the null model is equal to the score test.

(b) Can you modify these code segments to perform a score test of a 2-degree freedom alternative hypothesis, for example, the joint influence of z and x in the above example.

(c) Is it possible to implement a multivariate score test in SAS?

(d) Does PLINK implement the univariate score test?

6. Figure 3.6 is a so-called Manhattan plot of the results from the JAPC data as published by Cheng et al. [34]. Each point shows a *p*-value from a single test of association. Standard plots are on the $-\log 10$ scale so that a *p*-value of 1×10^{-6} is plotted as a 6, 1×10^{-8} is plotted as an 8, etc. The ordinate of the plot is chromosome number and location.

   Another very commonly produced plot is the quantile–quantile (QQ) plot plots, which often show the $-\log 10$ value of each sorted *p*-value plotted against its expectation given its rank. The basic idea (once the data have been read in) is as follows:

```
> M<-length(pvalues)
> x<- -log10(seq(1/M,1,1/M))
> plot(x,-log10(sort(pvalues)))
> abline(0,1)
```

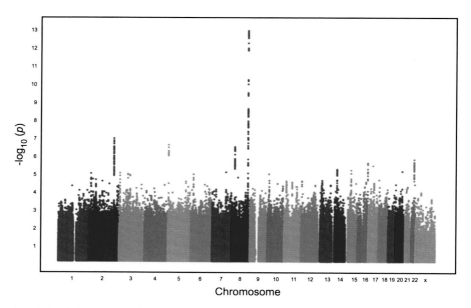

Fig. 3.6 Manhattan plot of single SNP associations in the LAPC data; from Cheng et al. [34], p. 849

Deviations from the $Y = X$ line, here *abline* (0, 1), can be indicative of many things including (1) significant "top hits" or (2) over dispersion perhaps due to population stratification.

(a) Describe the expected shape of the plot in both instances.
(b) With the results from the full PLINK analysis of the JAPC data create a QQ plot for the results in either R or SAS.
(c) A QQ plot can also be shown for the chi-square statistic rather than for the p-value. How would the code above be altered to do so?

Appendix

Proof of Equation (3.26). We have the OLS estimate of σ^2 equal to $\frac{1}{N-r} Y' \left(I - X(X'X)^{-1}X' \right) Y$. In order to simply the notation re-write this as

$$\frac{1}{N - r} Y'(I - \mathbf{P})Y,$$

where $\mathbf{P} = X(X'X)^{-1}X'$. Note that $\mathbf{PP} = \mathbf{P}$ and $(I - \mathbf{P})(I - \mathbf{P}) = (I - \mathbf{P})$ i.e. both P and $I - P$ are idempotent with trace equal to r and $N - r$ respectively. Now we take the expected value of the estimate. We have

$$E(\hat{\sigma}^2) = E\left\{\frac{1}{N-r}Y'(\mathbf{I}-\mathbf{P})Y\right\} = \frac{1}{N-r}\text{tr}\left\{(\mathbf{I}-\mathbf{P})E(YY')\right\}$$

$$= \frac{1}{N-r}\text{tr}\left\{(\mathbf{I}-\mathbf{P})\left[\text{Var}(Y)+E(Y)E(Y')\right]\right\}.$$

Note that

$$(\mathbf{I}-\mathbf{P})E(Y)E(Y') = \mathbf{X}\beta\beta'\mathbf{X}' - \mathbf{X}\beta\beta'\mathbf{X}'\mathbf{X}(\mathbf{X}'\mathbf{X})^{-1}\mathbf{X} = 0.$$

Thus the above expression simplifies to

$$\frac{1}{N-r}\text{tr}\left\{(\mathbf{I}-\mathbf{P})[\text{Var}(Y)]\right\}.$$

Since it assumed that $\text{Var}(Y) = \sigma^2\mathbf{I} + \gamma^2\mathbf{K}$, the above expression is equal to

$$\frac{1}{N-r}\text{tr}\left\{(\mathbf{I}-\mathbf{P})\left[\sigma^2\mathbf{I}+\gamma^2\mathbf{K}\right]\right\} = \frac{\sigma^2}{N-r}\text{tr}\left\{(\mathbf{I}-\mathbf{P})\right\} + \frac{\gamma^2}{N-r}\text{tr}\left\{(\mathbf{I}-\mathbf{P})\mathbf{K}\right\}$$

$$= \sigma^2 + \frac{\gamma^2}{N-r}\text{tr}\left\{(\mathbf{K}-\mathbf{P}\mathbf{K})\right\} = \sigma^2 + \frac{\gamma^2}{N-r}\text{tr}\left\{\left(\mathbf{K}-\mathbf{X}(\mathbf{X}'\mathbf{X})^{-1}\mathbf{X}\mathbf{K}\right)\right\}$$

$$= \sigma^2 + \frac{\gamma^2}{N-r}\left[\text{tr}\{\mathbf{K}\} - \text{tr}\left\{(\mathbf{X}'\mathbf{X})^{-1}\mathbf{X}'\mathbf{K}\mathbf{X}\right\}\right]$$

References

1. Armitage, P. (1955). Tests for linear trends in rates and proportions. *Biometrics, 11*, 375–386.
2. McCullagh, P., & Nelder, J. (1989). *Generalized linear models* (2nd ed.). Boca Raton, FL: CRC Press.
3. Moore, D. F. (1986). Asymptotic properties of moment estimates for overdispersed counts and proportions. *Biometrika, 73*(3), 583–588.
4. Liang, K. Y., & Zeger, S. L. (1986). Longitudinal data analysis using generalized linear models. *Biometrika, 73*(1), 13–22.
5. Hauck, W., & Donner, A. (1977). Wald's test as applied to hypotheses in Logit analysis. *Journal of the American Statistical Association, 72*, 851–853.
6. Schott, J. R. (1997). *Matrix analysis for statistics*. New York, NY: Wiley.
7. Kraft, P., Yen, Y. C., Stram, D. O., Morrison, J., & Gauderman, W. J. (2007). Exploiting gene-environment interaction to detect genetic associations. *Human Heredity, 63*, 111–119.
8. Maskarinec, G., Grandinetti, A., Matsuura, G., Sharma, S., Mau, M., Henderson, B. E., et al. (2009). Diabetes prevalence and body mass index differ by ethnicity: The Multiethnic Cohort. *Ethnicity and Disease, 19*, 49–55.

9. Frayling, T. M., Timpson, N. J., Weedon, M. N., Zeggini, E., Freathy, R. M., Lindgren, C. M., et al. (2007). A common variant in the FTO gene is associated with body mass index and predisposes to childhood and adult obesity. *Science, 316*, 889–894.

10. Hertel, J. K., Johansson, S., Raeder, H., Midthjell, K., Lyssenko, V., Groop, L., et al. (2008). Genetic analysis of recently identified type 2 diabetes loci in 1,638 unselected patients with type 2 diabetes and 1,858 control participants from a Norwegian population-based cohort (the HUNT study). *Diabetologia, 51*, 971–977.

11. Freathy, R. M., Timpson, N. J., Lawlor, D. A., Pouta, A., Ben-Shlomo, Y., Ruokonen, A., et al. (2008). Common variation in the FTO gene alters diabetes-related metabolic traits to the extent expected given its effect on BMI. *Diabetes, 57*, 1419–1426.

12. Smith, G. D., & Ebrahim, S. (2004). Mendelian randomization: Prospects, potentials, and limitations. *International Journal of Epidemiology, 33*, 30–42.

13. Reeves, J. R., Dulude, H., Panchal, C., Daigneault, L., & Ramnani, D. M. (2006). Prognostic value of prostate secretory protein of 94 amino acids and its binding protein after radical prostatectomy. *Clinical Cancer Research, 12*, 6018–6022.

14. Waters, K. M., Stram, D. O., Le Marchand, L., Klein, R. J., Valtonen-Andre, C., Peltola, M., et al. (2010). A common prostate cancer risk variant 5′ of MSMB (microseminoprotein-beta) is a strong predictor of circulating MSP (microseminoprotein) in multiple populations. *Cancer Epidemiology, Biomarkers and Prevention, 19*(10), 2639–2646.

15. Eeles, R. A., Kote-Jarai, Z., Giles, G. G., Olama, A. A., Guy, M., Jugurnauth, S. K., et al. (2008). Multiple newly identified loci associated with prostate cancer susceptibility. *Nature Genetics, 40*, 316–321.

16. Hung, R. J., McKay, J. D., Gaborieau, V., Boffetta, P., Hashibe, M., Zaridze, D., et al. (2008). A susceptibility locus for lung cancer maps to nicotinic acetylcholine receptor subunit genes on 15q25. *Nature, 452*, 633–637.

17. McKay, J. D., Hung, R. J., Gaborieau, V., Boffetta, P., Chabrier, A., Byrnes, G., et al. (2008). Lung cancer susceptibility locus at 5p15.33. *Nature Genetics, 40*, 1404–1406.

18. Greenland, S. (1980). The effect of misclassification in the presence of covariates. *American Journal of Epidemiology, 112*, 564–569.

19. Spielman, R. S., McGinnis, R. E., & Ewens, W. J. (1993). Transmission test for linkage disequilibrium: The insulin gene region and insulin-dependent diabetes mellitus (IDDM). *The American Journal of Human Genetics, 52*, 506–516.

20. Self, S. G., Longton, G., Kopecky, K. J., & Liang, K. Y. (1991). On estimating HLA/disease association with application to a study of aplastic anemia. *Biometrics, 47*, 53–61.

21. Weinberg, C. R. (1999). Methods for detection of parent-of-origin effects in genetic studies of case-parents triads. *The American Journal of Human Genetics, 65*, 229–235.

22. Piegorsch, W. W., Weinberg, C. R., & Taylor, J. A. (1994). Non-hierarchical logistic models and case-only designs for assessing susceptibility in population-based case–control studies. *Statistics in Medicine, 13*, 153–162.

23. Cornelis, M. C., Tchetgen, E. J., Liang, L., Qi, L., Chatterjee, N., Hu, F. B., et al. (2012). Gene-environment interactions in genome-wide association studies: A comparative study of tests applied to empirical studies of type 2 diabetes. *American Journal of Epidemiology, 175*, 191–202.

24. Mukherjee, B., Ahn, J., Gruber, S. B., & Chatterjee, N. (2012). Testing gene-environment interaction in large-scale case–control association studies: Possible choices and comparisons. *American Journal of Epidemiology, 175*, 177–190.

25. Mukherjee, B., & Chatterjee, N. (2008). Exploiting gene-environment independence for analysis of case–control studies: An empirical Bayes-type shrinkage estimator to trade-off between bias and efficiency. *Biometrics, 64*, 685–694.

26. Murcray, C. E., Lewinger, J. P., & Gauderman, W. J. (2009). Gene-environment interaction in genome-wide association studies. *American Journal of Epidemiology, 169*, 219–226.

27. Murcray, C. E., Lewinger, J. P., Conti, D. V., Thomas, D. C., & Gauderman, W. J. (2011). Sample size requirements to detect gene-environment interactions in genome-wide association studies. *Genetic Epidemiology, 35*, 201–210.
28. Wang, H., Haiman, C. A., Kolonel, L. N., Henderson, B. E., Wilkens, L. R., Le Marchand, L., et al. (2010). Self-reported ethnicity, genetic structure and the impact of population stratification in a multiethnic study. *Human Genetics, 128*, 165–177.
29. Purcell, S., Neale, B., Todd-Brown, K., Thomas, L., Ferreira, M. A., Bender, D., et al. (2007). PLINK: A tool set for whole-genome association and population-based linkage analyses. *The American Journal of Human Genetics, 81*, 559–575.
30. Dudbridge, F., & Gusnanto, A. (2008). Estimation of significance thresholds for genomewide association scans. *Genetic Epidemiology, 32*, 227–234.
31. Pe'er, I., Yelensky, R., Altshuler, D., & Daly, M. J. (2008). Estimation of the multiple testing burden for genomewide association studies of nearly all common variants. *Genetic Epidemiology, 32*, 381–385.
32. Siegmund, D., & Yakir, Y. (2007). *The statistics of gene mapping*. New York, NY: Springer.
33. Song, C., Chen, G. K., Millikan, R. C., Ambrosone, C. B., John, E. M., Bernstein, L., et al. (2013). A genome-wide scan for breast cancer risk haplotypes among African American women. *PLoS One, 8*, e57298.
34. Cheng, I., Chen, G. K., Nakagawa, H., He, J., Wan, P., Lurie, C., et al. (2012). Evaluating genetic risk for prostate cancer among Japanese and Latinos. *Cancer Epidemiology, Biomarkers and Prevention, 21*(11), 2048–2058.

Chapter 4
Correcting for Hidden Population Structure in Single Marker Association Testing and Estimation

Abstract Chapter 2 discussed both relatedness of study participants and hidden population structure in terms of the correlations induced between the number of copies, n_{iA} and n_{jA}, of a diallelic genetic variant carried by two individuals i and j. In Chap. 3 we discussed the requirement for association studies of unrelated subjects that the outcomes of interest, Y_i, be independent between study subjects. In this chapter we will expand on this initial discussion (1) to examine the impact of non-independence on the distribution of statistical tests for the influence of alleles (here a and A) on phenotype or disease risk, and (2) how non-independence between individuals' outcomes can arise as a direct result of correlation among the genotypes of study subjects due to hidden strata or relatedness or due to other factors (e.g., cultural/behavioral) that act as confounders of genetic associations. The chapter introduces several basic approaches for dealing with population structure in single marker association analyses and shows how all these methods deal, at least in part, with the fundamental problem of the analysis of correlated phenotypes. At the heart of these methods is the empirical estimation of a relationship matrix (more precisely a covariance structure matrix) that describes the relative relatedness of individuals. The statistical methods for dealing with covariances in estimation of single marker effects fall into three categories: *fixed effects* models utilizing adjustment for eigenvectors ("principal components") of this matrix; *random effects* methods dealing explicitly with the relationship matrix as a covariance matrix of random effects in extended *generalized linear modeling*; and *retrospective* methods, which invert the usual generalized linear modeling procedures so that the conditional distribution of the genetic markers given the phenotypes (rather than the reverse) is used for inference in genetic association studies. Our discussion of all these approaches is unified around the theme of dealing with false-positive associations that are due to unrecognized inflation of the variance of estimators relied upon in traditional regression methods when correlated data are analyzed. Finally the relative performance of the various methods is described in various settings.

D.O. Stram, *Design, Analysis, and Interpretation of Genome-Wide Association Scans*, Statistics for Biology and Health, DOI 10.1007/978-1-4614-9443-0_4, © Springer Science+Business Media New York 2014

4.1   Effects of Hidden Population Structure on the Behavior of Statistical Tests for Association

In this chapter the term population structure refers to all of the following three phenomena either separately or in combination: non-mixing subpopulation strata; incomplete admixture between formerly separated groups; and relatedness (IBD allele sharing) between subjects. The main concern of course is when population structure is "hidden," i.e., not directly known to the investigators in the study. Here much of our entire treatment of this subject is motivated by first deriving some results regarding the behavior of traditional estimates stemming from ordinary least squares analysis (OLS), when there exist nonzero correlations between outcomes. Specifically we derive below expressions for an expected "variance inflation" in regression parameter estimates due to ignoring correlations between outcomes when fitting models relating the mean of outcome Y_i to covariates X_i. By "variance inflation" we mean the difference between the true sampling variances of the regression parameter estimates compared to the variance estimates that derive naturally in OLS regression (see Chap. 3). While derived for OLS regression, we note that the similarity of the score statistics for testing for nonzero effects for other generalized linear models means that these same formulae can be relevant in other models such as logistic regression.

4.1.1   Effects on Inference Induced by Correlated Phenotypes

Consider (for the time being) the estimation of a linear model for a continuous phenotype Y_i, i.e., we seek to estimate the parameter vector β in the model:

$$E(Y_i|X_i) = X'_i\beta, \tag{4.1}$$

where Y_i is the outcome of interest for individual i and X_i is a r-vector of explanatory variables. Suppose that this mean model is correct, but that the covariance between Y_i and Y_j ($j \neq i$) of individual outcomes is nonzero. Specifically we assume that the $N \times N$ covariance matrix, Σ, for the vector of all observations $Y = (Y_1, Y_2, \ldots, Y_N)$ has the same special form discussed in Sect. 3.8.1, i.e.,

$$\text{Var}(Y) = \sigma^2 I + \gamma^2 \mathbf{K} \tag{4.2}$$

(we will see below that this covariance matrix structure is relevant in our discussion of the effects of both hidden relatedness and unknown population stratification). We now display some basic consequences of ignoring the (nonzero) covariances between individual outcomes when testing for the effect of the covariates, X_i, on the mean of the phenotype Y_i. Expanding the notation (as in Chap. 3, Sect. 3.4.8) a bit so that the $N \times r$ matrix, $\mathbf{X}$, has the covariate vector X_i as its ith row we write the ordinary least squares (OLS) estimate of β as

$$\hat{\beta} = \left(\mathbf{X}'\mathbf{X}\right)^{-1}\mathbf{X}'Y. \tag{4.3}$$

Since this expression is linear in Y and since $E(Y) = \mathbf{X}\beta$ it follows that the expected value of $\hat{\beta}$ is equal to the true value, β, a result that holds despite nonzero covariances between outcomes. While the covariances between outcomes do not affect the mean of the OLS estimator they do affect its sampling variance. Because of the linearity of $\hat{\beta}$ as a function of $\mathbf{Y}$ the sampling variance of $\hat{\beta}$ can readily be seen to be equal to

$$\begin{aligned} \text{Var}(\hat{\beta}) &= \left(\mathbf{X}'\mathbf{X}\right)^{-1}\mathbf{X}'\Sigma\mathbf{X}\left(\mathbf{X}'\mathbf{X}\right)^{-1} \\ &= \sigma^2\left(\mathbf{X}'\mathbf{X}\right)^{-1} + \gamma^2\left(\mathbf{X}'\mathbf{X}\right)^{-1}\mathbf{X}'\mathbf{K}\mathbf{X}\left(\mathbf{X}'\mathbf{X}\right)^{-1}. \end{aligned} \tag{4.4}$$

Suppose now that we ignore the covariance structure Σ and construct the usual OLS estimator of the variance–covariance matrix of. $\hat{\beta}$ This estimator is of form

$$\text{Var}_{\text{OLS}}(\hat{\beta}) = \hat{\sigma}^2(\mathbf{X}'\mathbf{X})^{-1} = \frac{Y'Y - Y'\mathbf{X}(\mathbf{X}'\mathbf{X})^{-1}\mathbf{X}'Y}{N - r}(\mathbf{X}'\mathbf{X})^{-1}. \tag{4.5}$$

Because expression (4.5) ignores the correlations between the components of $\mathbf{Y}$ it follows that $\text{Var}_{\text{OLS}}(\hat{\beta})$ is in general a biased estimate of the actual sampling variance given in expression (4.4). In fact using the result, given in Sect. 3.8.1, that $\hat{\sigma}^2$ for OLS regression has an expected value under model (4.2) of $(\sigma^2 + \gamma^2)$ $([\text{tr}\{\mathbf{K}\} - \text{tr}\{(\mathbf{X}'\mathbf{X})^{-1}\mathbf{X}'\mathbf{K}\mathbf{X}\}]/(N - r))$. we can write the expected value of $\text{Var}_{\text{OLS}}(\hat{\beta})$ as

$$\sigma^2(\mathbf{X}'\mathbf{X})^{-1} + \frac{\gamma^2}{N - r}(\mathbf{X}'\mathbf{X})^{-1}\left[\text{tr } K - \text{tr}\left\{(\mathbf{X}'\mathbf{X})^{-1}\mathbf{X}\mathbf{K}\mathbf{X}'\right\}\right]. \tag{4.6}$$

Therefore the expected error in variance estimation for $\hat{\beta}$ is equal to expression (4.4) minus (4.6) or

$$\gamma^2(\mathbf{X}'\mathbf{X})^{-1}\left[\mathbf{X}'\mathbf{K}\mathbf{X}(\mathbf{X}'\mathbf{X})^{-1} + \frac{\text{tr}\left\{(\mathbf{X}'\mathbf{X})^{-1}\mathbf{X}'\mathbf{K}\mathbf{X}\right\}}{N - r} - \frac{\text{tr } K}{N - r}\right]. \tag{4.7}$$

Consider the special case when $r = 2$ with the first column of $\mathbf{X}$ equal to a vector of 1s and where the second column, X, of $\mathbf{X}$ is the covariate of interest and X is orthogonal to the vector of 1s (i.e., its mean is zero). This corresponds to fitting a model with an intercept and a single slope parameter since "regressing out" the intercept corresponds to subtracting the mean of X from each element of X. In this case the $(2, 2)$ element of (4.7) (i.e., the inflation in the variance of the slope estimate) can with some straightforward but tedious algebra be shown to reduce to

$$\frac{\gamma^2}{X'X} \left[\frac{X'\mathbf{K}X}{X'X} \left(1 + \frac{1}{(N-2)} \right) - \frac{\text{tr}(\mathbf{K})}{N-2} + \frac{\mathbf{1}'\mathbf{K}\mathbf{1}}{N(N-2)} \right]. \tag{4.8}$$

Notice that for a fixed value of the variance of X [i.e., fixed $(X'X)$] this expression will be largest when $(X'\mathbf{K}X)/(X'X)$ is large and at its smallest when $X'\mathbf{K}X$ is small. If N is reasonably large we can simplify (4.8) a bit to be approximately

$$\frac{\gamma^2}{X'X} \left[\frac{X'\mathbf{K}X}{X'X} - \left(\frac{\text{tr}(\mathbf{K})}{N} - \text{Avg}(\mathbf{K}) \right) \right], \tag{4.9}$$

where $\text{Avg}(\mathbf{K})$ is the average value of $\mathbf{K}$, i.e., $\mathbf{1}'\mathbf{K}\mathbf{1}/N^2$.

The case when $\mathbf{K}$ is a correlation matrix with all diagonal elements equal to 1 (so that $\text{tr}(\mathbf{K}) = N$) is of special interest (it corresponds to relatedness but no hidden stratification or inbreeding). In this case (4.9) equals

$$\frac{\gamma^2}{X'X} \left[\frac{X'\mathbf{K}X}{X'X} - (1 - \text{Avg}(\mathbf{K})) \right]. \tag{4.10}$$

We can easily see that in some cases (i.e., when $(X'\mathbf{K}X)/(X'X) > 1 - \text{Avg}(\mathbf{K})$) the expected error in the variance estimation is positive, that is, $\text{Var}_{\text{OLS}}(\hat{\beta})$ underestimates the actual variability of $\hat{\beta}$ (the case of *inflation*, i.e., the true variance is larger than predicted). In other cases when $(X'\mathbf{K}X)/(X'X) < 1 - \text{Avg}(\mathbf{K})$ the true variance of $\hat{\beta}$ is overestimated by $\text{Var}_{\text{OLS}}(\hat{\beta})$. Having true variances that are inflated beyond what they are estimated to be when using OLS regression will clearly lead to anti-conservative tests and confidence intervals, whereas if the sampling variances are deflated (when $(X'\mathbf{K}X)/(X'X) < 1 - \text{Avg}(\mathbf{K})$) then this leads to exactly the opposite problem, i.e., confidence limits and tests will be over-conservative. Notice also that in the different types of population stratification that we have discussed each of the elements of $\mathbf{K}$ is positive so that the average value is positive as well. Moreover in most cases of interest (except in cases of extreme hidden stratification) the average value of $\mathbf{K}$ will be small and can be ignored in much of the remainder.

The discussion of principal components in this chapter noted that maximizing the quadratic form $X'\mathbf{K}X$ with respect to the vector X while keeping $X'X$ fixed gives as a solution the first eigenvector, V_1, of $\mathbf{K}$. A little algebra shows that this implies that any vector which is a scalar multiple of V_1 maximizes the ratio $(X'\mathbf{K}X)/(X'X)$ and that the maximum value of the ratio is equal to the first eigenvalue, λ_1 When $\mathbf{K}$ is a correlation matrix the first (i.e., largest) eigenvalue must be ≥ 1 since the sum of the eigenvalues of $\mathbf{K}$ equals the trace of $\mathbf{K}$ which here is equal to N. Thus if the explanatory variable X is close to the first eigenvector of $\mathbf{K}$ then the OLS variance estimate will tend to be an underestimate of the true sampling variance of $\hat{\beta}$; on the other hand if the explanatory variable is close to the last (smallest) eigenvector of $\mathbf{K}$ then $\mathrm{Var_{OLS}}(\hat{\beta})$ may well overestimate the true variability of $\hat{\beta}$ (i.e., if the last eigenvalue is less than $(1 - \mathrm{Avg}(K))$. By "close to" V_1 we mean that the dot product $X'V_1$ is large in magnitude while the dot products $X'V_2$, $X'V_3$, ..., $X'V_N$ are all small in magnitude. The dot products can be termed the *loadings* of the covariate vector X on the respective eigenvectors.

Finally consider the situation (highly relevant to the specific cases described below) when the vector X is itself a random variable with mean 0 (its mean having been subtracted) with a covariance matrix equal to $w\mathbf{K}$, with $w > 0$, and where all values of $\mathbf{K}$ are greater than or equal to zero (i.e., there are no "negative" relationships between individuals). Note from (4.10) that the expected difference in variances (true-estimated assuming independence) is positive when $X'\mathbf{K}X - X'X > - X'X\mathrm{Avg}(\mathbf{K})$. The expected value of the difference can be written as $\mathrm{tr}\{\mathbf{K}E(XX')\} - \mathrm{tr}\{E(XX')\}$ which can be simplified to

$$w(\mathrm{tr}(\mathbf{KK}) - \mathrm{tr}(\mathbf{K})). \tag{4.11}$$

Since $\mathrm{tr}(\mathbf{KK})$ is the sum of the eigenvalues of $\mathbf{KK}$ and since the eigenvalues of $\mathbf{KK}$ are the square of the eigenvalues of $\mathbf{K}$ (which are all positive and sum to N) it follows that $\mathrm{tr}(\mathbf{KK}) - \mathrm{tr}(\mathbf{K})$ is always greater than or equal to zero (with equality only when $\mathbf{K}$ is the identity matrix). Finally since the sum of all elements of $\mathbf{K}$, i.e., $\mathbf{1'K1}$, is (assuming positivity of the off diagonal elements) greater than or equal to the trace of $\mathbf{K} = \mathbf{1'1} = N$ it follows that the entire expression (4.11) must be greater than or equal to zero, and hence greater than $- X'X\mathrm{Avg}(\mathbf{K})$.

To reiterate what was just covered: we have shown that for a particular model for the variances and covariances of Y_i, i.e., $\sum = \sigma^2\mathbf{I} + \gamma^2\mathbf{K}$, on average the variance of $\hat{\beta}$ is underestimated by the OLS variance estimator $\mathrm{Var_{OLS}}(\hat{\beta})$ when using a single covariate which itself can be regarded a random variable with constant mean having a covariance matrix proportional to $\mathbf{K}$. Moreover the inflation underestimation is at its greatest in a given analysis when a specific realized value of the random covariate vector is proportional to the first leading eigenvector of $\mathbf{K}$.

In the following we will use this basic result to clarify a number of issues regarding the influence of between-subject correlation on hypothesis testing in OLS regression. Such results generally carry over to hypothesis testing for other models, i.e., when there are additional covariates, so that $p > 2$ in the linear predictor, and to other types of GLMs, e.g., logistic regression for case–control data. The implications of variance inflation are of course profound on inference; if we consistently underestimate the sampling variance of $\hat{\beta}$ due to unaccounted correlations between outcomes then the coverage properties of confidence intervals estimated for covariate effects will be adversely affected. Under the null hypothesis this implies loss of control of type I error rates and potentially many false-positive associations when the true effect of a covariate is equal to zero.

4.1.2   Influences of Latent Variables

When study outcomes, Y_i, are independent from subject to subject (conditional on covariates) hypothesis testing and confidence interval estimation in association testing and estimation will behave as expected. As indicated above, violations of the independence assumption can lead to loss of control of type I error rates for testing null hypotheses and biases in confidence interval coverage.

Consider the covariance matrix that is induced by the presence of a latent (unmeasured) factor U which affects the mean of Y_i. If the individual values of U_i are known for each subject we assume that the mean of Y_i can be written as

$$E(Y_i|X_i, U_i) = \mu + X_i\beta + \gamma U_i \qquad (4.12)$$

and that conditional on U_i and X_i the outcomes Y_i are independent with covariance matrix $\sigma^2 \mathbf{I}$. Now consider the issues that arise when U_i is an unobserved random effect. If the distribution of the unknown U_i depends upon the values of X_i then the results of fitting (4.12) may be seriously distorted; in particular if the mean of U_i depends on X_i then some of the information about Y_i that is captured by U_i will be misattributed to the effect of X_i. Also, however, from our above analysis for OLS regression we can see that even if the distribution of U_i does not depend on X_i at all there can be a failure of variance estimation which can lead to poorly performing confidence intervals and an excess of apparent (i.e., false positive) associations. Specifically if U_i is a random variable independent of X_i with variance–covariance matrix proportional to $\mathbf{K}$ then the model for the mean conditional on X only is $E(Y_i|X_i) = \mu + X_i\beta$ (with β taking the same value as in (4.12)), but the variance model is now equal to $\sigma^2 \mathbf{I} + \gamma^2 \mathbf{K}$ which is what was considered above. As before the variance of $\hat{\beta}$ will be underestimated by $\mathrm{Var}_{OLS}(\hat{\beta})$ when the covariate vectors load on the leading eigenvectors of $\mathbf{K}$. For the case of a single covariate $\mathbf{X} = (X_1, X_2, \ldots, X_N)'$ treated as a random vector the variance inflation will be positive on average when $\mathbf{X}$ has correlation structure similar to $\mathbf{K}$. A slightly modified version of this result still holds when other adjustment variables are included in the model. If an adjusted version of the variable of interest, $X_p = (X_{1p}, X_{2p}, \ldots, X_{Np})$, either (when thought of as a fixed effect) loads on the larger eigenvalues of $\mathbf{K}$ or (when regarded as random) has a correlation structure similar to $\mathbf{K}$ then inflation of the variance of $\hat{\beta}_p$ is expected relative to the OLS estimate of this variance. We describe what we mean by "adjusted version" of X_p further below.

4.1.3   Hidden Structure as a Latent Variable

In genetic association scans the effects of hidden population structure can be thought of as the latent variable, U, above, i.e., U_i is the effect on the mean phenotype that occurs due to the subpopulation membership of subject i. As described in Chap. 3 (and which is really a consequence of the same results that are given above), unrecognized strata (the presence of non- or incompletely mixing populations) induce pseudo-LD between markers that extends far beyond genomic regions actually relevant to disease and can mask true associations by the addition of noise. For any given outcome analyzed in a study (and many studies may examine more than one outcome) the role of hidden population structure may or may not be influential as a confounder, since this depends not only on the presence of hidden strata but also upon (1) whether the (mean) phenotype of interest varies in distribution among the strata and (2) whether (the mean of) the variable of interest (e.g., the allele count for a particular marker) also varies in distribution among the strata.

There are several ways in which population substructure can affect the distribution of phenotypes. For example, risk of certain diseases may differ by population strata because exposures differ among subpopulations. Such population differences in exposure may be unrelated to genetics except by accidents of history and culture affecting such factors as dietary preferences, occupational exposures, lifestyle choices made both voluntarily and as a response to external circumstances, etc. There are many examples of diseases having notable differences by race/ethnicity in their frequency, including diabetes, high blood pressure, heart disease, and certain cancers such as breast (strongly influenced by reproductive and hormonally related factors), where these ethnic differences in risk can be at least partly explained by different exposures to known risk factors [1]. In admixed populations the fraction of relatives (of a given study participant) who have derived from each recently mixing ancestral group may intuitively be a powerful factor driving culturally based exposures that influence disease risk in the study group. Since (1) the risks of a large number of common diseases are influenced by behavior and environmental factors and since (2) exposures and lifestyle choices related to disease are partly cultural and because (3) cultural similarities may correspond to genetic similarities, the potential exists for false genetic associations to arise due to the confounding of genetic variables with environmental determinants of disease.

4.1.4 Polygenes, Latent Structure, Hidden Relatedness, and Confounding

It is increasingly evident [2] that associations being detected by GWAS studies often have only limited effects on mean phenotype, even phenotypes which appear to be (from family studies) strongly genetically influenced. These include height [3], weight or obesity [4], lipid levels [5], blood pressure [6], and many others. In many of these phenotypes it would appear that a very large number of largely independent alleles each make very small contributions to the phenotype mean. For example, it has recently been shown that hundreds of variants [3] underlie the heritability of height in study populations. Phenotypes for which variability and heritability between individuals are influenced by the additive effect of many genes are termed *polygenic*.

When strongly polygenic effects are noted the *polygene* (which we can think of as a weighted sum of the many relevant alleles each weighted by its influence on phenotypic mean) itself acts as the confounder in studies of stratified or admixed populations and/or studies that include many relatives. If there is no hidden population structure in a study then the existence of even a powerful polygene itself has little influence upon the ability of a study to identify the influence of single variants related to risk. This is because true LD between the marker of interest and the other members of the polygene decays over a relatively short genetic distance and thus the variant or marker being tested for association with outcome is not at all (or only extremely weakly) associated with the remainder of contributors to the polygene. On the other hand when there is differentiation into hidden non-mixing substrata then the polygene can meet the requirements of a confounder; all markers will tend to have the same between person correlation structure inducing "pseudo-LD" between the polygene and the marker of interest being tested since the usual association tests (which assume no correlation) underestimate the variance of the estimated effects; standard tests for association between the marker of interest and the phenotype will be distorted because of the potential for the variance inflation and variance underestimation described above.

4.1.5   Hidden Non-mixing Strata

Here we explore the implications of the Balding–Nichols model (Sect. 2.4.1) for differentiation in population allele frequencies when there is a polygene present. Specifically if the polygene consists of a weighted sum of purely additive effects on the phenotype, so that for individual i the contribution of the polygene to phenotype mean or risk of disease is

$$g_i = \sum_k w_k n_{ik}. \tag{4.13}$$

The effect of the polygene g on the covariances of the individual outcomes Y_i is to induce a covariance matrix $\sum$ of form $\sigma^2 \mathbf{I} + \mathrm{Var}(\mathbf{g})$. From Chap. 2 (Homework problems), it is quite easy to show that the correlation between g_i and g_j for two different individuals will be the same as the correlation between the individual components n_{ik} and n_{jk} which is $2F_l/(1 + F_l)$ for pairs of individuals in the lth subpopulation and 0 for all other pairs (here, as in Chap. 2, F_l is the differentiation parameter between the lth subpopulation and the original ancestral population of the modern day groups). Therefore we may write the covariance matrix Σ as

$$\sigma^2 \mathbf{I} + \gamma^2 \mathbf{K}, \tag{4.14}$$

with $\gamma^2 = \sum_{j=1,\ldots,M} w_j^2 2p_j(1 - p_j)$. It is clear from above that the similarity between the covariance structure, $n_i(A)$, for the counts of a variant of interest and for Y_i can produce an excess of nominally significant false-positive associations between outcomes and any SNP that is differentiated by population. This in fact is again a special case of the analysis given at the beginning of this chapter: because g_i and $n_i(A)$ have the same correlation structure, both involving $\mathbf{K}$, then (when g_i is unmeasured) sampling variances for the effect of $n_i(A)$ on the mean of Y_i will tend on average to be underestimated. Moreover variance underestimation will be at the worst for those specific variants that align with the largest eigenvalues of $\mathbf{K}$. In this case (as seen below) this corresponds to those SNPs that are the most differentiated by population.

The following simulation in R should help to make these points clear.

```
# File polygene.r
set.seed(1003004) # so we get the same answer each time

L<-2 # number of strata
N<-1000 # number of subjects in each strata
M<-1000 # Number of SNPs composing the polygene
F<-0.02 # F for the differentiation between the L groups from an ancestral group
p<-runif(M+1) # p are the ancestral allele frequencies for the snps
              # composing the polygene and also for the SNP of interest
n<-rep(0,M+1) # the SNPs
w<-0.055      # this value for the constant weighting factor for each SNP makes
              # var(g) roughly equal to 1
g<-rep(0,N*L) # initialize the polygene, g
testSNP<-rep(0,N*L) # this stores the noncausal SNP that we will be testing
# generate SNP data from stratified population
for (l in 1:L){
        p_l<-rbeta(M+1,p*(1-F)/F,(1-p)*(1-F)/F) # modern day frequencies
                # for each gene in the polygene + the non causal test
        for (i in 1:N) {
                n=rbinom(M+1,2,p_l)
                g[((l-1)*N+i)]<-sum(n[1:M])*w
                testSNP[((l-1)*i+1)]<-n[M+1]
        }
}
# Generate the heritable outcome Y
mu<-0 # mean of Y doesn't matter what it is
Y<-mu+g+rnorm(N*L) #about half the variance of Y is
                   # due to the polygene g
R2<-cor(testSNP,Y)^2 # compute correlation between outcome and the SNP of interest
T2<-L*N*R2# perform Armitage test
pval<- 1-pchisq(T2,1)
```

In this simulation a total of $L = 2$ hidden strata are considered with differentiation parameters F_l both equal to 0.02. A polygene is generated as well as a test SNP and each SNP allele following the Balding–Nichols model described in Chap. 2. The weights for each component of the polygene are equal and are chosen so that on average approximately ½ the total variability of the individual phenotypes is due to the polygene. There is no LD between the SNP to be tested and any of the polygene members and it is not a causal SNP. If there was no hidden structure ($F = 0$ in the simulations) then there should be no association apparent between the test SNP and the outcome. However running this code once (with $F = 0.02$), i.e.,

```
> source("polygene.r")
> pval
> [1] 0.0005933753
```

gives a highly significant *p*-value for the association between the SNP count and the continuous phenotype which is very unlikely to be due to chance alone.

Note that the squared correlation between Y and the test SNP (calculated as)

```
> cor(testSNP,Y)^2
> [1] 0.0058883
```

means that this variant seems to explain about 1/2 of 1 % of the variability of the continuous variable Y despite having no causal association with Y. For many complex continuous phenotypes this seems to be about the magnitude of the correlation between outcome and many of the SNPs that have been found to be globally significant (c.f. [3] for height and [6] for blood pressure).

In fact here the correlations induced by the population stratification would be very difficult to differentiate between the correlations between the individual causal SNPs (elements of the polygene g) and the outcome Y assuming no population stratification. In this case (with the parameters chosen in the simulation) the true squared correlation of any single component, n, of the polygene, with the outcome Y will be equal to

$$\frac{\mathrm{Cov}(Y,n)^2}{\mathrm{Var}(Y)\mathrm{Var}(n)} = w^2 \frac{\mathrm{Var}(n)}{\mathrm{Var}(Y)}.$$

This value will be about equal to 0.00076 if n has 50 % frequency and is even smaller for smaller allele frequencies. These are fairly small signals to attempt to differentiate from the noise including the effects of population stratification without careful analysis.

Running the R code 50 times gives the highly overdispersed quantile– quantile plot (or QQ plot; see Chap. 3 Homework) shown in Fig. 4.1a. It is clear from the figure that hidden stratification and polygenic influences on phenotype can together produce false-positive associations that are far too large to be ignored when evaluating the results of genetic association studies. Similar results can easily be constructed for other types of phenotypes (e.g., disease in case–control studies), if we again assume that there are strong polygenic influences on disease.

4.1.5.1 Eigenvector Analysis

In the case of simple hidden strata the first few eigenvectors of the relationship matrix **K** can be shown to be equivalent to indicator variables for membership in the various strata. This is shown in Fig. 4.2 for the illustrative case of the presence of three distinct hidden strata each with sample size 100, 50, and 25 and the differentiation parameter, F_l, equal to 0.02 for all three populations. A plot of the eigenvalues (Fig. 4.2a) shows that only the first 3 eigenvalues are greater than 1 and all the others are just very slightly less than 1. The first eigenvector (with eigenvalue, λ_1, of 4.98) indicates whether a subject falls into population one versus the other

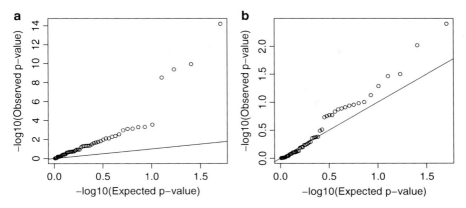

Fig. 4.1 Behavior of null test statistics in the presence of a strong and highly differentiated polygene affecting the mean of continuous phenotype Y. The figure shows the result of running the R code in file "polygene.r" 50 times. Shown is a quantile–quantile plot for the relationship between observed and expected p-values (on the log10 scale) for a test of zero correlation between Y and a noncausal SNP not in complete linkage equilibrium (in each population) with the components of the polygene g. (**a**) shows the QQ plot for $L = 2$ populations with $N = 1{,}000$ subjects and (**b**) with $L = 100$ populations each with $N = 20$ subjects

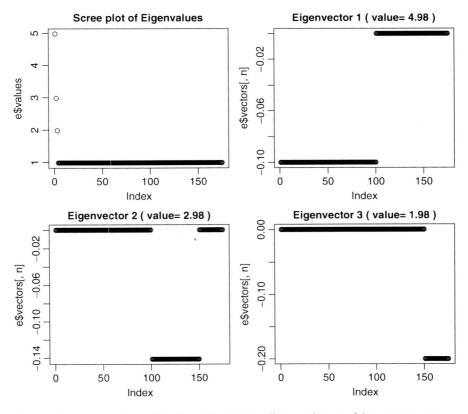

Fig. 4.2 Eigenvectors from a Kinship matrix corresponding to existence of three separate groups

two, eigenvector 2 does the same for population two ($\lambda_2 = 2.98$), and eigenvector 3 ($\lambda_3 = 1.98$) for population three. Thus the size of the hidden strata in the sample is reflected in the eigenvalue size. Later eigenvectors (with $\lambda < 1$) are not interpretable since the eigenvalues are equal to each other in which case eigenvectors are not unique.

From the above discussion above it follows that false-positive associations are particularly likely for a variant that has a frequency that is different in the largest population than in the combination of the two smaller populations, i.e., if it is correlated with the first eigenvector. False-positive associations are also more likely for variants that have different frequencies in the third population compared to the first two (i.e., most correlated with the third eigenvector) although (since the eigenvalue is smaller) the problem is less severe than in the first instance. On the other hand if the particular variant of interest is not informative about group membership then variance inflation is not present since all of the other eigenvalues are very close to 1.

There are aspects of the simulation which must be acknowledged as extreme. For example, the value of F used in the simulations is quite large compared to what would be expected in most studies and the assumption that the polygene consists of 1,000 components each with equal influence on phenotype mean is also something like a "worst-case" scenario—we expect that there will be some components of the polygene which will have considerably larger individual effects, even if many others have smaller effects, and these will be far more detectable than those with smaller individual influences. However the assumption of 50 % heritability of the phenotypic trait due to polygenic influences does not seem terribly high for many common phenotypes [2] and the sample size $N = 2,000$ used in the simulation is not as large as some of the very massive studies and meta-analyses that are now involved in finding genes for complex phenotypes such as height, blood pressure, lipid levels, and obesity [3–6].

4.1.5.2 Varying the Number of Strata

As the number of strata increases the problems associated with inference due to the presence of these strata tend to become less important all other things being equal. Altering the simulation experiment above so that there are 20 strata sampled each of size 100 (rather than 2 with 1,000 each) while keeping the other parameters the same as above produces a far less overdispersed plot shown as Fig. 4.1b. If the number of hidden strata is increased so that only a few subjects are in each strata then the variance inflation term is essentially zero even for very strong differentiation parameters. This can also be understood in terms of an eigenvector analysis of the matrix $\mathbf{K}$. As described above the leading eigenvectors can be thought of as indicator variables for each of the hidden strata. As the number of strata becomes larger and larger it becomes increasingly less likely that any single SNP will have a high allele frequency in just one strata and a low allele frequency in all others, or vice versa; however, this is exactly what is needed in order for a given SNP to be highly correlated with a leading eigenvector. Since the variance inflation term disappears as the correlation of SNP alleles with the leading eigenvectors decreases the OLS estimators of variance become more and more appropriate. This is not to say, however, that the problem goes away completely. For a large but fixed number of hidden strata, as sample sizes increase the pseudo correlations between phenotype and genotype become more and more statistically significant, even when the variance inflation is "almost" zero for a modest sample size. For the kinds of very large studies needed to obtain statistical significance when making hundreds of thousands (or millions) of separate tests correcting for population stratification remains important.

4.1.6 Admixture

There are many modern admixed populations throughout the world. In the USA these include African Americans, Hispanic populations, many Native American groups, and Pacific Islanders.

Studies of disease traits and other phenotypes in admixed populations are among the most susceptible to population structure, especially when studying populations in which very long separated continental groups are only partially mixed. Many reports of the apparent inflation of false-positive rates in (raw or unadjusted) analysis have been made for studies of admixed populations including schizophrenia [7] and Prostate Cancer [8] in African-American populations, diabetes in Native Americans [9], etc.

Although some admixed populations involve mixtures of several continental groups the focus here is the mixing of two long-separated ancestral groups. The covariances between markers for two individual members (i and j) of an admixed population are described in terms of the proportion, α, of ancestors that derive from a given long-separated population versus the other mixing population proportion $(1 - \alpha)$. We assume that admixture proportion varies between subject (so the α_i is not in general equal to α_j). Assuming that two long-separated populations are derived ultimately from a single ancestral population and that the differentiation parameters are both equal to F, then for subject i the variance of the allele count $n_i(A)$ for a given marker will be equal to $2p (1 - p)(1 + F(1 + 2 \alpha_i^2 - 2\alpha_i))$ (see Chen et al. [10]) where p is the frequency of the A allele in the original ancestral source population. The variance of $n_j(A)$ equals $2p (1 - p)(1 + F(1 + 2 \alpha_j^2 - 2\alpha_j))$ and the covariance between $n_i(A)$ and $n_j(A)$ is $4p (1 - p)F(1 + 2 \alpha_i \alpha_j - \alpha_i - \alpha_j)$. Thus assembling the entire covariance matrix for all the counts, $n_i(A)$, $i = 1, \ldots,$ N, of allele A the general form of the covariance matrix is equal to $2p(1 - p)\mathbf{K}$ where $\mathbf{K}$ is (as in the previous examples) the same for all markers.

4.1.6.1   Eigen Analysis of the Relationship Matrix
for Simple Admixture

We now examine the eigenvectors and eigenvalues of the **K** matrix that corresponds to admixture analysis of the data by Chen et al. [10] from the African-American Breast Cancer (AABC) GWAS study [8]. For this study Chen et al. inferred African-American ancestry for over 5,000 GWAS samples (using the STRUC-TURE program discussed briefly in Chap. 2). They estimated the average fraction of African ancestry in the AABC study as approximately 75–80 % of overall ancestry, with this average varying according to geographical location with study participants for the West Coast sites (Los Angeles, San Francisco) exhibiting about 5 % less African ancestry, on average, than study participants in the East or South of the USA. European ancestry constituted the majority of the remainder although there were smaller fractions (1–2 % on average) of Native American or Hispanic admixture apparent as well. Chen et al. suggested that the distribution of African ancestry for the sites participating in the AABC study could be modeled as a beta distribution with parameters $r = \alpha/h$ and $s = (1 - \alpha)/h$ with mean African ancestry α in the range from 0.75 to 0.80 and with h (a dispersion parameter) approximately equal to $1/7$.

Sampling from a beta distribution to form values of α_i for $N = 100$ subjects, constructing the $N \times N$ matrix **K** according to the values of α for each subject, and then plotting the first few eigenvectors of **K** against the simulated values of α_i, to produce Fig. 4.3, are performed using the following R program code given below

```
> # admixture.r
> # define function to compute the K matrix
> K_admixed<-function(a,F=0.1){#
>         N<-length(a)
>         K<-matrix(0,N,N)
>         for (i in 1:N){
>                 for (j in 1:N) {
>                         if(i == j) K[i,i] <- 1+F*(1+2*a[i]^2-2*a[i])
>                         else K[i,j] <- 2*F*(1+2*a[i]*a[j]-a[i]-a[j])
>                 }
>         }
> K
> }
> # simulate admixture fraction 100 subjects
> N <- 100
> a <- rbeta(N,.8/(1/7) ,(1-.8)/(1/7))
> #compute Relationship Matrix
> K <- K_admixed(a)
> e<-eigen(K)# extract eigenvectors and eigenvalues
> # plot the leading eigenvectors against admixture proportion
> par(mfrow=c(2,2))
> plot(a,e$vectors[,1], main=paste("Eigenvector 1 \n(value=",round(e$values[1],2),")"))
> plot(a,e$vectors[,2], main=paste("Eigenvector 2 \n(value=",round(e$values[2],2),")"))
> plot(a,e$vectors[,3],main=paste("Eigenvector 3 \n(value=", round(e$values[3],2),")"))
> plot(a,e$vectors[,4],main=paste("Eigenvector 4 \n(value=", round(e$values[4],2),")"))
```

Notice when running this code that the first two eigenvectors are the only two ones which have eigenvalues (displayed as *e$values*) greater than 1 (all the remaining eigenvalues fall in the range from 0.95 to 0.90). Both the leading eigenvectors are perfectly linear functions of admixture percentage α_i; the first

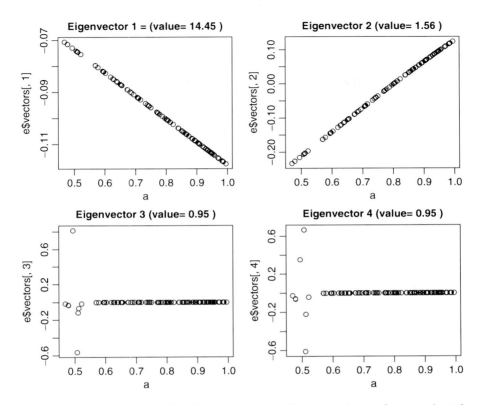

Fig. 4.3 Eigenvectors from a Kinship matrix corresponding to admixture of two continental groups (Africans and Europeans) as approximated by Chen et al.'s [10], p. 495, analysis of the AABC GWAS data

one is nearly equal to an indicator variable for African ancestry, while the second for non-African ancestry (and these are of course perfectly related). Note also that any marker that is strongly differentiated in frequency will tend to load on both of the first and second eigenvectors which are themselves extremely highly correlated (although their dot product is zero). We will see later on that when we estimate eigenvectors (using SNP data) in studies of simple simulated admixed individuals with two ancestral source populations that only one eigenvector related to ancestry will appear in the calculations and that eigenvectors of the estimated relationship matrix will not be correlated with each other (and will all be of zero mean).

No other eigenvectors have relationship to ancestry or have large eigenvalues. The implications of the analysis are (as expected) that when analyzing phenotypes with a mean that is related to fraction of African ancestry that false-positive associations are likely for markers which are informative about African ancestry.

4.1.7   Polygenes and Cryptic Relatedness

As expected very similar issues arise when study samples contain many relatives, which can happen in studies of small isolated and inbred populations [11]. Here we are concerned with situations where we do not in general know the relationship structure between participants in the study, i.e., situations where there is so-called *cryptic relatedness*. Cryptic relatedness can act as a confounder when a powerful polygene is present or when cultural patterns of environmental exposures mimic the genetic patterns.

4.1.7.1   Effects of Hidden Relatedness

Some of the most interesting examples to date of the use of small isolated inter-breeding populations as the source for GWAS studies are those that have been performed in the Micronesian island population of Kosrae. Naïve analysis of these data has been shown to produce many false positives [11] in association studies of quantitative outcomes such as BMI, plasma cholesterol, triglycerides, etc., and alternative data analysis strategies have been considered to deal with this variance inflation issue. Presumably this is because of relatedness between study subjects and possibly other aspects such as admixture with outside groups, e.g., Europeans [12].

For illustrative purposes we perform several simulations of this sort of relatedness on OLS estimation.

In small isolated inbreeding populations we expect that all individuals are at least somewhat related to each other. Interestingly, association analyses are not actually very much affected by low (or even high) levels of relatedness that is identical between all pairs of subjects, either in terms of power or in control of type I error rates. It is only when clusters of individuals are more related to each other than they are to others outside the cluster that relatedness begins to have adverse effects on association testing. The effect of a constant background level of relatedness between individuals can be determined by considering the eigenvectors of a $N \times N$ matrix $\mathbf{K}$ with ones on the diagonal and all off diagonals equal to a given value $b > 0$. It can be readily shown that this matrix has largest eigenvalue equal to $(N - 1)b + 1$ with all remaining eigenvalues equal to a constant $1 - b$. The leading eigenvector is constant with value $1/\sqrt{N}$ with all other eigenvectors orthogonal to this constant vector. The above analysis implies that the estimate of the mean of the phenotypes, i.e., $(1/N)\mathbf{1}'Y$, suffers from variance inflation because the "covariate" N-vector of ones, $\mathbf{1}$, is proportional to the first eigenvector of $\mathbf{K}$; note however that any covariate of zero mean will only load on the later eigenvectors and will not be overdispersed, since the later eigenvectors are all less than 1 and in fact are close to $\text{tr}(K) - \text{Avg}(K) \cong 1 - b$ in (4.9). In an analysis that fits both a mean and a slope it follows (from earlier discussion) that the usual variance estimate for the mean will be an underestimate of the true variance of this parameter estimate but not so for the slope parameter; its OLS variance estimate will be quite accurate.

We now consider a more complex situation in which there are levels of relatedness with each subject having a few first-degree relatives, a greater number of somewhat more distant relatives, and many more quite distant relatives as well as unrelated individuals.

Each of these simulations deals with a heritable trait that is influenced by a polygene, and the heritability of the outcome equal to 1/2, i.e., the model for the covariance of the outcome vector Y is that $\Sigma = \sigma^2 \mathbf{I} + \gamma^2 \mathbf{K}$ with $\sigma^2 = \gamma^2$. In each simulation null marker alleles are generated having covariance matrix equal to $\mathbf{K}$ while Y is generated as multivariate normal with mean zero and covariance matrix Σ.

In order to generate SNP and outcome data with a covariance pattern of this type we introduce the r function *Sim_SNP_related* in the file *Sim_SNP_related.r*. This function simulates SNP data on a single chromosome from an arbitrary pedigree of related individuals and allows for admixture and hidden stratification as well. In order to use this function in the simulations we first must define a pedigree matrix, called *pedigree*, and specify SNP allele frequencies for each chromosome and for each population (when admixture or hidden stratification is considered) as well. For example, in order to simulate sets of siblings a *pedigree* matrix would be of form:

```
> pedigree<-matrix(c(1:4,c(0,0,1,1),c(0,0,2,2),rep(1,4),rep(1,4)),4,5)
> colnames(pedigree)<-c("iid","fid","mid","fpop","mpop")
```

```
> pedigree
     iid fid mid fpop mpop
[1,]   1   0   0    1    1
[2,]   2   0   0    1    1
[3,]   3   1   2    1    1
[4,]   4   1   2    1    1
```

Here the rows of the pedigree matrix correspond to individuals; the columns are individual id (iid), father's id (fid), mother's id (mid), fathers' population (fpop), and mothers' population (mpop).

The second and third columns (the 1 and 2s) on rows 3 and 4 indicate that the father and mother of subjects 3 and 4 are subjects 1 and 2, respectively. Those pedigree members (i.e., the first two) with no parents in the pedigree are "founders" indicated by the pair (0 0) for father and mother ids. The fpop and mpop refer to the population group (here all set to population 1) that a parent not in the pedigree originates from. Thus the pedigree matrix can specify multiple groups and/or admixture by specifying different values of fpop and mpop for different individuals. Note that if, for a given subject, a parent of that subject is in the pedigree (so that columns 2 and/or 3 are not equal to zero) then the population (columns 4 and/or 5) for that parent is ignored. The remainder of the code needed to call *Sim_SNP_related* to create an array of simulated SNP data (*SNPs_chr1* below) is

```
> nsnps_per_chr=100; # suitable for a small GWAS simulation
> nchr=22
> npops=1 # number of populations this can be changed to simulate hidden strata or admixture
> freqs=array(runif(nsnps_per_chr*nchr,.05,.95),c(npops,nchr,nsnps_per_chr))
>         # this generates SNPs allele frequencies (random)
>         # first index for array freqs is for population,
>         # second for chromosome, third for SNP
>         # Here we only simulate common SNPs for a single population
> recomb=1 # allows 1 potential recombination per chromosome
```

The call to *Sim_SNP_related*

```
> SNPs_chr1<-Sim_SNP_related(chr=1,nout=c(3,4))
```

generates SNP count data (0, 1, or 2 copies) for a single chromosome (chromosome here 1 with 100 SNPs). The nout variable indicates that data for subjects 3 and 4 (the siblings) are to be returned and stored in the *SNPs_chr1* array. In a typical simulation the *Sim_SNP_related* function is called many times to generate data for one or more (diploid) chromosomes for many subjects.

A more complex structure is used in the next example. Here we assume that some of the pedigrees are from one population (all with background relationship coefficient, b, equal to 0.03215 between nominally unrelated subjects), and others are from a second population (with same b). The following code generates a dataset of 400 individuals 200 from each of the two populations, within each population each individual is related to 7 other individuals, 1 sibling and 6 first cousins.

```
> set.seed(321256)# to get same results each run
> source("sim_snp_related.r")
> pedigree<-matrix(c(c(1:18),rep(0,6),rep(1,4),7,7,4,4,9,9,6,6,rep(0,6),
>        rep(2,4),3,3,8,8,5,5,10,10,rep(1,18),rep(1,18)),18,5)
>
> # use Balding Nichols model to generate the different allele
> #frequencies for the different populations
> nsnps_per_chr=100;
> nchr=22
> npops=2
> F=.016338; # differentiation factor corresponds to a correlation of
>         # 2F/(1-F)=0.03215 within pops
> M=nchr*nsnps_per_chr;
> p=runif(nsnps_per_chr*nchr,.05,.95)
>     # freqencies in original population
> freqs=array(0,c(npops,nchr,nsnps_per_chr))
> for (L in 1:npops) freqs[L,,]<-rbeta(M,(1-F)*p/F,(1-F)*(1-p)/F) # freqs in modern populations
> #
>         SNPs<-Sim_SNP_related(chr=1,nout=11:18)
> #
> # Set up simulation loops
> #
> nfamilies=50 #
> clustersize=8 # number of related subjects contributing data from each family
> nsubjects=nfamilies*clustersize
> SNPs<-matrix(0,nsubjects,M)
> for (i in 1:nfamilies) { # main loop
> # update populations that each founder comes from
>         pedigree[,4]<-1 + (i>nfamilies/2) # first half from first population
>         pedigree[,5]<-1 + (i>nfamilies/2) # second half from second population
>         for (j in 1:nchr) {
>                 SNPs[((i-1)*clustersize+1):(i*clustersize),((j-1)
>                 *nsnps_per_chr+1):(j*nsnps_per_chr)]
>                 =Sim_SNP_related(chr=j,nout=11:18)
>         }
> }
```

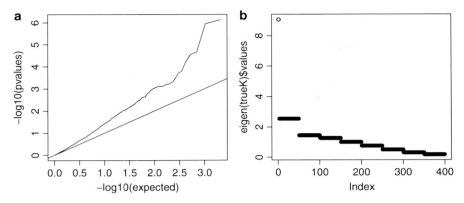

Fig. 4.4 Complex simulated data: (**a**) QQ plot of association statistics; (**b**) eigenvalues of true *K* matrix; (**c**) eigenvalues of estimated *K* matrix; and (**d**) QQ plot after adjusting for one or ten principal components

Next an outcome is generated according to a polygenic model involving a set of 100 randomly chosen "causal" SNPs. A polygene consisting of the unweighted sum of (randomly chosen) risk alleles is computed and used to simulate a (for illustrative purposes) highly heritable phenotype (Y) with 90 % of the outcome variance explained by the polygene. Then association statistics are computed for the noncausal SNPs.

```
> # choose SNPs to make up a polygene g #
> causal<-sort(sample(1:M,100))
> notcausal<-(1:M)[-causal]
> g<-rowSums(SNPs[,causal])
> # generate outcome y
> R2 <- .9 # desired fraction of polygenic variance of Y
> vare<-(1-R2)/R2*var(g)
> y<-g+rnorm(nsubjects,g,sqrt(vare))  # generates observed y
> #
> # Perform association tests
> #
> T2<-rep(0,length(notcausal)) # F stat for association (can treat as chisq)
> ij=0
> for (i in notcausal) {
>     ij=1+ij
>         ci<-cor(SNPs[,i],y)
>         T2[ij]<-(nsubjects-2)*ci^2/(1-ci^2) # F test
> }
> pvalues<-sort(pchisq(T2,1,lower.tail=F))
> x<-seq(1/length(notcausal),1,1/length(notcausal))
> plot(-log10(x),-log10(pvalues),type="l",lty=1)
> abline(0,1)
> abline(-log10(.05/length(notcausal)),0,lty=3) #Bonferroni criterion
```

A QQ plot of the association statistics is given as Fig 4.4a.

For this model we can calculate the true covariance structure matrix for the SNP data. The *R* code

```
> trueK<-2*0.016338*diag(2)%x%(rep(1,200)%*%t(rep(1,200))))
> kf<-matrix(c(1,.5,rep(.125,6),.5),8,8)
> trueK<-trueK+diag(50)%x%kf
```

generates the true value of K and a plot of the eigenvalues of this matrix is given in Fig. 4.4b

```
> plot(eigen(trueK)$values)
```

Here the first two eigenvectors of the true K are both very nearly equal to indicator variables for the two populations from which the founders are drawn from. Now however there are many other eigenvalues >1 which has implications about the success of certain of the methods for correcting for population structure described below.

4.2   Correcting for the Effects of Hidden Structure and Relatedness

In the remainder of this chapter four different approaches to adjusting for the effects of population stratification and cryptic relatedness will be considered. These include *genomic control*, adjustment for *principal components*, *variance components methods*, and a *retrospective* approach for adjustment. Here our main interest is on the analysis of studies of nominally unrelated subjects with unknown pedigree structure so that other approaches such as *family-based association testing* [13, 14] are not usually applicable.

4.2.1   Genomic Control

The simplest approach to addressing the effects of between-person correlations in outcome variables, whether due to hidden structure, admixture, or to cryptic relatedness between subjects, is based upon empirical examination of the behavior of test statistics for a large number of markers and an adjustment of the level of evidence required before a marker can be considered "significant" in a particular analysis. This approach, known as *genomic control* [15, 16], specifically adjusts for widespread overdispersion of the chi-square statistics computed from the Armitage trend test (Chap. 5) by simply estimating an overdispersion factor, usually denoted λ, from the collective behavior of chi-square tests for association with phenotype for marker allele count variables. Genomic control (similar to all empirical methods) requires that many markers be genotyped; rather than dealing with the correlation structure of the genotypes in some way (which is the key to the other methods discussed) genomic control directly addresses the behavior of test statistics, T_k^2, from the

Armitage trend test (here $k = 1, 2, \ldots, M$ denotes marker). In particular genomic control adopts an altered model for the distribution of one degree of freedom chi-square tests under the null hypothesis so that $T_k^2/\lambda \sim \chi_1^2$. The overdispersion parameter λ is estimated under the assumption that the majority of markers are null, that is, not associated with the phenotype or disease of interest. In fact the most commonly used estimate of λ is simply equal to the observed median of the T_k^2 statistics divided by 0.455 which is the median of the central χ_1^2 distribution. The genomic control method of adjustment simply corresponds to the division of each observed trend statistic, T_k^2, by the estimate $\hat{\lambda}$ based on all the observed T_k^2. The original paper [15] related genomic control to several possible sources of correlations between outcomes (e.g., hidden relatedness, strata, and admixture) and indicated that the null distribution of the Armitage test under population structure could often be approximated in this manner. It should be intuitively clear that the calculation of a reliable $\hat{\lambda}$ requires a considerable number of unlinked null markers. If only a few markers are available and especially if many of these markers are in high LD with each other then the estimate of λ is highly variable. In the extreme case, when most markers are located in regions associated with the phenotype of interest then $\hat{\lambda}$ will be biased upward by the presence of true non-null associations.

There have been many criticisms of the use of genomic control as a method for controlling for the effects of population structure in GWAS studies, chief among these is the complaint that the method never reorders associations [17], i.e., the most significant association before correction always remains the most significant after correction, even in situations when other methods are much more selective. From our perspective genomic control ignores the correlation of specific SNPs with the leading eigenvectors of Σ on determining whether specific associations are likely to be overdispersed or not when a applying a uniform correction for all SNPs.

Another potential problem with this method is that it can behave strangely asymptotically; in particular the power of a study that relies only upon genomic control may not increase in the expected way as the study sample size, N, increases [10] (see also Chap. 7). Intuitively this is because the correction factor λ may depend on sample size, N, and $\lambda - 1$ can in some cases increase linearly with sample size which is the same rate that the noncentrality parameter increases when testing for a given true association; this means that the effective increase in sample size per subject added to the study becomes smaller and smaller as $N \to \infty$, and the power for testing a given true non-null hypothesis may reach an asymptotic value that is less than one. This is discussed again in Chap. 7.

Despite these concerns the estimated overdispersion factor, $\hat{\lambda}$, is a very important and widely used summary statistic for describing the success of other approaches to dealing with hidden population structure. The calculation of $\hat{\lambda}$ before and after other correction methods have been applied is an easy and intuitive method of judging whether adequate correction for hidden population strata has been achieved by these other methods; the closer that $\hat{\lambda}$ is to the null value of 1 the better that population structure has been accounted for, at least in terms of control for false-positive association under the assumption that the majority of associations must be null.

4.2.2   Regression-based Adjustment for Leading Principal Components

The first sections of this chapter have stressed the importance of the eigenvector/eigenvalue structure of the covariance matrix for individual phenotypes in determining the behavior of tests for marker/phenotype associations under the null hypothesis of no effect. Two basic results are (1) that when the outcomes have a special structured covariance matrix, $\Sigma = \sigma^2 I + \gamma^2 K$, covariates which load heavily on the first few eigenvectors of the matrix K will tend to appear to be falsely associated with the phenotype because of underestimation of the variance of the effect estimates and (2) that under a model in which the phenotype means are affected by population substructure either due to cultural influences or because of the presence of a polygene, the markers will have a covariance matrix which is proportional to K allowing us to estimate this matrix. These two results motivate the so-called principal components method of adjustment for population stratification.

The exposition of the principal components method as described in an influential paper by Price et al. [17] is as follows. Recall that the discussion of principal components in Chap. 4 describes extracting the leading eigenvectors of the $N \times N$ relationship matrix $\hat{K}$ having off-diagonal elements equal to $(1/M) \sum_{k=1}^{M} z_{ik} z_{jk}$ and diagonal elements equal to $(1/M) \sum_{k=1}^{M} z_{ik}^2$ for $i \neq j = 1, \ldots, N$ with $z_{ik} = (n_{ik} - 2p_k)/\left(\sqrt{2p_k(1 - p_k)}\right)$. These eigenvectors (referred to as principal components by Price et al.) were in Chap. 2 used to qualitatively describe population structure for various populations in graphical plots. Consider now the use of the principal components as adjustment variables in GLMs relating genotype counts to phenotype mean or disease risk.

As originally described the correction method of Price et al. starts (as does the genomic control method) with the Armitage trend test, T^2, for association between phenotype and a marker count variable, computed as $T^2 = N r^2$ where N is the sample size and r is the usual sample estimate of the correlation between phenotype and genotype. Next both the phenotype values, Y_i, and the genotype counts, n_{ik}, for a specific marker k are transformed so that they are orthogonal to each of the L leading eigenvectors, V_l. This orthogonalization is done by computing the residuals of the linear regression first of the phenotype values $Y = (Y_1, Y_2, \ldots, Y_N)'$ on the leading eigenvectors $V_1, V_2, \ldots, V_L$ and then computing the residuals for each of the genotype counts $\mathbf{n}_k = (n_{1k}, n_{2k}, \ldots, n_{Nk})'$ after regression on the same set of eigenvectors. Denoting the residuals for each of these as Y_{adjusted} and $\mathbf{n}_{k\ \text{adjusted}}$, an adjusted Armitage trend test for the association between marker k and phenotype is computed as

$$T^2_{\text{adjusted}} = (N - L) r^2_{\text{adjusted}}, \tag{4.15}$$

where r_{adjusted} is the usual sample correlation between Y'_{adjusted} and $\mathbf{n}'_{k\ \text{adjusted}}$.

Note that to the degree that the eigenvectors of the true relationship matrix $\mathbf{K}$ and its estimated value $\hat{\mathbf{K}}$ coincide, the eigenvector adjustment process described above produces adjusted genotype count vectors which load only on the lower eigenvectors of $\mathbf{K}$. From our earlier discussion of variance estimation in the OLS model we conclude that variance inflation (and hence false-positive associations) arising from correlations between outcomes due to population substructure should be reduced if eigenvector-adjusted phenotype and genotype count variables are used in the analysis.

While we have only carefully described the situation for linear regression with one variable in the model those results translate to the following types of analyses:

1. Use of F-tests in multiple linear regression for testing for a nonzero association between a single continuous outcome and counts of a single variant including the first L eigenvectors as adjustment variables as well as other (non-genetic adjustment variables).
2. Score tests in logistic regression for the null hypothesis of no effect of genotypes, adjusting for the first L eigenvectors.
3. Use of the adjusted Armitage test, $(N - L)r^2_{\text{adjusted}}$, for either binary or continuous phenotype variables.

These results extend to logistic regression because of the correspondence (described in Sect. 3.4.7) between score tests for logistic regression and OLS regression applied to binary phenotypes when the effect of the variable of interest is small. Thus type I error properties under the null hypothesis of no association will be similar whether one uses OLS regression or logistic regression to analyze the binary disease endpoint.

Note again that the adjusted Armitage trend test corresponds very closely to testing in OLS regression when the sample size N is large and true effect sizes are small. In OLS regression the F-test for the influence of a single variable after adjustment for L other variables (plus an intercept term) can be written as $F = (N - L - 2)r^2_{\text{adjusted}}/(1 - r^2_{\text{adjusted}})$. Since the F distribution with 1 df in the numerator converges, as the denominator of degrees of freedom increases, to a chi-square with 1 df, the two tests (T^2 and F) will be similar for large N and small r^2.

4.2.3   Implementation of Principal Components Adjustment Methods

Principal components methods involve first the estimation of the relationship matrix $\mathbf{K}$, then the eigenvector eigenvalue decomposition of the estimate, $\hat{\mathbf{K}}$, and the choice of which of the leading eigenvectors to use as adjustment variables.

4.2.3.1 Estimation of K

Estimation of the relationship matrix has already been discussed in Chap. 2, although certain practical details have not been mentioned. For example, we have not discussed what to do when certain subjects are missing genotypes for a given marker included in the analysis; nor have we discussed the distortions in eigenstructure of the estimate of $\mathbf{K}$ that occur due to the inclusion of large number of markers that are in high LD with each other, or the effects on the estimate of not knowing true (ancestral) values of allele frequencies and making due instead with estimated frequencies. Finally we have not considered questions regarding the number of markers needed for an analysis or the uncertainty of estimation of $\mathbf{K}$ based on a given set of markers. As above the estimated relationship matrix $\hat{\mathbf{K}}$ has its i, j element (for i and j from 1 to N) equal to

$$\hat{k}_{ij} = 1/M \sum_{k=1}^{M} \frac{(n_{ik} - 2\hat{p}_k)(n_{jk} - 2\hat{p}_k)}{2\hat{p}k(1 - \hat{p}_k)}. \tag{4.16}$$

Deletion of either all subjects with any missing genotype data or of all markers with any missing samples is not usually practical when constructing $\mathbf{K}$ since virtually every genotyping platform has some degree of genotyping failure rate for each of the hundreds of thousands of markers required for genome-wide study. An ad hoc approach of substituting in 0 to replace $(n_{ik} - 2\hat{p}_k)$ when n_{ik} is missing is much more widely used than the alternative of using pairwise deletion only (which could produce non-positive semi-definite estimates). Clearly if very large numbers of markers are missing data for large numbers of subjects then this could lead to gross distortions in $\hat{k}_{ij}$ and presumably in the eigenstructure of $\hat{\mathbf{K}}$ as well. Enforcing a requirement that markers that are to be included in the calculation of $\hat{k}_{ij}$ be missing for only a small fraction of participants (from 1 to 5 %) ensures that the added zeros do not dominate the estimation of the matrix.

Another important question is the degree to which LD between markers may distort the eigenvector structure. If there are large numbers of markers that are all in high LD with each other then some of the eigenvectors may be distorted. For example, the most common large-scale chromosomal inversion in humans occurs on chromosome 9 with a frequency of from 1 to 3 %. Because inversion suppresses recombination in heterozygotes [18] mutations appearing on the inversion are in high LD over the entire length of the inversion. Markers on that inversion can have significant effects on the estimation of the strength of genetic relationship between individuals carrying the inversion with individuals carrying the inversion appearing to be more closely related than they would otherwise be, all other things being equal. In terms of the calculation of $\hat{k}_{ij}$ it should be clear that if there is high correlation between a string of markers then sums such as (4.16) will be more variable than if each marker is independent. For this reason principal components analysis is usually carried out using a "thinned" set of markers, imposing a restriction that nearby markers not be in high linkage disequilibrium. A common criterion is to preclude any marker that has an $R^2 > 0.2$ with any already chosen marker within several hundred kb in order to avoid overestimation of relatedness [19, 20]. Generally however purely local LD (with just a few nearby SNPs in high LD with each marker) will have little effect on the leading eigenvectors since these are sensitive to the larger patterns in the data.

Having to estimate p_k for each marker has several effects on the estimation of $\mathbf{K}$. First of all the estimate of the elements of $\mathbf{K}$ using (4.16) produces an estimate with rank at most equal to $N - 1$ rather than N. Rakovski and Stram note that since the sum $\sum_i^N (n_{ik} - 2\hat{p}_k)$ equals zero for each marker this implies that a vector of ones is in the null space of $\hat{\mathbf{K}}$ and therefore $\hat{\mathbf{K}}$ is not invertible (an issue for the retrospective approach to the analysis of case–control data detailed below). This has implications for the eigenvector structure of $\hat{\mathbf{K}}$ compared to $\mathbf{K}$. For example, Fig. 4.3 showed the true eigenvector structure for an admixed sample of subjects; in this figure both eigenvector 1 and eigenvector 2 of the true value of $\mathbf{K}$ are perfectly correlated with the admixture fraction α as described above. However if we simulate a sample of SNP markers according to the same model so that

1. Allele frequencies for two related populations are chosen using Balding–Nichols beta binomial model.
2. An admixture fraction α_i is chosen for subject i from the beta distribution having parameters α/h and $(1 - \alpha)/h$ for i from 1 to N and then.
3. For each subject a total of M SNP allele counts are generated with fraction α_i coming from the first ancestral population and fraction $(1 - \alpha_i)$ from the second.

Then computing $\hat{\mathbf{K}}$ using the SNP data (with $M = 10,000$ and $N = 100$) and plotting the first 4 of the resulting eigenvectors against admixture proportion α_i gives the plot shown in Fig. 4.5. In this plot there is only one eigenvector that is correlated with admixture fraction compared to two in Fig. 4.3. The "loss" of eigenvector 2 seen in Fig. 4.3 is due to the fact that $\hat{\mathbf{K}}$ is of rank $N - 1$. The original first two eigenvectors were perfectly correlated with each other (although their dot product was 0); however since the vector $\mathbf{1}$ is in the null space of $\hat{\mathbf{K}}$ all the eigenvectors with eigenvalues greater than zero must have mean equal to zero. Therefore the correlation between eigenvectors of $\hat{\mathbf{K}}$ must be exactly equal to zero and hence the loss of a second eigenvector that is also correlated with ancestry. Such a loss however is not relevant to the use of the eigenvectors as adjustment variables since it is in any event impossible to include two perfectly correlated variables as adjustment variables in a regression analysis. Using only one adjustment variable that is (almost) perfectly correlated with ancestry will still ensure that (residual) loadings of the covariate of interest on either of the two eigenvectors with eigenvalues >1 of the true $\mathbf{K}$ will be near zero.

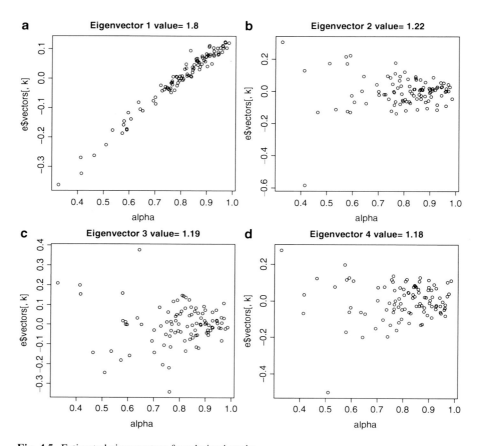

Fig. 4.5 Estimated eigenvectors for admixed study

4.2.3.2 Choosing the Number of Eigenvectors to Include as Adjustment Variables

Several rules for choosing eigenvectors to be used as adjustment variables for phenotypic analysis have been described. Roughly speaking these fall into two categories: methods based only on the eigenstructure structure of the marker data and methods that also take into account the behavior of the phenotype data as well. For example, one rule is to simply include a fixed number of eigenvectors; ten is often used following a precedent established by Price et al. [17]. A second approach is to use statistical criteria related to the statistical significance of a given eigenvector. For example, Patterson et al. [21] employed the Tracy–Widom [22] statistic to determine a set of L eigenvectors which had eigenvalues greater than the remainder of eigenvalues, with the number L proposed as the number of leading eigenvectors to be adjusted for in association analysis. From our analysis it would appear that a simpler approach for choosing L would simply be the number of eigenvalues that are greater than 1, since it is the loading of covariates upon the corresponding eigenvectors that leads to variance inflation.

In our experience [10] with genotypes from a large GWAS breast cancer risk in an admixed, African-American, population, neither of these two criteria yielded particularly helpful suggestions for the number of eigenvectors to use as adjustment equations in association analysis. Starting with approximately 5,000 cases + controls approximately 660 eigenvectors were greater than 1 and approximately 400 of these were nominally significantly elevated, compared to the remainder, using the Tracey–Widom statistic as computed by the program SMARTPCA [21]. The very large number of eigenvalues greater than 1 may be a finite sample issue. Since the trace of the $\hat{\mathbf{K}}$ matrix computed for these data was quite close to N the average value of the trailing eigenvalues is just under one. Using a finite number of SNPs in estimating the eigenvalues sampling error in $\hat{\mathbf{K}}$ could easily send many estimated values over one just due to chance alone. It is unclear why there were so many significant eigenvectors reported from the Tracey–Widom statistic implemented in SMARTPCA; this may be a consequence of LD being lengthened by incomplete admixture (personal communication, Nick Patterson, Broad Institute, Cambridge, MA).

In any given analysis specific eigenvectors may or may not be associated with disease. Including a variable that is not associated with disease as an adjustment variable usually has little effect on the conclusions of an analysis regarding the association of the alleles of interest with the phenotype being examined, so long as the number of such variables used is not large and so long as the adjustment variable is not highly correlated with the independent variable of interest. Therefore rather than trying to use the eigenstructure of the $\hat{\mathbf{K}}$ matrix alone to determine which eigenvectors should be used as adjustment variables it is often far more parsimonious to simply include just those eigenvectors that appear to be predictive of the phenotype of interest at some level of significance. In this fashion the choice of eigenvectors for adjustment will be treated as an ordinary variable selection problem. In the African-American breast cancer data described by Chen et al., only a single eigenvector, namely, the first, highly correlated with fraction of African ancestry, was significant in the breast cancer analysis, and this association was mainly restricted to a specific subtype (estrogen receptor negative disease) known to be more common in African-American women.

To summarize, the adjustment for principal components is probably the most commonly used approach for the inclusion of information about ancestry available from a GWAS to adjust association statistics for the presence of either hidden non-mixing groups as well as admixture between historically separate populations. The PC method has been widely applied to both case–control data and to analysis of continuous phenotypes.

For more complicated structure involving levels of hidden relatedness between individuals the PC method does not work well [23]. To take an extreme example (which is discussed also in Chaps. 3 and 7) a study in which cases are matched to sibling controls cannot be analyzed as if the siblings are unrelated even if large numbers of eigenvectors (e.g., 1 per sibship) are included in the regression model. In general the principal components based methods are less well equipped to deal with cryptic relatedness than is either genomic control or the next two types of analyses to be considered.

4.2.4   Random Effects Models

This section revisits the analysis of continuous phenotypes Y_1, Y_2, ..., Y_N for which a model for the mean phenotype is written as

$$E(Y_i) = \beta_1 X_{i1} + \beta_2 X_{i2} + \cdots + \beta_{r-1} X_{i,r-1} + \beta_r X_{ir}. \tag{4.17}$$

In addition we assume that the variance/covariance matrix for the vector of outcomes $Y = (Y_1, Y_2, \ldots, Y_N)'$ is of form

$$\Sigma = \sigma^2 \mathbf{I} + \gamma^2 \mathbf{K}. \tag{4.18}$$

Our interest is when one of the variables (for example, the last one, X_r) corresponds to the allele count $n(A)$ of a variant, A, of interest being tested for association with phenotype Y and where the other X variables relate phenotype means to measured exposures or other host factors (age, race, body mass index, etc.) that we would like to adjust for in the model. Since the goal of a GWAS study is to evaluate the effect of each of many variants by fitting model (4.17) many times, X_r will take many different sets of values namely (in turn) $\mathbf{n}_k = (n_{1k}, n_{2k}, \ldots, n_{Nk})'$, $k = 1, 2, \ldots, M$ for the allele counts of the kth variant being tested.

Implicitly we are assuming that the $\mathbf{K}$ matrix in (4.18) driving the covariance between outcomes is actually proportional to the variance–covariance matrix for each $\mathbf{n}_k$. As described above this model is reasonable for polygenic phenotypes or for phenotypes in which cultural factors are related to environmental determinants (exposures, lifestyle choices, etc.) and where cultural similarities in these determinants mimic genetic similarities.

From Chap. 3 if each of $\mathbf{K}$, σ^2, and γ^2 are known then the best linear unbiased estimate, $\hat{\beta}_{\text{BLUE}}$, of β can be written as

$$\hat{\beta}_{\text{BLUE}} = \left(\mathbf{X}' \Sigma^{-1} \mathbf{X} \right)^{-1} \mathbf{X}' \Sigma^{-1} Y \tag{4.19}$$

with

$$E(\hat{\beta}_{\text{BLUE}}) = \beta$$

and

$$\mathrm{Var}\left(\hat{\beta}_{\mathrm{BLUE}}\right) = \left(\mathbf{X}'\mathbf{\Sigma}^{-1}\mathbf{X}\right)^{-1}. \tag{4.20}$$

For large values of N (the number of observations) Wald tests for the parameter of interest: that is, testing whether $\beta_r = 0$ by dividing $\hat{\beta}_r 2$ by the (r, r)th element of $(\mathbf{X}'\mathbf{\Sigma}^{-1}\mathbf{X})^{-1}$ will have appropriate size (e.g., type I error will be controlled) and generally will have good power. This will hold even when the true values of σ^2 and γ^2 are replaced by consistent estimates of these quantities.

4.2.4.1 Introduction to Estimation of Random Effects Models

If the matrix $\mathbf{K}$ is known, then the problem of estimating σ^2 and γ^2 is a special case of fitting a so-called linear structured covariance matrix model; Anderson (e.g., [24]) and other statisticians defined these models and introduced estimating equations that provide maximum likelihood estimates, when phenotypes are normally distributed, for all parameters in the mean and variance functions. Estimating equations for the parameters in such models (here σ^2 and γ^2) have been noted [25] to be equivalent to performing a series of weighted least squares regression of elements of the sample covariance matrix $(Y - \mathbf{X}\beta)(Y - \mathbf{X}\beta)'$ upon the elements of the matrices in the covariance model, here $\mathbf{I}$ and $\mathbf{K}$ (see Yang et al. [26] for an application that stresses such a regression procedure in the context of estimating the heritability of height). Once σ^2 and γ^2 have been estimated large sample inference (based on a Wald test) about the influence of $\mathbf{n}_k$ on phenotype Y is performed by dividing the rth element of the vector $\hat{\beta}_{\mathrm{BLUE}}$ to (the square root of) the $r \times r$ element of $\mathrm{Var}\left(\hat{\beta}_{\mathrm{BLUE}}\right)$ and comparing this ratio to critical values for a normal random variable (or the square of the ratio to the critical values for a χ_1^2)

Variance components models for genetic analysis originally were introduced for the analysis of continuous traits when the genealogical relationships between study subjects are known. These methods have a long history starting with work by Fisher [27]. In a recent example Pilia et al. [28] examined the heritability of cardiovascular and personality traits among 5,610 participants, for whom pedigree information was available, recruited from four towns in the Sardinian province of Nuoro. In this study there were over 34,000 relative pairs identified with an average kinship coefficient of 0.1625. The program POLY (http://www.sph.umich.edu/csg/chen/public/software/poly/) was used to compute (by analysis of IBD sharing from the pedigree information) the components of the relationship matrix and to estimate heritability, by solving the estimating equations needed to estimate σ^2 and γ^2 for the quantitative traits of interest. This program allows additional components of variance to be included in the model for the covariance matrix of the phenotype, for example, to take account of effects of especially strong shared environment for very close relatives such as siblings, genetic dominance components, interaction (epistatic) components, etc. These are incorporated into the general model by inclusion of additional (known) covariance matrices in the covariance model so that the variance–covariance matrix of the phenotypes becomes equal to

$$\mathbf{\Sigma} = \sigma^2 \mathbf{I} + \sum_{r=1}^{R} \gamma_r^2 \mathbf{K}_r. \qquad (4.21)$$

Again the $\mathbf{K}_r$ are assumed to be known from first principles (rather than estimated from marker or other data) and the variance components γ_r^2 are estimated in the analysis. For example, in order to estimate a genetic dominance component as well as an additive component of heritability, one can fit a model

$$\mathbf{\Sigma} = \sigma^2 \mathbf{I} + \gamma_1^2 \mathbf{K}_{\text{add}} + \gamma_2^2 \mathbf{K}_{\text{dom}},$$

in which the elements of $\mathbf{K}_{\text{add}}$ are equal to the additive kinship coefficients, or $z_1 + 1/2 z_2$, for all pairs of subjects and where the elements of $\mathbf{K}_{\text{dom}}$ equal z_2. (The z_1 and z_2 are the probabilities of sharing either one or two alleles identically by descent and are calculated for each pair of subjects, Chap. 2). It can be shown that z_2 is greater than zero only when related individuals have paths of coancestry through both of their respective parents, as have full sibs and double first cousins [29].

A general algorithm for estimation of linear structured covariance models of this form as described by Anderson involves the repeated inversion of large matrices (of order $N \times N$), once for each iteration. Because of the time and computer resources required for these computations it is not realistic to estimate σ^2 and the γ^2 parameters in (4.18) or (4.21) separately for each marker being tested. Instead these parameters are estimated just once, at the beginning of the scan, and these initial values retained. For each marker the BLUE estimate, $\hat{\beta}_{\text{BLUE}}$, of the mean parameters as well as its variance estimate is constructed and tests performed, cf. Kang et al. [30], using the same estimate of Σ. This procedure is quite effective at providing valid tests and unbiased estimates so long as no single marker explains a large fraction of the variability of the genetic component and moreover closely corresponds to a score test of the null hypothesis of no effect on phenotype mean for a given marker [30].

4.2.4.2   Software for Genetic Applications

The historical, rarely now used, program BMDP5v [31] was the first widely available general purpose program that could fit general structured covariance matrix models such as those of interest here. The currently very widely used SAS (Cary, NC) procedure PROC MIXED can fit linear structured covariance matrix models for fairly large problems (thousands of individuals). Specialty software that can be used for genetic association analysis of quantitative traits includes programs such as PAP, ACT, SEGPATH, SOLAR, SAGE, MENDEL, and MERLIN [32]. These programs generally rely upon knowledge of the genealogy of the sample in order to compute the relationship matrix and other covariance matrices corresponding to other terms (dominance components, shared environment among close relatives, etc.) in order to deal with covariance structures such as (4.21). More recently programs such as EMMAX (below) have been described which incorporate estimation of a covariance structure matrix based on the observed SNPs for use in the variance components analysis.

4.2.4.3   Estimation of K

Empirical estimation of the covariance structure matrix $\mathbf{K}$ by observing the correlation structure of large numbers of SNP alleles has been discussed already above. Several other choices have been considered; for example, EMMAX [30] permits the use of either a (normalized) IBS matrix (a simple count of the number of alleles shared for pairs of individuals summed overall all markers and normalized to have diagonals equal to ones) or the matrix with elements $\hat{k}_{ij}$ as in (4.16) (termed the Balding–Nichols matrix by Kang et al.). Their analysis found that use of either estimate appeared to have similar control for type I error rates and power characteristics.

4.2.4.4   Control of Confounding Using Random Effects Models for Case–Control Data

Generalized linear models which include predictor variables Z associated with random effects w, i.e.,

$$g\big(E(Y|\mathbf{X},\mathbf{Z})\big) = \mathbf{X}\beta + \mathbf{Z}w, \tag{4.22}$$

with w treated as random mean zero quantities with a covariance matrix that is known up to some set of parameters, can be used as a starting point both for the correction of association tests for population stratification (our interest here) and (see Chap. 8) for tests for the aggregate effects of many (typically rare) variants as in the sequence kernel (SKAT) tests described by Wu et al. [33]. The influence of hidden structure, admixture, or other relatedness together with the action of a polygene (or culturally based behaviors or exposures which mimic such polygenetic effects) can (as with the linear models described above) be modeled as

$$g\big(E(Y|\mathbf{X},\mathbf{Z})\big) = \mathbf{X}\beta + g. \tag{4.23}$$

Here, as before, we assume that the covariance matrix of g equal to $\gamma^2\mathbf{K}$ with the $\mathbf{K}$ equal to a known or the estimated relationship matrix. Direct incorporation of the random term g with this covariance matrix, and maximum likelihood estimation of the parameters β and γ^2 for generalized linear models is provided by certain well known statistical software programs (SAS Proc GLIMMIX, R packages GLMM and lme4). These general purpose programs, however, are quite slow (requiring iterative inversion of an NxN matrix for example) and are not generally suitable for large-scale genetic analysis involving hundreds of thousands of markers.

Kang et al. [30] discussed the application of standard random effects regression (for quantitative traits) to binary outcomes (case–control) data for the testing of effects and came to the conclusion that applying to case–control data using same software used for quantitative traits worked reasonably well. This is partially justified by noting the similarities of the Armitage trend test to both F-tests for the significance of variables in OLS regression and to score tests in logistic regression. This may be the most feasible approach to apply random effects methods to case–control data for genome-wide association testing. Such calculations are of most interest in situations (such as the presence of many highly related subjects) where the fixed effects principal components methods tend to fail.

4.2.5 Retrospective Methods

Up to this point we have considered models in which phenotype means or case–control status probabilities are described conditionally upon marker genotype. It is possible and potentially useful to think about this problem from the other direction, i.e., by investigating the distribution of marker counts given case–control status. In many cases modeling the mean of genotypes given case–control status will yield equivalent or nearly equivalent inference as does modeling disease status given marker genotype; some classic results on use of retrospective versus "prospective" methods are given by Prentice and Pyke [34]: in addition, retrospective analyses can be extended to cases in which both the genotypes and phenotypes for different individuals are not independent of each other. This approach leads to a development of methods for the analysis of case–control studies that allow for non-independence due to population stratification and hidden relatedness in a more natural manner than simply applying methods designed for quantitative data directly to case–control data as suggested above. A classic paper by Bourgain et al. [35] applied retrospective analyses to analysis of genetic associations when pedigree structure is known, and these have been more recently adapted to large-scale association testing when pedigree structure is not known, e.g., [36, 37].

To give a very simple example when so-called retrospective analysis agrees with a more familiar case–control analysis, consider a sibling matched case–control study. The sibling-based case–control design and certain other family-based designs provide highly effective protection against the effects of population stratification [38]. Matching full siblings on disease status ensures that every case has a control with exactly the same ancestry so that differences in ancestry between cases and controls cannot lead to an excess of false-positive associations. When using conditional logistic regression (Chap. 5) of 1:1 matched data with only one variable of interest, i.e., a genotype count, $n(A)$ for a specific allele the conditional likelihood readily reduces to

$$\prod_{i=1}^{N_{\text{pairs}}} \frac{\exp(n_{i1}\beta)}{\exp(n_{i1}\beta) + \exp(n_{i0}\beta)}, \tag{4.24}$$

where the index i indicates matched pair (here sibship), and the index of 1 or 0 refers to case and control status, respectively.

It is easy to see that that the score statistic for testing $\beta = 0$ is equal to

$$\frac{1}{2} \sum_{i=1}^{N_{\text{pairs}}} (n_{i1} - n_{i0}),$$

and the information is

$$\frac{1}{2} \sum_{i=1}^{N_{\text{pairs}}} (n_{i1} - n_{i0})^2.$$

So that the score test is simply

$$\frac{\left[\sum_i (n_{i1} - n_{i0}) \right]^2}{\sum_i (n_{i1} - n_{i0})^2}. \tag{4.25}$$

This test is closely related to the square of the usual paired t-test for testing whether there is a difference in the mean counts for cases and controls. Specifically we can rewrite (4.25) as

$$\frac{\overline{\delta}^2}{\frac{\hat{\sigma}_\delta^2}{N_{\text{pairs}}} \left(\frac{(N_{\text{pairs}}-1)}{N_{\text{pairs}}} + \frac{\overline{\delta}^2}{N_{\text{pairs}}} \right)},$$

where $\delta_i = n_{i1} - n_{i0}$, $\overline{\delta} = \frac{1}{N_{\text{pairs}}} \sum_{i=1}^{N_{\text{pairs}}} \delta_i$, and $\hat{\sigma}_\delta 2$ is the usual sample variance estimate computed from the δ_i. Therefore as N_{pairs} increases the score test rapidly approaches $T^2 = N_{\text{pairs}} \left(\overline{\delta}^2 / \hat{\sigma}_\delta^2 \right)$, which is the square of the usual paired-t test.

Now consider this same problem from a slightly different angle. We construct the vector, $\mathbf{n}$, of counts of allele A of length $2N_{\text{pairs}}$ as $\mathbf{n} = (n_{1,1}, n_{1,0}, n_{2,1}, n_{2,0}, \cdots, n_{N_{\text{pairs}},1}, n_{N_{\text{pairs}},0})'$ and we adopt the following retrospective model for $\mathbf{n}$:

$$E(\mathbf{n}) = \mu + \mathbf{c}\beta, \tag{4.26}$$

where the vector $\mathbf{c}$ (also of length $2N_{\text{pairs}}$) contains ones and zeros indicating case and control status, respectively, i.e., we are now modeling the mean allele count for controls as equal to μ and the mean allele count for cases as $\mu + \beta$; note that if the disease outcome is rare then μ should equal twice the allele frequency, p. Now consider a model for the variance–covariance matrix of $\mathbf{n}$ reflecting the sibling design. Assuming that individuals from different sibships are independent of each other then $\text{Var}(\mathbf{n})$ will be equal to $2p(1 - p)\mathbf{K}$, with $\mathbf{K}$ a block diagonal matrix having blocks equal to $\begin{pmatrix} 1 & 0.5 \\ 0.5 & 1 \end{pmatrix}$ and all other elements equal to zero, where p is the allele frequency of A (and is equal to $1/2\mu$). Letting the $2N_{\text{pairs}} \times 2$ matrix $\mathbf{C}$ have first column equal to a vector of 1s and second column equal to $\mathbf{c}$ then the BLUE estimate of μ and β will be computed (Chap. 3) as

$$\begin{pmatrix} \hat{\mu} \\ \hat{\beta} \end{pmatrix} = \left(\mathbf{C}'\mathbf{K}^{-1}\mathbf{C}\right)^{-1}\mathbf{C}'\mathbf{K}^{-1}\mathbf{n}. \tag{4.27}$$

The variance–covariance matrix of the estimates will be

$$\text{Var}\begin{pmatrix} \hat{\mu} \\ \hat{\beta} \end{pmatrix} = 2p(1 - p)\left(\mathbf{C}'\mathbf{K}^{-1}\mathbf{C}\right)^{-1}. \tag{4.28}$$

In (4.27) the matrix $(\mathbf{C}'\mathbf{K}^{-1}\mathbf{C})^{-1}\mathbf{C}'\mathbf{K}^{-1}$ reduces to the $2 \times 2N_{\text{pairs}}$ matrix with elements

$$\frac{1}{N_{\text{pairs}}}\begin{bmatrix} 0 & 1 & 0 & 1 & \ldots & 0 & 1 \\ 1 & -1 & 1 & -1 & \ldots & 1 & -1 \end{bmatrix},$$

and the variance matrix $(\mathbf{C}'\mathbf{K}^{-1}\mathbf{C})^{-1}$ equals

$$\frac{2p(1 - p)}{N_{\text{pairs}}}\begin{bmatrix} 1 & -0.5 \\ -0.5 & 1 \end{bmatrix}.$$

A test of $\beta = 0$ with an asymptotic χ_1^2 distribution can be computed as $\left(\hat{\beta}^2\right)/\left(\text{Var}(\hat{\beta})\right)$ or

$$N_{\text{pairs}}\frac{\overline{\delta}^2}{2p(1 - p)}. \tag{4.29}$$

Since

$$\text{Var}(\delta_i) = \text{Var}(n_{i,1}) + \text{Var}(n_{i,0}) - 2\text{Cov}(n_{i,0}, n_{i,1}) = 2p(1 - p),$$

this test is equivalent to $T^2 = N_{\text{pairs}}\left(\overline{\delta}^2/\sigma_\delta^2\right)$, which is the paired t-test with a slightly different variance estimate, i.e., $2\hat{p}(1 - \hat{p})$ after substitution of p with $\hat{p}$.

The point of this exercise is to establish the idea that retrospective tests that take account of the correlation structure of the allele counts of interest are often equivalent to more familiar tests performed in studies designed specifically to deal with population structure. Another example [36, 39] of this is the analysis of affected-offspring + parents (trio) data. Rakovski et al. show that if each trio is unrelated that the retrospective regression method produces a test very similar to the transmission-disequilibrium test [40] often used to analyze affected-offspring trios (see also Chap. 3, Sect. 3.6.2).

4.2.5.1   The Bourgain Test

A general retrospective approach to using the correlation structure of allele counts to analyze case–control data in the presence of relatedness between subjects was proposed by Bourgain et al. [35]. The basic idea generalizes the procedure just used. The model for the mean of the allele counts for a specific variant being tested remains the same as above, that is, $E(\mathbf{n}) = \mu + \mathbf{c}\beta$. In the setting in which Bourgain et al. introduced the test, it was assumed that the kinship coefficients between individuals (as well as inbreeding coefficients) could be computed on the basis of pedigree information. Bourgain et al. motivated this test by considering a study of asthma occurrence taking place among the Hutterites, an isolated North American religious population whose entire population can be traced back to 90 ancestors in the 1780s/1800s. The complete genealogy of 719 different study participants was constructed from a Hutterite pedigree of over 12,000 individuals. The covariance matrix of the counts, $\mathbf{n}$, of a given allele was assumed to be equal to $2p(1 - p)\mathbf{K}$ with

$$\mathbf{K} = \begin{bmatrix} 1 + h_1 & 2\phi_{12} & \cdots & 2\phi_{1N} \\ 2\phi_{12} & 1 + h_2 & \cdots & 2\phi_{2N} \\ \vdots & \cdots & \cdots & \vdots \\ 2\phi_{1N} & 2\phi_{2N} & \cdots & 1 + h_N \end{bmatrix}. \tag{4.30}$$

Bourgain et al. consider the simultaneous estimation of both parameters, μ and β, using methods that correspond to the use of the BLUE estimates of (4.27) to provide estimates of both these parameters (and hence $p = \mu/2$ as well).

4.2.5.2   An Empirical Bourgain Test

Several authors [36, 37, 39] have considered the use of empirical estimates, calculated from GWAS data, of an approximate relationship matrix, $\hat{\mathbf{K}}$, when genealogical data are absent for substitution into the BLUE estimation procedure described above. Astle et al. [39] explored the substitution of $\hat{\mathbf{K}}$ of (4.16) for $\mathbf{K}$ in (4.27) and (4.28) as a method of correcting for any of hidden relatedness or hidden stratification and/or admixture in the analysis of case–control studies. A few practical issues have to be dealt with in order to consider the use of this test. First as noted above the maximum rank of $\hat{\mathbf{K}}$ is equal to $N - 1$ since the vector of 1s lies in the null space of $\hat{\mathbf{K}}$. Thus $\hat{\mathbf{K}}^{-1}$ does not exist. As noted by Rakovski and Stram [36] the use of a generalized inverse of $\hat{\mathbf{K}}$ in place of $\mathbf{K}^{-1}$ in (4.27) allows for the estimation of β only if μ (and hence $p = \mu/2$) is treated as known (set, for example, to its naïve estimate, ignoring population stratification) rather than a parameter to be estimated in the course of the fitting procedure.

A second important issue is the amount of computation involved when using this test on a genome-wide basis. Note that if no SNPs are missing any data then the matrix $(\mathbf{C}'\mathbf{K}^{-1}\mathbf{C})^{-1}\mathbf{C}'\mathbf{K}^{-1}$ in (4.27) needs to be computed only once. The estimate $\hat{\beta}$ is then computed for each marker in turn by post-multiplying this matrix by each count vector $\mathbf{n}$. Similarly $(\mathbf{C}'\mathbf{K}^{-1}\mathbf{C})^{-1}$ in (4.28) remains constant during the calculations as well and only $\hat{p}$ needs to be calculated separately for each SNP. In a real study all SNPs will be missing some data and it is best to avoid performing many-fold calculations of the inverse of the submatrix of $\hat{\mathbf{K}}$ that corresponds to those subjects with data. Using formulae for partitioned matrices is one possible approach, and this reduces the computation of the inverse of the submatrix to that of inverting a matrix of the same size as the number of subjects missing that marker. Another is to simply substitute the expected value, $2p$, for any missing count values. Thornton and McPeek [37] provide other suggestions and in particular try to exploit case–control status information and the marker count values of known relatives, when dealing with missing data.

4.3   Comparison of Correction Methods by Simulation

In order to compare the methods given above, i.e., genomic control, principal components, variance components, and the retrospective approach we develop a sequence of simulated data using the *R* routine *Sim_SNP_related* described above to generate random SNP data under conditions of relatedness, population structure, and/or very recent admixture. For illustrative purposes the simulated phenotypes are highly heritable and driven by a polygene consisting of 100 randomly selected SNP alleles (the causal alleles) from among 2,200 simulated markers. In each simulation all noncausal SNPs are tested for association (to estimate type 1 error rate) as well as the causal alleles (in order to estimate power for each approach). We implement each of the correction methods in *R*, following the general approaches described by Price et al. [17] for principal components correction, Kang et al. [30] (EMMAX program) for the mixed model, and Rakovski and Stram [36] for the retrospective model. We also consider a hybrid approach that both adjusts for significant principal components and corrects for any remaining overdispersion using genomic control (a PC + GC approach)

The first simulated dataset consists of a combination of close and distant relatedness between individuals (the presence of both hidden strata and inclusion of close relatives). We compare genomic control to principal components (controlling for eigenvectors that are significantly related to the generated phenotype) and to the mixed model approach. The mixed model uses the R function *EMMAX_mimic* (defined in the *linStructCov.r* file) to fit the mean and variance parameters in the model $E(Y) = \mu$ and $\text{Var}(Y) = \sigma^2 Y + \gamma^2 \hat{\mathbf{K}}$ with $\hat{\mathbf{K}}$ estimated as in expression (16) above.

Consider a simulation experiment in which there is weak relatedness between large groups of individuals but very close relatedness for some family members. Weak relatedness is simulated as the presence of two different non-mixing populations with (ancestral) differentiation parameter F in the Balding–Nichols model to a value ($F = 0.0163$) that gives a correlation between individuals within the two populations of $2F/(1 + F) = .03215$, which is the level expected for second cousins. Within each population there are 50 families for which eight members are genotyped so that each individual has one sibling and six cousins in the study. The results of a typical simulation are shown as a series of QQ plots in Fig. 4.6. Figure 4.6a gives the distribution of $(-\log 10)$ p-values for the noncasual SNPs either uncorrected or corrected for significant principal components from a single simulation realization. Notice that there is a very strong overdispersion of p-values in the uncorrected analysis ($\lambda = 2.62$) and also overdispersion after PC correction ($\lambda = 1.13$); this reflects that it is both population stratification and also relatedness that is being simulated here. Figure 4.6b shows the QQ plot for the noncausal SNPs using the mixed model approach, indicating good protection against type 1 error. Finally Fig. 4.6c shows the results of running the mixed and PC correction method on the 100 causal SNPs. Because there was overdispersion in Fig. 4.6a for the PC method the chi-square statistics were divided by the corresponding genomic control factor $\lambda = 1.13$ (the hybrid PC + GC approach described above). In the PC method (for this single simulation run) a total of 12 principal components (ranging from numbers 1 to 219) were nominally significantly associated with outcome (at $p = 0.05$); however, it was the first principal component (highly correlated with population membership) that was the most significant. In this single simulation it appears that the PC+GC approach is similar to the mixed model approach both in terms of type 1 error control (Fig. 4.6b) and power; it will take much more simulation work to really evaluate whether they are consistently similar strategies (the R code used is called *sim1*.r, see Homework).

4.3.1   Comparison of the Mixed Model and Retrospective Approach for Binary (case–control) Outcomes

A second simulation modifies the above in two ways. First the differentiation parameter F is increased to a very large value (0.1) for illustrative purposes, and second a truncated version of y (split at the median) is used as the outcome variable. The implementation of the retrospective method is provided by function *retro* defined in *retrospective.r*. The simulations described are implemented in *sim2*.r. Figure 4.7a

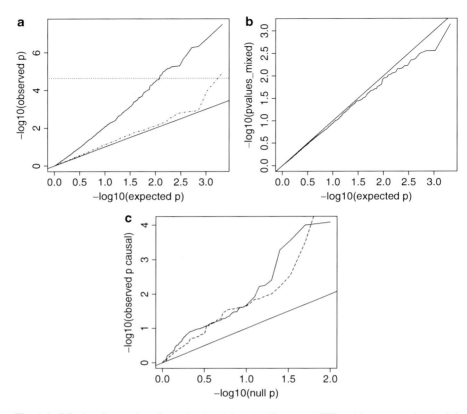

Fig. 4.6 QQ plots for *p*-values from simulated data: (**a**) Noncausal SNPs with no correction (*solid line*) and correction for significant principal components (*dashed line*). (**b**) Noncausal SNPs using the mixed model (EMMAX) method. (**c**) Causal SNPs using the mixed method (*solid lines*) and combination of PC correction and genomic control (*dashed line*). Also shown for reference is the Y=X line (*solid*)

shows the null distribution for both the mixed model and retrospective method applied to the data, both appear (in this simulation) to be adequately following a null chi-square distribution. Figure 4.7b shows a very similar dispersion of the tests of the causal SNPs indicating that both tests appear to have similar power.

4.3.2   Conclusions

Of the four different methods considered two of them, the mixed model and retrospective approach, appear to be general purpose algorithms in the sense that whether the cause of overdispersion of tests is due to either hidden population structure or hidden relatedness or both the methods seem to have good type 1 error

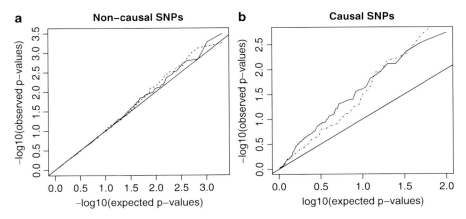

Fig. 4.7 Comparisons of mixed model and retrospective approaches to analysis of case–control data. (**a**) QQ plot for noncausal SNPs showing mixed model (*solid line*) retrospective (*dashed line*) and the unadjusted Armitage test (*dotted line*). (**b**) QQ plot for causal SNPs

properties and similar power. In a sense they lie in between the PC method and the genomic control method. The PC method works well when large-scale hidden structure is present or for correcting for the effects of recent admixture (but see Chap. 8 for more discussion of association testing using admixed populations). The genomic control method works best when individual study members are related to some fraction of other study participants.

From a practical standpoint there are many advantages to the PC and genomic control methods compared to the mixed or retrospective models, in their simplicity and wide availability. While special software may be required (such as EIGENSTRAT) to compute principal components for large numbers of individuals, once they have been computed implementation is very easy. Moreover in many cases (and this can be seen with further experimentation with *Sim_SNP_related*) the hybrid PC + GC method (genomic control applied after significant PCs have been included in the model) can be used to adequately control for both hidden structure and hidden relatedness. This was illustrated in Fig. 4.6c where the hybrid (PC + GC) correction gave only slightly less significant results than the mixed model, and in most simulations the hybrid method was very competitive with the mixed model (or retrospective) approach (Homework).

4.4   Behavior of the Genomic Control Parameter as Sample Size increases

As discussed also in Chaps. 3 and 7, if the genomic control parameter, λ, increases with sample size then this can have a serious effect on study power; for example, if this increase is linear study power can reach an asymptote below 1 (Chap. 7). On the other hand, if λ remains constant as sample size increases then the power of tests will continue to increase with sample size in an expected fashion. We consider here a simple structured population problem, i.e., one in which there are a number of non-mixing populations within the study population and consider what happens to the variance of the estimated slope in OLS regression as sample size increases. Two possibilities are allowed, the first is when the number of groups stays constant as sample size increases and the fraction of members from each group in the whole study also stays constant, and the second is when the number of groups increases at the same rate as sample size keeping the number of individuals from any given group constant. The first situation is similar to a typical population stratification or admixture problem affecting a population-based study, i.e., increasing the study size (by drawing from the same admixed or stratified population) does not alter the fraction of study individuals who are "related" (i.e., in the same strata) to any specific individual. The second situation is more typical of having included closely related individuals in a study. As the study size increases the number of individuals that a given participant is closely related to remains relatively constant so that the fraction who are related to that participant decreases with sample size. In order to examine these two cases more closely we discuss the following simplification of this problem.

Suppose that Y_{ij} denotes the outcome observed for individual j in group i and that Y_{ij} has a mean that depends on a variable x_{ij} (e.g., a genotype count for that individual) but that the Y_{ij} given x_{ij} are not independent of the outcome of other group members. In particular assume that Y_{ij} follows the random intercept model $Y_{ij} = \mu + \beta x_{ij} + a_i + e_{ij}$ for $i = 1, 2, \ldots, N, j = 1, 2, \ldots, n_i$ with $\mathrm{Var}(e_{ij}) = \sigma^2$ and $\mathrm{Var}(a_i) = \gamma^2$. Then $E(Y) = \mu + \mathbf{X}\beta$ with block constant variance–covariance matrix $\mathrm{Var}(Y) = \sigma^2 I + \gamma^2 \mathbf{I}_n \otimes \mathrm{diag}(11'_{n_i})$ ($\otimes$ denotes the Kronecker product), where $\mathbf{X}$ is a matrix with rows equal to $(1, x_{ij})$ for (i,j) as above. It is relatively easy to show in this situation that the variance of the OLS estimate of $\hat{\beta}$ is equal to

$$\frac{\sigma^2}{\sum_{ij}(x_{ij} - \overline{x})^2} \left(1 + \frac{\gamma^2}{\sigma^2} \frac{\sum_{i=1}^{N}\left\{ \left[\sum_{j=1}^{n_i}(x_{ij} - \overline{x}) \right]^2 \right\}}{\left[\sum_{ij}(x_{ij} - \overline{x})^2 \right]} \right).$$

Now (as in population stratification problems where x is a SNP count variable) we assume that the covariance matrix of the predictor variable is similar to that of Y. Specifically suppose that x_{ij} can also be written as a random intercept model $x_{ij} = f + w_i + \varepsilon_{ij}$ with $\mathrm{Var}(w_i) = \nu^2$ and $\mathrm{Var}(\varepsilon_{ij}) = \tau^2$. Now the question is what happens to the variance of $\hat{\beta}$ as (1) the number of groups, N, grows but group sizes n_i do not and (2) the number of groups stays constant but the group sizes grow. The term

$$\frac{\gamma^2}{\sigma^2} \frac{\sum\limits_{i=1}^{N}\left\{\left[\sum\limits_{j=1}^{n_i}(x_{ij}-\bar{x})\right]^2\right\}}{\left[\sum_{ij}(x_{ij}-\bar{x})^2\right]}, \tag{4.31}$$

acts as an overdispersion term. If this term is large then variances will be underestimated in OLS regression, so that genomic control parameter will be greater than 1.

To simplify things we consider the ratio of the expectations of the numerator and denominator of (4.31) (rather than the expectation of the ratio itself). The key issue here is to understanding the expectation of $\left[\sum_{j=1}^{n}(x_{ij}-\bar{x})\right]^2$. This is equal to the variance of $\sum\limits_{j=1}^{n_i}(x_{ij}-\bar{x})$ which can, with a bit of work, be written as

$$(\tau^2 + n_i\nu^2)\left(1 - \frac{2n_i}{n_{tot}}\right) + \left(\frac{n_i}{n_{tot}}\right)^2\left[n_{tot}\tau^2 + \nu^2\sum_i n_i^2\right]. \tag{4.32}$$

Assuming all n_i are equal to n then the entire numerator has expectation

$$N(\tau^2 + n\nu^2)\left(1 - \frac{2n}{n_{tot}}\right) + N\left(\frac{n}{n_{tot}}\right)^2\left[n_{tot}\tau^2 + N\nu^2 n^2\right] = (N - 2 + n)(\tau^2 + n\nu^2)$$

while the denominator has expectation $(\tau^2 + \nu^2)(nN - 1)$. Therefore expectation of the denominator is linear in both the number of blocks, N, and the size of the blocks, n, while the expectation of the numerator is linear in the total number of blocks but quadratic in n. This implies if the number of blocks increases but the block size does not the overdispersion term (and hence the genomic control λ, which corrects for overdispersion) will tend to a constant value, while if the size, n, of the blocks increases the overdispersion term, and λ, increases linearly with n.

This finding generalizes to more complex situations (e.g., involving relatedness and admixture as well as hidden stratification), which can be seen empirically by further exploration with *Sim_SNP_related*. The basic principle is that if the fraction of pairs of individuals that are "related" stays constant with sample size (as in admixture or simple population stratification) as the sample size increases then the genomic control λ will tend to increase with sample size. If on the other hand if the fraction of pairs that are related to each other decreases (even if the total number of related individuals increase) then the genomic control parameter will not increase.

4.5   Removing Related Individuals as Part of Quality Control, Is It Needed?

The design of most GWAS studies targets unrelated individuals as study members. Looking at estimated relatedness (i.e., by estimating IBD probabilities z_0, z_1, and z_2; see Chap. 2) in the course of data cleaning for quality control is important in order to find sample mix-ups that have led to unintended duplicate samples or to find evidence of sample contamination a hallmark of which is that one or more participant samples appear to be related to a large number of other study samples. Removal of unintended duplicates and potentially contaminated samples is of course well advised. In the course of data quality control however it is not uncommon to find that some pairs of individuals appear to be genuinely but unexpectedly related to each other. In fact the discovery of pairs of identical twins (verified by record search or recontact) is not unheard of, and almost all studies find sets of siblings, parent–offspring pairs, and other close relationships (e.g., avuncular, half-sibs) that are not possible to classify strictly on the basis of IBD probabilities. It is commonly recommended practice (for example, see the National Human Genome Research Institute, GENEVA project [41] website https://www.genevastudy.org and the material therein) to remove samples in order to break up first- and second-degree relative pairs for analyses that are to be performed assuming all individuals are unrelated. A simulation study in *R* (*sim3.r*) looks at the necessity of doing so in a small sized GWAS. In this simulation 500 pairs of individual genotypes are generated (again using *Sim_SNP_related*) with 400 of the pairs being strictly unrelated to each other; the remaining participants consist of 10 parent–offspring pairs, and 30 pairs each of siblings, half-siblings, and avuncular relations. Removal of 100 individuals (from 100 related pairs) leaves 900 subjects, keeping them in leaves 1,000 individuals but with the possibility that we may have to correct for overdispersion using genomic control (or other methods). Using a setup similar to *sim1.r* above (e.g., a continuous outcome Y with 50 % polygenic heritability), the result of 100 replications is shown in Fig. 4.8. Even with this small simulation it is evident that (1) overdispersion caused by even 10 % of individuals being closely related to another study member is small (average GC parameter was $\lambda = 1.038$ for the full dataset compared to $\lambda = 1.022$ for the unrelated individuals only); (2) that type 1 error was well preserved by genomic control; and (3) that the mean power was a few percent higher using all individuals (with GC adjustment) than only the unrelated samples (where no GC was applied).

These results are suggestive that keeping subjects in the study, even when nominally related to other members, may have either little influence on power, or may provide power gains, relative to their removal. Moreover the implications of the previous section are that in this situation we would not expect the GC parameter to tend to increase with sample size (which of course can be verified by further simulation work; see Homework) so that the results here from this very small simulation will remain consistent as sample sizes increase.

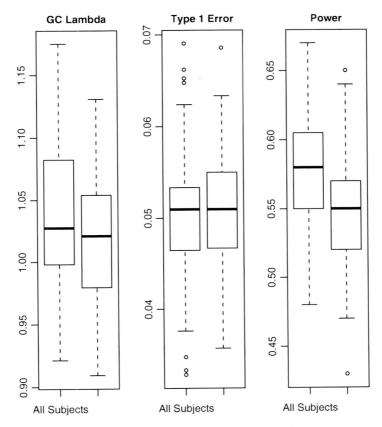

Fig. 4.8 Results of third simulation experiment (*sim3.r*). One hundred simulations were performed. Type 1 error rate is computed using the fraction of noncausal SNPs (2,100 used in each simulation) with nominal association at $p \leq 0.05$, and power is computed using the fraction of causal SNPs found to be significantly associated (at $p \leq 0.05$)

4.6 Chapter Summary

This chapter has reviewed the effects of population structure, namely, hidden relatedness, stratification, and admixture on association estimation and testing using a unified eigenvector-based approach. Three different types of procedures including *fixed effects*, *random effects*, and *retrospective* modeling, for dealing with hidden population structure, have been introduced and motivated. General theoretic analyses as well as some simulation experiments have been used to describe the problems associated with and the utility of each of these types of correction methods. Fixed effects approaches, specifically principal components analysis, for the analysis of genetic associations for both binary (case–control) outcomes, and quantitative phenotypes appear to be highly effective at dealing with the problem of admixture and gross hidden stratification. Hidden relatedness can require other approaches and the use of random effects modeling as well as retrospective modeling (for quantitative and case–control outcomes, respectively) can be helpful in such settings, as illustrated here. Another reasonable and easy to implement method is to control for gross stratification by the PC method but allow for additional relatedness using genomic control.

Homework

1. In the normalization process described by Price et al. and discussed in Sect. 4.2.2 the eigenvectors are orthogonal and assume that there is no missing data. Show that this implies that performing the linear regression of Y on leading eigenvectors V_j for $j = 1, \ldots, L$ is equivalent to computing $Y_{adjusted} = Y - Y'V_1 - Y'V_2 - \cdots - Y'V_L$ and similarly for the linear regression of each n_k on the leading eigenvectors. What is necessary to modify here in the presence of missing data?
2. In the method of Price et al. is it really necessary to adjust both Y and n_k? Suppose we only adjust $\mathbf{n}_k$ but leave Y alone when calculating the Armitage tests, what effects does this have on the false-positive rate for the Armitage test now constructed as $(N - L)\text{Cor}(n_{k,\text{adjusted}}, Y)^2$ rather than $(N - L)\text{Cor}(n_{k,\text{adjusted}}, Y_{\text{adjusted}})^2$. Are the false-positive rates similar for these two tests? Similarly if we only adjust Y and not n_k, does this also give similar results? Modify *sim1.r* (Supplementary material) so that these possible correction methods are included.
3. Consider the Model

$$Y_i = \sum_{k=1}^{r} \beta_k + \sum_{k=1}^{N} \alpha_k V_k$$

with V_k equal to the k eigenvector of $\mathbf{K}$. Show that when the α_k are treated as independent random variables with mean 0 and $\text{Var}(\alpha_k) = \gamma^2 \lambda_k$, this model is equivalent to model (4.17) for the means combined with model (4.18) for the variances. Therefore the models described in Sect. 4.2.4 can be thought of as a random effects version of the fixed effects principal components regression presented in Sect. 4.2.2.
4. Show that performing a simple linear regression of Y_{adjusted} on each $n_{k,\text{adjusted}}$ is equivalent (in terms of inference about the influence of genotype on phenotype) to a multiple linear regression of Y on n_k and the leading eigenvectors $V_j, j = 1, \ldots, L$.
5. Perform other simulation experiments using the *sim1.r*, *sim2.r*, and *sim3.r* programs. For example, make additional runs of *sim1.r* to determine whether the GC + PC method is indeed competitive (on the basic of power) with the mixed model method in this complicated simulation. How does the GC parameter increase with sample size:

   (a) If there is no correction for principal components.
   (b) If the leading principal component (first) is included.

Data and Software Exercises

The following are based on the availability (from dbGaP) of the JAPC data from Cheng et al. If these data are not handy please substitute any other large-scale association study dataset that is available:

1. In the JAPC data are any of the first 10 principal components, computed as part of Homework in Chap. 2, predictive of prostate cancer?
2. Use PLINK, with the—*logistic* flag or other software to adjust for leading eigenvectors and red the QQ and Manhattan plots from Chap. 3 Homework.
3. Download and install the EMMAX software to fit variance model (4.18) to the JAPC data and perform single SNP analysis for each SNP.

   (a) Read the results into SAS or R and make QQ plots to compare with those in 2.
   (b) Should leading eigenvectors be adjusted for, i.e., included in the mean model (4.17).

References

1. Pike, M. C., Kolonel, L. N., Henderson, B. E., Wilkens, L. R., Hankin, J. H., Feigelson, H. S., et al. (2002). Breast cancer in a multiethnic cohort in Hawaii and Los Angeles: Risk factor-adjusted incidence in Japanese equals and in Hawaiians exceeds that in whites. *Cancer Epidemiology, Biomarkers and Prevention, 11*, 795–800.
2. Manolio, T. A., Collins, F. S., Cox, N. J., Goldstein, D. B., Hindorff, L. A., Hunter, D. J., et al. (2009). Finding the missing heritability of complex diseases. *Nature, 461*, 747–753.
3. Lango Allen, H., Estrada, K., Lettre, G., Berndt, S. I., Weedon, M. N., Rivadeneira, F., et al. (2010). Hundreds of variants clustered in genomic loci and biological pathways affect human height. *Nature, 467*, 832–838.
4. Speliotes, E. K., Willer, C. J., Berndt, S. I., Monda, K. L., Thorleifsson, G., Jackson, A. U., et al. (2010). Association analyses of 249,796 individuals reveal 18 new loci associated with body mass index. *Nature Genetics, 42*, 937–948.
5. Chambers, J. C., Zhang, W., Sehmi, J., Li, X., Wass, M. N., Van der Harst, P., et al. (2011). Genome-wide association study identifies loci influencing concentrations of liver enzymes in plasma. *Nature Genetics, 43*, 1131–1138.
6. Ehret, G. B., Munroe, P. B., Rice, K. M., Bochud, M., Johnson, A. D., Chasman, D. I., et al. (2011). Genetic variants in novel pathways influence blood pressure and cardiovascular disease risk. *Nature, 478*, 103–109.
7. O'Donovan, M. C., Craddock, N., Norton, N., Williams, H., Peirce, T., Moskvina, V., et al. (2008). Identification of loci associated with schizophrenia by genome-wide association and follow-up. *Nature Genetics, 40*, 1053–1055.
8. Haiman, C. A., Chen, G. K., Blot, W. J., Strom, S. S., Berndt, S. I., Kittles, R. A., et al. (2011). Genome-wide association study of prostate cancer in men of African ancestry identifies a susceptibility locus at 17q21. *Nature Genetics, 43*, 570–573.
9. Knowler, W. C., Williams, R. C., Pettitt, D. J., & Steinberg, A. G. (1988). Gm3;5,13,14 and type 2 diabetes mellitus: An association in American Indians with genetic admixture. *American Journal of Human Genetics, 43*, 520–526.

10. Chen, G. K., Millikan, R. C., John, E. M., Ambrosone, C. B., Bernstein, L., Zheng, W., et al. (2010). The potential for enhancing the power of genetic association studies in African Americans through the reuse of existing genotype data. *PLoS Genetics, 6*, e101096.
11. Lowe, J. K., Maller, J. B., Pe'er, I., Neale, B. M., Salit, J., Kenny, E. E., et al. (2009). Genome-wide association studies in an isolated founder population from the Pacific Island of Kosrae. *PLoS Genetics, 5*, e1000365.
12. Bonnen, P. E., Lowe, J. K., Altshuler, D. M., Breslow, J. L., Stoffel, M., Friedman, J. M., et al. (2010). European admixture on the Micronesian island of Kosrae: Lessons from complete genetic information. *European Journal of Human Genetics, 18*, 309–316.
13. Rabinowitz, D., & Laird, N. (2000). A unified approach to adjusting association tests for population admixture with arbitrary pedigree structure and arbitrary missing marker information. *Human Heredity, 50*, 211–223.
14. Laird, N. M., Horvath, S., & Xu, X. (2000). Implementing a unified approach to family-based tests of association. *Genetic Epidemiology, 19*(Suppl 1), S36–S42.
15. Devlin, B., & Roeder, K. (1999). Genomic control for association studies. *Biometrics, 55*, 997–1004.
16. Devlin, B., Roeder, K., & Wasserman, L. (2001). Genomic control, a new approach to genetic-based association studies. *Theoretical Population Biology, 60*, 155–166.
17. Price, A. L., Patterson, N. J., Plenge, R. M., Weinblatt, M. E., Shadick, N. A., & Reich, D. (2006). Principal components analysis corrects for stratification in genome-wide association studies. *Nature Genetics, 38*, 904–909.
18. Kirkpatrick, M. (2010). How and why chromosome inversions evolve. *PLoS Biology, 8*. doi: 10.1371/journal.pbio.1000501.
19. Zou, F., Lee, S., Knowles, M. R., & Wright, F. A. (2010). Quantification of population structure using correlated SNPs by shrinkage principal components. *Human Heredity, 70*, 9–22.
20. Hoggart, C. J., O'Reilly, P. F., Kaakinen, M., Zhang, W., Chambers, J. C., Kooner, J. S., et al. (2012). Fine-scale estimation of location of birth from genome-wide single-nucleotide polymorphism data. *Genetics, 190*, 669–677.
21. Patterson, N., Price, A. L., & Reich, D. (2006). Population structure and eigenanalysis. *PLoS Genetics, 2*, e190.
22. Tracy, C., & Widom, H. (1994). Level-spacing distributions and the Airy kernel. *Communications in Mathematical Physics, 159*, 151–174.
23. Price, A. L., Zaitlen, N. A., Reich, D., & Patterson, N. (2010). New approaches to population stratification in genome-wide association studies. *Nature Reviews Genetics, 11*, 459–463.
24. Anderson, T. W. (1973). Asympotically efficient estimation of covariance matrices with linear structure. *The Annals of Statistics, 1*, 135–141.
25. Goldstein, H. (1986). Multilevel mixed linear model analysis using iterative generalized least squares. *Biometrika, 73*, 43–56.
26. Yang, J., Benyamin, B., McEvoy, B. P., Gordon, S., Henders, A. K., Nyholt, D. R., et al. (2010). Common SNPs explain a large proportion of the heritability for human height. *Nature Genetics, 42*, 565–569.
27. Fisher, R. A. (1918). The correlation between relatives on the supposition of Mendelian inheritance. *Transactions of the Royal Society of Edinburgh, 52*, 399–433.
28. Pilia, G., Chen, W. M., Scuteri, A., Orru, M., Albai, G., Dei, M., et al. (2006). Heritability of cardiovascular and personality traits in 6,148 Sardinians. *PLoS Genetics, 2*, e132.
29. Falconer, D. S., & Mcackay, T. F. C. (1996). *Introduction to quantitative genetics*. Harlow: Longman.
30. Kang, H. M., Sul, J. H., Service, S. K., Zaitlen, N. A., Kong, S. Y., Freimer, N. B., et al. (2010). Variance component model to account for sample structure in genome-wide association studies. *Nature Genetics, 42*, 348–354.
31. Jennrich, R. I., & Schluchter, M. D. (1986). Unbalanced repeated-measures models with structured covariance matrices. *Biometrics, 42*, 805–820.

32. Almasy, L., & Warren, D. M. (2005). Software for quantitative trait analysis. *Human Genomics, 2*, 191–195.
33. Wu, M. C., Kraft, P., Epstein, M. P., Taylor, D. M., Chanock, S. J., Hunter, D. J., et al. (2010). Powerful SNP-set analysis for case–control genome-wide association studies. *American Journal of Human Genetics, 86*, 929–942.
34. Prentice, R., & Pyke, R. (1979). Logistic disease incidence models and case–control studies. *Biometrika, 66*, 403–411.
35. Bourgain, C., Hoffjan, S., Nicolae, R., Newman, D., Steiner, L., Walker, K., et al. (2003). Novel case–control test in a founder population identifies P-selectin as an atopy-susceptibility locus. *American Journal of Human Genetics, 73*, 612–626.
36. Rakovski, C., & Stram, D. O. (2009). A kinship-based modification of the Armitage trend test to address population structure and small differential genotyping errors. *PloS One, 4*, e5825.
37. Thornton, T., & McPeek, M. S. (2010). ROADTRIPS: Case–control association testing with partially or completely unknown population and pedigree structure. *American Journal of Human Genetics, 86*, 172–184.
38. Gauderman, W. J., Witte, J. S., & Thomas, D. C. (1999). Family-based association studies. *Journal of the National Cancer Institute Monographs, 31–37*.
39. Astle, W., & Balding, D. J. (2009). Population structure and cryptic relatedness in genetic association studies. *Statistical Science, 24*, 451–471.
40. Spielman, R. S., McGinnis, R. E., & Ewens, W. J. (1993). Transmission test for linkage disequilibrium: The insulin gene region and insulin-dependent diabetes mellitus (IDDM). *American Journal of Human Genetics, 52*, 506–516.
41. Cornelis, M. C., Tchetgen, E. J., Liang, L., Qi, L., Chatterjee, N., Hu, F. B., et al. (2012). Gene-environment interactions in genome-wide association studies: A comparative study of tests applied to empirical studies of type 2 diabetes. *American Journal of Epidemiology, 175*, 191–202.

Chapter 5
Haplotype Imputation for Association Analysis

Abstract This chapter discusses extending association analyses to include a larger set of hypotheses beyond just the single markers that have been genotyped in a particular study. This chapter first reviews haplotype frequency estimation and *imputation*. It gives the details of EM estimation and haplotype imputation for a small number of SNPs using data from unrelated subjects and then considers the extension of this method to larger number of SNPs. The partition-ligation EM algorithm is detailed as a method of obtaining haplotype count estimates for individuals in an association study for a moderate number of SNPs.

The problem of haplotype-specific risk estimation and incorporation of SNP haplotype analysis into generalized linear regression models is considered in some detail; first a simple substitution of imputed for true haplotypes into association testing is described. Since this method ignores uncertainties in the estimation of the haplotype frequencies that underlie the imputation of haplotypes, the chapter also considers simultaneous maximum likelihood estimation of all parameters (risk estimates and haplotype frequency estimates), so that haplotype uncertainty is formally taken account of in the construction of hypothesis tests and confidence intervals. For case–control data, a full likelihood-based approach also must take into account ascertainment of cases and controls as haplotype frequencies in the sample may not reflect haplotype frequencies in the population, specifically for haplotypes that are associated with risk.

The substitution of expected (imputed) haplotype count for unobserved true haplotype count in regression analysis is a special case of the "expectation-substitution" method described in the statistical literature on the subject of regression parameter estimation when measurement errors occur in the explanatory variables. It is known to have reasonable statistical properties in many analyses, especially for forming tests of the null hypothesis (of no haplotype-specific effects). However under the alternative hypothesis, the validity of the expectation-substitution method can be questioned, and joint estimation as well as ascertainment correction

D.O. Stram, *Design, Analysis, and Interpretation of Genome-Wide Association Scans*, 183
Statistics for Biology and Health, DOI 10.1007/978-1-4614-9443-0_5,
© Springer Science+Business Media New York 2014

(for case–control sampling) may be considered. This and other problems in haplotype-specific risk estimation are discussed.

Finally some special requirements of imputing SNPs or haplotypes in heterogeneous populations are described.

5.1   The Role of Haplotypes in Association Testing

Haplotype analysis is used to extend the number of hypotheses that are tested during association analysis. Haplotypes, by which is meant the arrangement of alleles on chromosomal segments, contain information about variants that are in LD with the measured marker alleles, but which were not genotyped directly. If a causal variant (consisting of a single mutation) occurs within a region of limited recombination and then (through selection or random drift) becomes common, the SNP haplotype that this variant fell on necessarily also becomes common. Since there may have been no single SNP that uniquely defined that haplotype from all others (see Fig. 5.1), it follows that haplotype-based association testing may be a more powerful approach to detecting the effect of the (unmeasured) causal variant than will the analysis of any of the single SNPs that make up the observed haplotypes. In the figure, the second (causal) SNP falls exclusively on the (0 1) haplotype of the first and third SNPs and so is perfectly associated with that haplotype while not being perfectly correlated with either the first or the third SNP. If we only measured the first and third SNPs, then we should see a stronger haplotype association than any single SNP association.

The above illustration serves as a heuristic rationale for the use of *haplotype-block-based* analysis. Haplotype blocks [1, 2] are simply regions of limited recombination between SNPs demarked by regions with higher levels of historical recombination. Several algorithms can be used to define such blocks, and are most notably implemented in the graphical program Haploview [3]. Haplotype-specific association analysis is often thought of as being restricted to such blocks since the likelihood of picking up an association from an unmeasured variant is much smaller when the measured SNPs are nearly independent (i.e., NOT in the same haplotype block). Since the same comment applies to single SNP associations, the only realistic approach to finding risk variants in regions of high

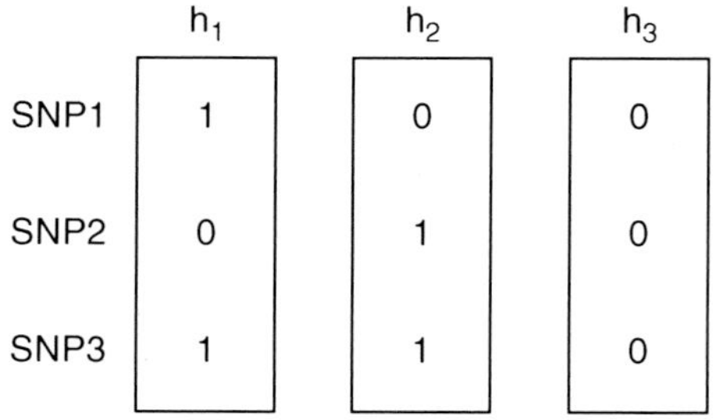

Fig. 5.1 Three SNP haplotypes

recombination is simply to genotype every known variant in the region and hope that there are no unknown causal variants there.

In addition, haplotypes can also be causal variants themselves. In a very well worked out example, Nackley et al. [4] reported that three common haplotypes involving two synonymous and one non-synonymous SNPs in the COMT gene code for differences in COMT enzymatic activity and are associated with pain sensitivity. Strong evidence that it was the haplotypes rather than the individual SNPs that influenced the activity was found in functional analysis of RNA loop structures and enzymatic activity; one of the low-activity haplotypes has been associated with preeclampsia in a Norwegian cohort [5]. Haplotype associations (sometimes called *cis-interactions*) have been found to be stronger than associations with the individual markers in many instances, e.g., [6–11]; however (as with most single marker associations) the functional basis for the haplotype effects underlying the associations is yet to be understood.

5.2   Haplotypes, LD Blocks, and Haplotype Uncertainty

Haplotypes are observed with uncertainty (for the autosomes) even if all the SNPs (or other variants) are genotyped without error. The degree of uncertainty in haplotype imputation correlates both with the number of SNPs making up the haplotype of interest and upon the extent of historical recombination that has occurred between the SNPs.

A formal calculation of the squared correlation, R_h^2, of the estimates, $E(\delta_h|G_i)$, with the true counts, δ_h, of haplotype h carried by each subject is described briefly below [12]; this quantity will be less than one if recombinant haplotypes have nonzero frequency p_h. In regression analysis haplotype uncertainty reduces the effective sample size (or noncentrality parameter) of a haplotype-based association analysis (compared to a study that could genotype haplotypes directly) approximately in proportion to R_h^2. For very small numbers of SNPs in linkage equilibrium (but near enough so that the possibility of contemporary recombination can be ignored) or for larger numbers of markers that are in high linkage equilibrium, the predictability of common haplotypes is generally quite high.

5.3   Haplotype Frequency Estimation and Imputation

5.3.1   Small Numbers of SNPs

Start by considering haplotype frequency estimation from genotype data for unrelated participants under the assumption of Hardy–Weinberg equilibrium applied to the haplotypes. An EM implementation of maximum likelihood estimation [13] involves the calculation for each possible haplotype, h, of an estimate of the *haplotype dosage*, $\delta_h(H)$, which is the count of the number of copies of h contained in the true (but generally unknown) pair of haplotypes H carried by that individual (i.e., $\delta_h(H) = 0$, 1, or 2).

Starting with an initial set $\left(p_{h_1}, p_{h_2}, \ldots, p_{h_{2m}}\right)^0$ of haplotype frequency estimates, in each iteration of the EM, the expectation step estimates (the superscript indicates iteration number), for each subject, i, (for $i = 1, \ldots, N$), the expected haplotype dosage $\delta_{h,i}(H)$ conditionally on the genotype data G_i for each subject treating the current estimates of the haplotype frequencies as if they were known. Assuming HWE, the expected haplotype dose estimates are computed for each haplotype h as

$$E\left(\delta_h \mid G_i\right) = \frac{\displaystyle\sum_{H \sim G_i} \delta_h(H) p^k_{h_1} p^k_{h_2}}{\displaystyle\sum_{H \sim G_i} p^k_{h_1} p^k_{h_2}}, \tag{5.1}$$

where $H \sim G_i$ denotes the set of haplotype pairs $H = (h_1, h_2)$ that are compatible with the observed genotype data G_i (so that $h_1 + h_2 = G_i$). Next the haplotype frequency estimates, p^k_h, are updated in the maximization step as

$$p^{k+1}_h = \frac{1}{2N} \sum_{i=1}^N E\left(\delta_h \mid G_i\right).$$

This process is then repeated iteratively. Upon convergence of the algorithm, the haplotype dosage estimates, $E(\delta_{h,i} \mid G_i)$, can be used in association analysis, to form score tests for haplotype-specific effects [14, 15] as described below.

Haplotype imputation using fewer SNPs than were considered when defining the haplotypes can also be considered; the aim is to infer haplotypes seen in reference data, such as the HapMap, using the genotypes of tagging SNPs (for candidate gene analyses) or the SNPs available on a GWAS platform. The only modification to (5.1) that is needed is to have the symbol h represent the haplotype of interest as seen in the reference data while G_i represents just the measured genotypes.

5.3.2   Haplotype Uncertainty

As mentioned above, even if haplotype frequencies are known, and all SNPs are genotyped, there remains uncertainty in haplotype prediction (for the autosomes) using measured data. One measure of haplotype uncertainty applied separately to each haplotype is the haplotype R^2_h measure which is the variance of $E(\delta_h \mid G_i)$ computed over the distribution of genotypes divided by the unconditional variance of δ_h which is $2p_h(1 - p_h)$ under Hardy–Weinberg equilibrium. Under HWE

$\mathrm{Var}\{E(\delta_h|G_i)\}$ can be calculated formally from the haplotype frequencies.[1] Table 5.1 shows the details of the calculation for two SNPs.

In Table 5.1, the top row lists the possible genotype counts, $G = (n_1, n_2)$, for the first and second SNP, respectively, and each entry in the second row lists the (unordered) pair or pairs of haplotypes that are consistent with the genotype counts above it. p_0 to p_3 are the haplotype frequencies for haplotypes (0,0), (0,1), (1,0), and (1,1), respectively. Notice that the only pair of genotypes where there remains any uncertainty about which pair of haplotypes is present is the double pair of heterozygotes, $G = (1,1)$, where the haplotype pairs $\{(0,0), (1,1)\}$ and $\{(0,1), (1,0)\}$ are both consistent with the observed data. The third row gives the probability of observing each of the genotypes and the last four rows give the expected values for each of the four haplotype counts δ_h, given the genotype counts in row 1. For the first haplotype count, δ_0, the variance is calculated as $E_G[(E\{\delta_{h0}(H|G\})^2] - E(\delta_{h0}(H))^2$ with

$$E\{E(\delta_{h0}(H))\} = 2 \times (p_0^2) + 1 \times (2p_0p_1) + 1 \times (2p_2p_0)$$
$$+ ((p_3p_0)/(p_2p_1 + p_3p_0)) \times (2(p_2p_1 + p_3p_0)),$$

which is easily shown (after substituting $p_3 = 1 - p_0 - p_1 - p_2$) to equal $2p_0$. And

$$E\left(\delta_{h0}(H)^2\right) = 4 \times (p_0^2) + 1 \times (2p_0p_1) + 1 \times (2p_2p_0) + ((p_3p_0)/(p_2p_1 + p_3p_0))^2$$
$$\times (2(p_2p_1 + p_3p_0)).$$

So that the variance is

$$\mathrm{Var}\{E(\delta_{h_0}|G)\} = 2p_0 \frac{(p_1^2p_2 - p_0p_1 + p_1p_0^2 + p_2^2p_1 - p_2p_0 + p_2p_0^2 + p_0 - 2p_0^2 + p_0^3)}{p_0^2 + p_0p_1 + p_2p_0 - p_2p_1 - p_0},$$

(here p_3 does not appear since it has been replaced with $1 - p_0 - p_1 - p_2$).

Notice if either of p_1 or p_2 is zero (or if $p_3 = 1 - p_0 - p_1 - p_2$ is zero), the variance of $E(\delta_{h_0}|G)$ will be $2p_0(1 - p_0)$ so that R_h^2 will be equal to 1. Otherwise the variance will always be less than $2p_0(1 - p_0)$ (and $R_h^2 < 1$).

The uncertainty of haplotype count prediction can be extended to haplotypes involving more than 2 SNPs and to the situation when not all SNPs that make up the haplotypes are measured. Figure 5.2 (adapted from Stram et al.) gives a plot of haplotype R_h^2 for haplotypes involving N SNPs in the special case when all SNPs have frequency ½ and are in complete linkage equilibrium. At 7 SNPs, the certainty of haplotype count estimation is quite low with R_h^2 near 0.3. Figure 5.3 shows R_h^2 for

---

[1] Note that HWE for the haplotypes implies HWE for each SNP individually. However it does not imply that there is no linkage disequilibrium for the SNPs; linkage disequilibrium is dependent upon the haplotype frequencies p_h which can take any positive values summing to 1.

Table 5.1 Details of the calculation of $\mathrm{Var}[E\{\delta_h(H_i)|G_i\}]$ and R_h^2 for two SNPs

Genotype, G	(0, 0)	(0, 1)	(0, 2)	(1, 0)	(1, 1)	(1, 2)	(2, 0)	(2, 1)	(2, 2)
Haplotype pair, H	{(0,0), (0,0)}	{(0,0), (0,1)}	{(0,1), (0,1)}	{(1,0), (0,0)}	{(1,0), (0,1)} {(1,1),(0,0)}	{(1,1), (0,1)}	{(1,0), (1,0)}	{(1,1), (1,0)}	{(1,1), (1,1)}
$P(G)$	p_0^2	$2p_0p_1$	p_1^2	$2p_2p_0$	$2(p_2p_1 + p_3p_0)$	$2p_3p_1$	p_2^2	$2p_3p_2$	p_3^2
$E(\delta_{h0}(H)|G)$	2	1	0	1	$\dfrac{p_3p_0}{p_2p_1 + p_3p_0}$	0	0	0	0
$E(\delta_{h1}(H)|G)$	0	1	2	0	$\dfrac{p_2p_1}{p_2p_1 + p_3p_0}$	1	0	0	0
$E(\delta_{h2}(H)|G)$	0	0	0	1	$\dfrac{p_2p_1}{p_2p_1 + p_3p_0}$	0	2	1	0
$E(\delta_{h3}(H)|G)$	0	0	0	0	$\dfrac{p_3p_0}{p_2p_1 + p_3p_0}$	1	0	1	2

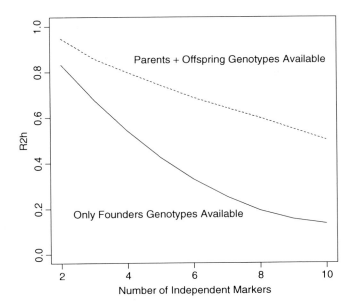

Fig. 5.2 R_h^2 for predicting haplotype h0 in the case of n independent SNPs each with frequency $= \frac{1}{2}$

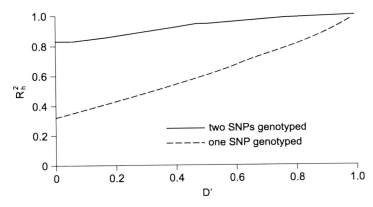

Fig. 5.3 R_h^2 for predicting haplotypes composed of two SNPs each with allele frequency of 1/2 according to standardized linkage disequilibrium coefficient D' when (**a**) two SNPs are genotyped or (**b**) when only one SNP is genotyped

two SNP haplotypes when only one of the pair of SNPs are measured, as a function of the D' statistic (which is 1 if at least one of p_0 to p_3 are zero) between the SNPs. If D' is 1, then (in the special case of SNPs both with frequency equal to $\frac{1}{2}$) genotyping only one SNP predicts haplotype counts perfectly, but with only about 30 % certainty ($R_h^2 \cong 0.3$) for $D' = 0$.

5.4 Haplotype Frequency Estimation for Larger Numbers of SNPs

If the number of SNPs, m, is large, a brute force EM algorithm used to estimate haplotype frequencies is very slow, since with 2^m possible haplotypes there are $(2^m + 1)2^{m-1}$ possible haplotype pairs, H, which are (in a naïve implementation) being summed over for each subject. However given the genotypes, G_i, for an individual, the size of the set of haplotype pairs, $[H|H \sim G_i]$, which are compatible with that data depends upon the number of heterozygous SNPs for that individual not on total m of SNPs being considered. For example, if genotype counts for 6 SNPs for a given individual are equal to $G_i = (0, 1, 2, 2, 1, 0)$, then in (5.1) only haplotype pairs of form $H = \begin{bmatrix} (0, \{1, 0\}, 1, 1, \{1, 0\}, 0) \\ (0, \{0, 1\}, 1, 1, \{0, 1\}, 0) \end{bmatrix}$ need to be considered in the summation, leaving just four pairs left. Since typically about 30–40 % of common SNPs will be heterozygous for a given subject, this alone reduces the computational burden noticeably.

5.4.1 Partition-Ligation EM Algorithm

In regions of limited recombination where the number of haplotypes is small, most of the haplotype frequency estimates p_h will rapidly approach zero in the EM algorithm. This observation suggests a simple divide-and-conquer strategy that can be used to extend the number of markers that can be utilized. This algorithm (called the *partition-ligation EM algorithm* [16]) applies the EM algorithm in "chunks" (partitions) of 5–10 markers and then performs a stitching together (ligation) of adjoining partitions, by running the EM algorithm again. In the ligation EM algorithm, the summation in (5.1) is over the cross product of the haplotypes in each partition that are estimated to have nonzero probability from the earlier EM steps. This method can be effective in estimating haplotype frequencies for 20 or more SNPs in high LD.

5.4.2 Phasing Large Numbers of SNPs

As we will see in the discussion of SNP imputation, large-scale SNP imputation using current software packages generally requires that reference panel data be phased (i.e., haplotype pairs assigned to each study participant) to begin the process. From the previous discussion, it is clear that phasing of large numbers of genotypes for a panel unrelated individuals must be inherently unreliable. For example, if as few as 7 very common SNPs are in linkage equilibrium, then the estimate of the number of copies (0, 1, or 2) of any given haplotype that are carried is predicted quite poorly (as indicated by R_h^2 in Fig. 5.2). This is overcome to some degree if data from nuclear families is available—for example, if parents and a single child are genotyped, then a doubly heterozygous parent has uncertain haplotype counts only if the child's genotypes are also doubly heterozygous and the other parent is heterozygous for at least one of the two SNPs. A calculation of haplotype uncertainty under the same assumptions as Fig. 5.2 (1–10 independent SNPs) but with sibling data also available can be done readily by simulation, by first generating independent binomial data as genotypes for the parents and then following Mendel's laws to generate random genotypes for the offspring. Running an imputation program that uses the genotype data for the children as well as the parents allows empirical estimation of the variance, $\text{Var}(E(\delta_h|G))$, of the dosage estimate for a given haplotype and comparison to the expected $2p_h(1 - p_h)$. This is shown as the dotted line in Fig. 5.2 which plots the estimate of R_h^2 computed for the parents for haplotype imputation for from 2 to 10 very common SNPs. The implication of Fig. 5.2 is that once ten or more very common SNPs in linkage equilibrium are included in the set of SNPs to be phased haplotype identification is not highly accurate. Despite this inherent uncertainty, we will see that imputed long-range phased haplotypes for the HapMap or 1000 Genomes data are routinely used as a starting point for SNP imputation.

5.5 Regression Analysis Using Haplotypes as Explanatory Variables

5.5.1 Expectation Substitution

Haplotype association testing using the expectation-substitution method for studies of unrelated subjects involves three basic steps: [1] the estimation of haplotype frequencies for all the haplotypes of the SNPs of interest; [2] the formation of estimated haplotype dosage variables, $E(\delta_h|G_i)$, for each individual i with measured genotypes G_i; and then [3] the use of these dosage variables, which we abbreviate as $\hat{\delta}_{h,i}$, as (continuous) predictor variables in the generalized linear model analysis. That is, we simply use our standard model to fit the *generalized linear regression model* (or *GLM*)

$$g[E(Y_i)] = \mu + \beta_h \hat{\delta}_{h,i}, \tag{5.2}$$

to estimate haplotype-specific effects for carriers of a 1 or more copies of a single haplotype compared to all other haplotypes (here, g is the link function, as in logistic or linear regression).

More generally estimation of all haplotype effects involves fitting the model

$$g[E(Y_i)] = \mu + \sum_h \beta_h \hat{\delta}_{h,i},\tag{5.3}$$

with the sum over the haplotypes with nonzero estimated probability.

Notice that the expectation-substitution method is extremely simple and convenient: once the haplotype dosage variables are estimated for each subject, they are used as ordinary continuous variables in generalized linear models in order to fit associations with phenotypes and disease. As just described, the models are estimating the change in mean phenotype or in log odds of disease that is associated with a one-copy increase in δ_h, i.e., we are fitting an additive or log additive model to the phenotype means or log odds, respectively. As described in Chap. 3, there may also be interest in other types of models, i.e., dominant, recessive, or unconstrained two degrees of freedom (codominant) models. Before we discuss the (minor) changes to the expectation-substitution approach that are needed to fit such models, we first consider the impact that uncertainty in the haplotype frequency estimation will have upon testing and estimation in these models.

The expectation-substitution method used both in general statistical analysis [17] and in haplotype analysis [15, 18] typically has extremely good control of the type I error rate. So long as errors in dosage estimation are *non-differential*, control of type I error rates will be preserved. The assumption of *non-differential errors* means that the haplotype dosage estimates are not predictive of disease except to the degree that they are *surrogate variables* for the true haplotype dosages. For example, in analysis of binary traits ($D = 0$ or 1), we assume that

$$\Pr(D = 1|\hat{\delta}_{h,i}, \delta_{h,i}) = \Pr(D = 1|\delta_{h,i})\tag{5.4}$$

where $\delta_{h,i}$ denotes the value of the true haplotype count δ_h for individual i. The assumption of non-differential errors can be violated if, for example, we perform haplotype frequency estimation separately for the cases and controls in a case–control study, since then the random error in haplotype frequency estimation will cause consistent differences in the estimates of $E(\delta_h|G_i)$ between cases and controls. It is important therefore to use all the data simultaneously (combining cases and controls) when haplotype frequencies are estimated.

It turns out that not only does the expectation-substitution method give correct type I error rates when $\hat{\delta}_{h,i}$ is substituted for $\delta_{h,i}$, but doing so can be shown [15] to be equivalent to performing a score test that the regression parameter β_h in (5.4) is zero in a model in which both the haplotype frequencies and the regression parameters are estimated simultaneously by maximum likelihood (ML). Thus for testing purposes, expectation substitution should have near-optimal characteristics.

Expectation-substitution methods have been noted in the exposure measurement error literature to have some biases both in effect and confidence interval estimation when used away from the null hypothesis. These biases are most important when the exposure is very influential (i.e., the magnitude of β_h is large) and where there is considerable error in the parameters (here the haplotype frequency estimates) that relates the observed data to the true exposure of interest. Rosner et al. [19] give a correction to the standard errors of an effect estimate which can be used when calibration study data is available. For haplotype analysis, simple corrections to improve the standard errors for regression parameters have not been worked out and would seem to be difficult to derive. Instead a number of authors [20–22] have considered maximum likelihood estimation of both the haplotype frequency estimates and the risk parameters in general linear regression involving haplotypes, with the hope that these methods will have better statistical properties than the expectation-substitution method.

Note that while the range of the values that $E(\delta_h|G_i)$ takes is from 0 to 2, this expectation is not necessarily equal to an integer value. Only if R_h^2 is precisely equal to 1 for that haplotype will all values be integer (0, 1, and 2). Allowing $E(\delta_h|G_i)$ to take non-integer values helps to correct for the uncertainty of haplotype estimation by removing attenuation bias.

5.5.2 Fitting Dominant, Recessive, or Two Degrees of Freedom Models for the Effect of Haplotypes

The EM algorithm can be used to compute the expectation of functions of the haplotype count; for example, we can fit a generalized linear model using a codominant (2 degrees of freedom) coding as

$$g(E(Y_i)) = \mu + \beta_1 I(\delta_{h,i} = 1) + \beta_2 I(\delta_{h,i} = 2), \tag{5.5}$$

where $I(\cdot)$ is the indicator function by replacing the indicator functions with their expectations given the observed genotype data, as

$$g(E(Y_i)) = \mu + \beta_1 E\{I(\delta_{h,i} = 1)\} + \beta_2 E\{I(\delta_{h,i} = 2)\}. \tag{5.6}$$

The expectations of the indicator functions are computed, when the EM algorithm converges, as

$$E\{I(\delta_{h,i} = 1)\} = \frac{\displaystyle\sum_{H \sim G_i} I\big(\delta_h(H) = 1\big) p_{h_1} p_{h_2}}{\displaystyle\sum_{H \sim G_i} p_{h_1} p_{h_2}} \quad \text{and}$$

$$E\{I(\delta_{h,i} = 2)\} = \frac{\displaystyle\sum_{H \sim G_i} I\big(\delta_h(H) = 2\big) p_{h_1} p_{h_2}}{\displaystyle\sum_{H \sim G_i} p_{h_1} p_{h_2}}, \tag{5.7}$$

respectively. Fitting dominant or recessive models can be performed by constraining β_1 to either equal β_2 or zero, respectively.

Alternative approaches that seem attractive but which can introduce problems are based upon first estimating the *phase* of the diploid genotype data. As described above, there are a number of programs (fastPHASE [23], BEAGLE [24], PHASE [25]) which provide estimates of the two haplotypes that each individual carries. The EM estimate as described above is not estimating haplotype phase per se. The expectations described above provide an estimate of the conditional probability that a person carries haplotype h_1 given G_i and an estimate of the conditional probability that a person carries h_2 but not the joint conditional probability that the individual carries h_1 and h_2. In order to estimate this joint probability, (5.1) needs to be adjusted to compute the expectation of the product of two indicator functions as in

$$E\{I(\delta_{h_1,i} = 1) \times I(\delta_{h_2,i} = 1)|G_i\} = \Pr\{[I(\delta_{h_1,i} = 1) \times I(\delta_{h_2,i} = 1)] = 1|G_i\}$$

$$= \frac{\sum_{H \sim G_i} I(\delta_{h_1}(H) = 1)I(\delta_{h_2}(H) = 1)p_{h_1}p_{h_2}}{\sum_{H \sim G_i} p_{h_1}p_{h_2}}.$$

$$(5.8)$$

Essentially phasing programs like fastPHASE estimate these probabilities for many pairs of haplotypes and then nominate the haplotype pair with the greatest probability as the *phased data* for subject i.

It is tempting to apply a program such as fastPHASE over the region of interest and then to use the estimated pair of haplotypes, $\hat{H}_i$, as if they were actually equal to the unknown H_i and to treat δ_h as known when fitting models (5.2) or (5.5). However this approach introduces attenuation bias (bias of the regression parameter estimates towards zero) and can also reduce power to reject a false null hypothesis relative to the expectation-substitution approach [18, 26]. In general, the use of phased data when fitting models in (5.4) or (5.5) for association analysis produces less reliable estimates than the regression substitution method.

5.5.2.1 Global Test for Haplotype Effects

Haplotype dosages estimated for the haplotypes in a given region can be used in several different ways to construct tests and assign significant levels to the results of the analysis. Besides the testing for the effects (on phenotypes) of single haplotypes, global tests of the null hypothesis can be constructed by fitting all haplotype dosage variables simultaneously. For example, suppose that in a given region or haplotype block there are r haplotypes and we wish to examine whether any of the haplotypes are (linearly) related to the phenotype. The model we are interested in is

$$g(E(Y_i)) = \mu + \beta_1 \delta_{h_1 i} + \beta_2 \delta_{h_2 i} + \cdots + \beta_r \delta_{h_r i} \tag{5.9}$$

and the null hypothesis of interest is $\beta_1 = \beta_2 = \cdots = \beta_r = 0$. This hypothesis can be tested by comparing the log likelihood of the null model (with only μ) to that of the full model, fit by expectation substitution. Several practical issues arise in this testing. First the model of (5.9) is (not surprisingly) over-parameterized. Specifically for each subject, the sum of the haplotype dosage variables is equal to 2, so that imposing a constraint is needed to make the model identifiable. A typical analysis such as [27] drops the most common haplotype from the model so that the mean phenotypes of carriers of one or more of the all the less common haplotypes are compared to carriers of two copies of the most common haplotype which serves as the baseline comparison group (now captured by the estimate of μ). When haplotypes are made up of more than just a few, SNPs certain of the haplotypes are likely to be present but in low frequency. Since power to detect the effects of rare haplotypes can be limited (and also convergence problems may arise in the IRWLS algorithm used to fit a model that includes very sparse covariates), it may not be useful to include all rare haplotypes in model (5.9) individually. If the terms β_j that correspond to rare haplotypes are simply dropped from the model, then whatever effect that these haplotypes have is mixed into the effect of the baseline (most common) haplotype. Separating the effects of the rare haplotypes from the common haplotypes is accomplished by computing the sum of all haplotype counts for haplotypes of less than some frequency and using this sum as a composite (rare haplotype) effect. Thus for practical purposes, if h_1 is the most common haplotype and h_k through h_r are all rare haplotypes, then model (5.9) can be modified as

$$g(E(Y_i)) = \mu + \beta_2 \delta_{h_2, i} + \beta_3 \delta_{h_3, i} + \cdots + \beta_{k-1} \delta_{h_{k-1}, i}$$
$$+ \beta_{\text{rare}} \left(\delta_{h_k, i} + \delta_{h_{k+1}, i} + \cdots + \delta_{h_r, i} \right).$$

Here all the β estimates relate to the differences in phenotype expected value compared to individuals carrying two copies of the most common haplotype.

5.6   Dealing with Uncertainty in Haplotype Estimation in Association Testing

5.6.1   Full Likelihood Estimation of Risk Parameters and Haplotype Frequencies

We now consider maximum likelihood methods for jointly estimating the regression parameters in the (additive) model:

$$g[E(Y_i)] = \mu + \sum_h \beta_h \delta_{h,i}, \tag{5.10}$$

where $\delta_{h,i}$ is the count (0, 1, or 2) of copies of haplotype h carried by subject i. For the time being, we ignore issues of population structure or relatedness among subjects and concentrate on studies in which both HWE equilibrium (for all haplotype counts and hence all markers as well) and independence (between Y_i and Y_j for $i \neq j$) can be assumed.

Assuming initially that there has been no explicit sampling on case–control status the likelihood to be maximized is

$$
\begin{aligned}
\prod_i \Pr(Y_i, G_i) &= \prod_i \sum_H \Pr(Y_i, G_i, H_i) \\
&= \prod_i \sum_H \Pr(Y_i|H, G_i)\Pr(H, G_i) = \prod_i \sum_{H \sim G_i} \Pr(Y_i|H)\Pr(H),
\end{aligned}
$$

here the likelihood is a function of both the haplotype frequency parameters p_h and the regression parameters in model (5.10). Under HWE $\Pr(H)$ is simply $p_{h_1}p_{h_2}$ as in (5.1). The removal of G_i from $\Pr(Y_i|H, G_i)$ and $\Pr(H,G_i)$ follows because any genotype count can be constructed as the sum of the counts of the haplotypes that contain the alleles counted in G_i.

A generalized EM algorithm [20], which is based upon formulae described in [28] which can be used to maximize this likelihood, involves the following steps:

1. Given an initial set of parameter estimates for each of the parameters μ and each pair of haplotype frequencies p_h and haplotype effects β_h, a calculation of the conditional expected value of the vector of score statistics for the regression parameters is performed. This expectation is obtained by first computing, for each subject i, the score contributions, $S_i(\mu, \beta|G_i)$ as a weighted average of $S_i(\mu, \beta|H)$ with the weights being equal to $\Pr(H|G_i, Y_i; \mu, \beta, \mathbf{p})$ (where $\mathbf{p}$ is the set of haplotype frequencies) which are computed as:

$$\Pr\{H = (h_1, h_2)|G, Y)\} = \frac{I(H \sim G)\Pr(Y|H)p_{h_1}p_{h_2}}{\sum_{H' \sim G} \Pr(Y|H')p_{h_1}p_{h_2}}. \tag{5.11}$$

2. Computing a pseudo information matrix $\iota'(\mu, \beta)_i$ as the weighted average over all possible H of the contributions of individual i to the information matrix $\iota(\mu, \beta|H)_i$ given H with the weights again equal to $\Pr\{H = (h_1, h_2)|G, Y)\}$.
3. Summing over i to compute the total score vector $S(\mu, \beta)$ and pseudo information matrix $i'(\mu, \beta)$.
4. Updating the parameter vector as $(\mu^{\text{new}}, \beta^{\text{new}})^{\text{T}} = (\mu^{\text{new}}, \beta^{\text{old}})^{\text{T}} + i'(\mu^{\text{old}}, \beta^{\text{old}})^{-1} S(\mu^{\text{old}}, \beta^{\text{old}})$.

We call $l'(\mu,\beta)$ a pseudo information matrix since computing the proper information matrix in the course of an EM algorithm involves additional calculation as described in [28]. Since the expectation given in (5.11) depends upon the imperfectly known population haplotype frequencies, updating of these frequencies with each new estimate of β_h formally becomes part of the step (4) as well. The updating of the haplotype frequencies is now modified from those given in (5.1) as

$$p_h^{\text{new}} = \frac{1}{2N}\sum_i E\big(\delta_h(H)\big|G_i,Y_i\big) = \frac{1}{2N}\sum_{i=1}^{n}\sum_{H\sim G_i}\delta_h(H)\Pr\big(H\big|Y_i,G_i;\alpha^{\text{old}},\beta^{\text{old}},p^{\text{old}}\big).$$

5.6.2   Ascertainment in Case–Control Studies

Case–control sampling leads to the enrichment of cases with high-risk haplotypes (those where $\beta_h > 0$) thereby distorting our estimates of haplotype frequencies p_h and possibly violating the assumption of Hardy–Weinberg equilibrium in the combined data. In order to deal with the complications due to case–control sampling, we adopt a simplistic "view" of the way in which case–control data has been ascertained [20]. This approach is appropriate when 1) frequency matching, rather than individual matching, of cases to controls is utilized and 2) the disease rate in the underlying population is known. We make here the simplifying assumption that cases in the underlying population were chosen randomly with known probability π_1 and that controls were chosen randomly with known probability π_0. Thus an approximation to the full likelihood of the case–control dataset [29] is

$$\prod_i \Pr\big(Y_i,G_i\big|\text{subject } i \text{ is sampled}\big) = \prod_i \frac{\pi_{Y_i}\Pr\big(Y_i\big|G_i\big)\Pr(G_i)}{\pi_1\Pr(Y=1)+\pi_0\Pr(Y=0)}. \tag{5.12}$$

By summation over the haplotypes, this can be written as

$$\frac{\prod_i \pi_{Y_i}\sum_{H\sim G_i}\Pr\big(Y_i\big|H_i\big)\,p_{h_2}p_{h_2}}{\left[\sum_{\text{all } H}\big\{\pi_1\Pr\big(Y=1\big|H\big)\,p_{h_1}p_{h_2}+\pi_0\Pr\big(Y=0\big|H\big)\,p_{h_1}p_{h_2}\big\}\right]^N}. \tag{5.13}$$

In order to estimate simultaneously all parameters in the likelihood (5.13), we first estimate initial values for all the p_h by using the standard EM algorithm (if there are large numbers of SNPs, we use an implementation of the partition-ligation EM algorithm of [16]). This is equivalent to maximizing (5.13) with an initial value of $\beta = 0$. Then we drop from further consideration all haplotype frequency parameters which are estimated in this first stage that have smaller estimated frequency than a fixed positive constant (we used $\varepsilon = 0.001$ for the calculations for the example below). We then construct the full score and full information matrix for all remaining parameters. This is done by using the Louis formulae for the likelihood in the numerator in (5.13) and then by subtracting the first and (minus the) second derivatives of the log of the denominator from the appropriate elements of the resulting score and information. These calculations allow for a full Newton–Raphson update for all parameters simultaneously which can be used iteratively to compute the final ascertainment-corrected estimates. Inverting the matrix of second derivatives can be problematic when there are numerous low-frequency haplotypes being considered. It is for this reason that we drop the lowest-frequency haplotypes from the computations.

A number of other authors [21, 22, 30] have discussed maximum likelihood or related approaches to haplotype analysis for case–control studies; the main difference between the approach outlined above and the other examinations has to do with the details of case–control ascertainment, for example, the analysis of individually matched rather than frequency matched case–control involves analysis of the conditional likelihood function rather than the unconditional, ascertainment-corrected likelihood described above.

5.6.3   Example: Expectation-Substitution Method

This section uses data originally published in Stram et al. [20]. The data are for a nested case–control study of a candidate gene (CYP17) in breast cancer. The expectation substitution uses a partition-ligation version of the EM algorithm (originally written in Fortran 90) called from an R function named "expected_haplotypes." This function takes genotype count data from unrelated individuals and returns an object that contains (1) a list of haplotypes with nonzero frequency, (2) the frequency of each such haplotype, and (3) the estimated haplotype count data for each haplotype for each individual. To see how this works, we first reproduce the haplotype frequency estimates for the controls in the study as given in Stram et al. The dataset CYP17_breast_WH_cases_and_controls.dat can be read into R as follows:

```
> source("expected_haplotypes.r")
> x<-read.table("Cyp17_WHCases_and_Controls.dat")
> IDs<-as.character(x[,1]) # ID variable
> cc<-x[,2] # the second column is case control status
> nsnps<-dim(x)[2]-3
> SNPTable<-as.matrix(x[,4:(nsnps+3)])
> # select the controls only for analysis
> controlh<-expected_haplotypes(IDs[cc==0],SNPTable[cc==0,])
```

The return value (here *controlh*) is a list with elements *controlh$hfreqs* (a sorted list of haplotype frequencies), *controlh$ids* (which gives back the IDs used in the call), and *controlh$haps* which provides the predicted haplotype counts for each subject. We can view the haplotype frequencies by entering:

```
> controlh$hfreqs
               [,1]
h000000 0.3806501323
h111001 0.2275617725
h000010 0.1819039683
h110101 0.0945781746
h000001 0.0414222222
h011001 0.0340137566
h111000 0.0125899471
h010000 0.0076760582
h001001 0.0068908730
h000011 0.0065330688
h101011 0.0020357143
h010011 0.0018878307
h100000 0.0012752646
h100001 0.0009822751
```

Recomputing the haplotype frequencies using the cases and controls in order to use the predicted haplotypes in a model for case–control status is accomplished as:

```
> h_all<-expected_haplotypes(IDs,SNPTable)
```

Upon examination of *h_all$hfreqs*, we see that there are now four haplotypes with estimated frequency greater than 5 % and these constitute 88 % of all segregating haplotypes. Using each of these haplotypes in turn to fit regression models is accomplished as:

```
> summary(glm(cc~h_all$haps[,1],family=binomial()))
> summary(glm(cc~h_all$haps[,2] ,family=binomial()))
> summary(glm(cc~h_all$haps[,3]) ,family=binomial())
> summary(glm(cc~h_all$haps[,4]) ,family=binomial())
```

The results show modestly significant results for haplotype h000000 (log OR = -0.26119, std err. = 0.11530, $p = 0.0235$) comparing carriers of this (most common) haplotype to all others. The global test for the significance of any of the first 4 haplotypes can be accomplished by first fitting the null model and calculating the deviance (978.24) and then the deviance of the model that includes the haplotypes (2–4) and adds an additional variable calculated as the sum of all rare haplotypes so that haplotypes (2–4) will be compared to the most common haplotype. This is accomplished as:

```
> rare<-rowSums(h_all$haps[,5:20])
> summary(glm(cc~h_all$haps[,2:4]+rare,family=binomial()))
```

The change in deviance from the null model is equal to $978.24–970.38 = 7.86$ on 4 df ($p = 0.097$) so that again the evidence for any haplotype effect is only modest. There is some indication of risk associated with carrying the third most common haplotype (h000010) compared to the most common (h000000)

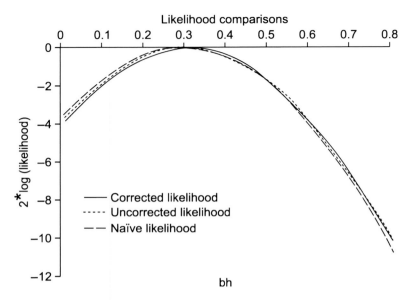

Fig. 5.4 Comparisons of three profile likelihoods based on the approaches described in the text. The naïve likelihood refers to the profile likelihood from the expectation-substitution method

($p = 0.0205$), but enthusiasm for this finding is tempered by the fact that the overall test is not strongly significant.

A detailed analysis of profile likelihoods from three different methods to fit the first model (comparing haplotype h000000 to all the other haplotypes) to these data is given in Stram et al. [20]. The three methods compared are:

1. Expectation substitution.
2. Full likelihood analysis without any case–control sampling ascertainment correction.
3. Full likelihood analysis including the ascertainment correction (5.13) with selection probabilities $\pi_0 = 0.002$ for controls and $\pi_1 = 1$ for cases.

Figure 5.4 is from that paper. The profile likelihoods at each point on the curves are obtained from these data by holding the log odds ratio parameter, β_{00000}, corresponding to h000000, fixed at the value given on the x-axis while maximizing out the other parameters in the model, and then calculating the log likelihood of that maximized model which is then displayed on the y-axis. For the expectation-substitution method, the only other parameter is the intercept parameter μ which incorporates "all other" haplotypes. For the two full likelihood methods, the estimates of the haplotype frequencies p_h are also being simultaneously maximized out as the value of β_{000000} is fixed at each point shown on the x-axis.

Note that, for this example at least, there is no important difference between the three likelihoods or between inferences using them. The far simpler expectation-substitution approach appears to have provided an adequate analysis including appropriate standard errors in this instance. Simulation studies tend to support this general finding, i.e., that there is little evidence of bias in the expectation-substitution method for dealing with haplotype imputation. Simulation work [26] tends to show that acceptable type I error coverage and good coverage of confidence intervals under both the null and alternative hypotheses are retained by the expectation-substitution method.

5.7 Haplotype Analysis Genome-Wide

Consider now the problem of performing haplotype risk estimation, where haplotypes are made up of contiguous SNPs either in haplotype blocks, which may be defined in a number of different ways, or are grouped together using windowing methods.

5.7.1 Studies of Homogeneous Non-admixed Populations

As in Chap. 4, correction for population structure, admixture, and possibly for hidden relatedness between subjects is an important issue in single SNP analysis, and these considerations carry over into haplotype analysis. Within homogeneous populations, Hardy–Weinberg equilibrium can be assumed for most markers and marker haplotypes so that (5.1) applies for the population (except possibly for haplotypes under strong selective pressures). Note that in case–control studies, it can generally be assumed that HWE holds for the controls (especially for a rare disease) but not for the cases, because selection of high-risk haplotypes could have distorted the underlying haplotype frequencies. However, as mentioned previously, ignoring this distortion in allele frequencies still leads to valid tests of the null hypothesis, for the simple reason that under the null, HWE will hold for the combination of cases and controls, so that using the expectation-substitution method gives an appropriate score test [14, 15].

If genome-wide SNP data is available, then either a block-based or sliding window-based method can be considered in order to look for contiguous SNPs, the haplotypes of which are predictive of (unknown) variation related to phenotypes or disease.

The block-based approach of Gabriel et al. [2], which is the most common method used to visualize LD blocks, has an important drawback when it comes to defining groups of SNPs to be used in haplotype association; specifically many SNPs are declared by the algorithm to not be in blocks at all. However minor adjustments in the details of the block definition (specifically the values of D' and confidence intervals computed for D' used in the algorithm implemented in

Haploview) can cause SNPs outside blocks to be included in blocks or the reverse. For example, in Fig. 5.5 one third of the common SNPs in a small region in chromosome 8q24 for the CEU population are found with the default Gabriel et al. block definitions in Haploview to be outside of blocks. Relatively minor adjustments will determine whether these SNPs are included in blocks or not, and overall this region appears to be of relatively high LD.

An alternative to a block-based approach is windowing, in which a window of a certain size—the number of contiguous markers to be included in the window—is determined and then either overlapping or nonoverlapping windows are placed over the region of interest. Within each window, haplotype frequencies are estimated and the expectation-substitution method is used to investigate haplotype-specific risk. An inflexible window size (especially if it is quite short) will produce many correlated tests when it is run over regions of very high linkage disequilibrium, but if the window size is too large, then haplotypes in regions in low LD will each be of very low frequency. A more flexible approach is to allow the window size to be larger in regions of high linkage disequilibrium and smaller in regions of low LD. A compromise approach is to define haplotype blocks according to some reasonable criteria but to include, using a windowing method, SNPs outside of blocks using a short window size.

Overlapping (sliding) and nonoverlapping windows have been considered as an approach for discovery of haplotype effects. While offering a more comprehensive examination of each region, the downside to using sliding or otherwise overlapping windows in haplotype analysis is the increase in computation time and the increases in difficulty in obtaining type I error bounds for global significance. The Bonferroni method certainly will be poorly performing in such a setting since overlapping windows will have very similar haplotypes. Adjustments to the Bonferroni method using permutation methods and approximations [31–34] are possible.

5.7.2   The Four-Gamete Rule for Fast Block Definition

A very simple approach to estimating haplotype blocks is based upon the four-gamete rule. This rule is one of the methods implemented in Haploview for block definition, and it is also extremely simple to compute in R or in other appropriate languages. As described above, we can show that the presence of all four possible haplotypes (a-b, A-b, a-B, and A-B) of two SNPs (with alleles a and A and b and B, respectively) is evidence (under an infinite sites approximation) for the occurrence of recombination between these two loci. A very quick way of checking, using the genotype data alone without having to impute haplotypes, whether there is evidence of recombination is to form the 3×3 table of minor allele counts for each SNP as given in Table 5.2.

Note that if any of n_{00}, n_{01}, or n_{10} are nonzero, then this implies that haplotype a-b must be present. Similarly, if any of n_{10}, n_{20}, and n_{21} are nonzero, then haplotype A-b must be present. Extending this to the other "corners" of the table leads to the rule that

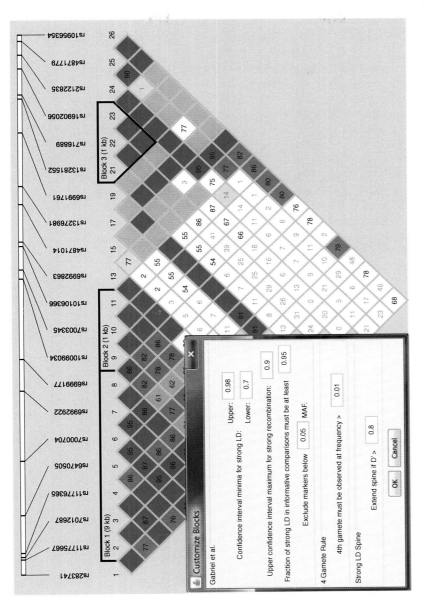

Fig. 5.5 Haploview plot of LD pattern for 26 SNPs in region 8q24. Block definitions are based on the Gabriel et al.'s default criteria shown in the *Customize Blocks dialog box*. Minor modifications in the default parameters determine whether or not SNPs labeled as 13–19 or 24–26 are included in the *block* now encompassing only SNPs 20–22. Data based on HapMap phase 2 CEU participants

Table 5.2 Genotype data for two SNPs; the body of the table contains counts of the number of individuals with the listed genotype combination

	Genotypes for SNP 1		
Genotypes for SNP 2	Aa	aA	AA
bb	n_{00}	n_{10}	n_{20}
bB	n_{01}	n_{11}	n_{21}
BB	n_{02}	n_{12}	n_{22}

if all of the quantities $(n_{00} + n_{10} + n_{01})$, $(n_{10} + n_{20} + n_{21})$, $(n_{21} + n_{22} + n_{12})$, and $(n_{01} + n_{12} + n_{02})$ are greater than zero, then all four haplotypes must be present and therefore a recombination can be assumed to have occurred. This "four corners" rule can be checked rapidly while blocks are being defined. Note that the frequency of haplotype a-a is at least equal to $(2n_{00} + n_{10} + n_{01})/2n$ with the only uncertain contribution being the number of copies of haplotype a-b that contributed to n_{11} since individuals in this cell have uncertain haplotypes (either (a-b, A-B) or (a-B, A-b)). A reasonable relaxation of the four-gamete rule allows the minimum of $(2n_{00} + n_{10} + n_{01})/2n$ and the other similar quantities for the other haplotypes to be nonzero but "small," while blocks are extended from an initial starting point. Checking all pairs of SNPs in this fashion as blocks are extended is thus a simple, easy to implement, and quite fast block formation rule.

5.7.3   Multiple Comparisons in Haplotype Analysis

The global test based on fitting model (5.9) is useful because it can help us (in the course of a windowing or haplotype-block-based analysis) to identify regions of interest for which more detailed examination may subsequently be undertaken. Considering regions in which there is no recombination between markers (i.e., in an idealized haplotype block), three useful facts are worth noting. First of all if the haplotype-type frequencies are known (and consistent with no recombination), then there is no haplotype uncertainty; all the dosage variables for all the haplotypes will take integer values 0, 1, or 2 equal to the true haplotype counts. Secondly the likelihood ratio test constructed for a global test of no haplotype effects will be precisely the same test as the likelihood ratio test of no SNP effects, i.e., the likelihood obtained fitting model (5.9) will be the same as the likelihood obtained by fitting the model

$$g(E(Y_i)) = \mu + \beta_1 G_{i1} + \beta_2 G_{i2} + \cdots + \beta_s G_{is} \qquad (5.14)$$

where s is the number of SNPs in the region and G_{ij} are the genotype counts for SNP j for subject i. This model may also be over-parameterized, not because of the inclusion of μ, but because some of the markers may be perfectly correlated with each other. Specifically for a given set of s SNPs, there can be at most $s + 1$ nonrecombinant haplotypes (and there are often far less in long haplotype blocks), so that in the absence of recombination, the degrees of freedom obtained by fitting equation (5.14) will be equal to $r - 1$ just as when fitting model (5.9).

Bearing this in mind, a reasonably fast haplotype-block-based search for haplotype effects may be considered genome-wide as follows:

1. Use the four-gamete rule to define haplotype blocks as in the previous algorithm.
2. Compute likelihood ratio or score tests for model (5.14) using standard regression software.
3. For haplotype blocks for which the global test is significant (see below), examine haplotype effects more carefully by first imputing dosage variables for all haplotypes and then fitting models such as (5.9) or (5.2).

If only SNPs showing no (or little) evidence of historical recombination are to be considered in genome-wide haplotype analysis, then (as follows from the above discussion) the effective number of tests in a haplotype analysis is very similar to the effective number of tests that are performed using SNP markers alone (i.e., after taking account of LD). Thus similar criteria for global significance ($p < 10^{-8}$ or so) is likely to be useful for block-based haplotype analysis.

5.8 Multiple Populations

Haplotype analysis in multiple populations raises some interesting issues. Since LD structure changes, sometimes dramatically, between long-separated populations, the indirect use of haplotype analysis to search for unknown variants that may be in higher LD with SNP haplotypes than with individual SNPs may be attenuated in power by the inclusion of multiple groups. Even if the same unobserved variant is present and biologically related to phenotype or disease susceptibility in all groups, it may not be associated with the same haplotype or group of haplotypes in each group. On the other hand as emphasized below, haplotypes of known variants themselves may be disease- or phenotype-related biologically, and therefore it is worth discussing the issue of multiple ethnic groups for haplotype analysis.

A standard approach taken in such papers as Haiman et al. [27], who analyzed data from the CYP19 gene (like CYP17, CYP19 is a candidate gene for breast cancer), is to estimate haplotype frequencies separately for each racial/ethnic group included in a given analysis. This may be important since HWE, which underlies the EM algorithm, is violated when data for multiple populations are combined. To give some idea of the importance of this, we compare two different methods for predicting haplotype frequencies for African-American participants in the sub-study used for haplotype discovery in Haiman et al. First we use the 70 - African-American subjects with dense genotyping for this gene to estimate the haplotype frequencies for the African Americans and produce the haplotype frequency estimates for these same subjects for 22 SNPs in "block 1" of this gene. *R* code to do this using the data for CYP19 is shown below:

```
> AA<-read.table("aa.dat")
> AA_IDs<-as.character(AA[,1])
> nsnps<-22
> AA<-AA[,1:(25+nsnps)] # drop all but 22 SNPs of actual interest
> AA_SNPTable<-as.matrix(AA[,4:(nsnps*2+3)])
> ha<-expected_haplotypes(AA_IDs,as.matrix(AA_SNPTable),code=2)
> # code=2 means 2 numbers per SNP
```

We next perform haplotype imputation using a total of 5 ethnic groups (whites, African Americans, Latinos, Japanese Americans, and Native Hawaiians) in one run (rather than separately) to compute haplotype comparing the haplotype imputations on the African-American data from this run with the imputations from the "African-American-only" data derived above:

```
> All<-read.table("all.dat") # read data for 5 ethnic groups
> IDs<-as.character(All[,1])
> race<-as.character(All[,2]);
> nsnps<-22
> All_SNPTable<-as.matrix(All[,4:(nsnps*2+3)])# 22 SNPs read with 2 columns
per SNP
> hall<-expected_haplotypes(IDs,All_SNPTable,code=2)
> AAlist<-(race=="A") # select the African Americans
> # The most common AA haplotype is the 2nd most common in the overall data
so
> plot(ha$haps[,1],hall$haps[AAlist,2]) # plots the two dosage estimates for
the same haplotype
```

Figure 5.6 shows the resulting plot. While the two dosage estimates are similar for most individuals, in several instances the estimates are quite different, emphasizing that haplotype imputation is sensitive to population stratification. However

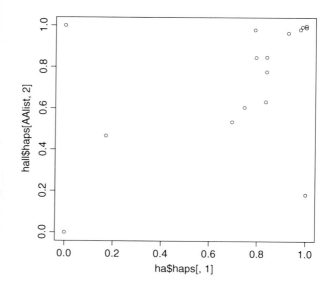

Fig. 5.6 Plot of predicted number of copies of the most common haplotypes in the African-American group, using either (*x*-axis) only the African-American group as the reference or (*y*-axis) all five ethnic groups combined

the overall correlation between the two imputations is high at about 0.92; there is a large mass at (0, 0) that is not obvious in this plot. Looking through additional plots (see file *haplotype_predictions.r*) finds that other common haplotypes are similarly predicted for this example, i.e., when changing the reference panel from only African Americans to all groups combined, the estimates of δ_h for the common haplotypes h are generally similar but with some outlying values. In this example, the haplotypes being imputed consisted of 22-SNP haplotypes, and this is probably more SNPs that would customarily be examined in this way.

5.9   Chapter Summary

Haplotype analysis is an important part of association testing since haplotype analysis can be sensitive to unmeasured variants for which single SNP analysis may miss. Haplotype imputation for common haplotypes among a set of SNPs with limited historical recombination can be highly accurate and a variety of methods are applicable to this problem. Limitations exist on the ability of any algorithm to reconstruct haplotypes in regions of high recombination rates or for very long haplotypes especially if family data is not available.

We have emphasized relatively simple EM-based techniques that permit fitting of regression parameters for generalized linear model estimation including logistic or normal regression analysis for studies of unrelated subjects. The problem of accounting for uncertainty in haplotype imputation given only genotype data for unrelated subjects has similarities to other measurement error problems in epidemiological analysis, and simple methods that work reasonably well in that setting are useful generally here as well.

Most of the above discussion has treated haplotypes as surrogates for unmeasured variants, but of course haplotypes may themselves be the causal variants. Two or more potentially causal variants may themselves only have an effect, or their effects may be enhanced, if they fall upon the same chromosome (e.g., [4]).

It is possible that causal haplotypes could include SNPs that are not in very high linkage disequilibrium with each other, and so the restriction of interest to haplotypes only made up of neighboring SNPs (as in haplotype block or windowing methods) may be too strict. A search over wide regions in the genome for such long-range haplotype effects would by necessity have to involve only 2 or possibly 3 SNPs since using any more vastly increases the number of comparisons to be tested and would increase the uncertainty in haplotype estimation. Nevertheless it would be interesting to consider, in a scan, estimation of phenotype or risk effects of all two or three SNP haplotypes of all SNPs that lie within a centimorgan or so of each other. While this is a large number of haplotypes, it is much smaller than the number of pairwise or three-way interactions between all SNPs in the human genome which has sometimes been considered [35–37]. Moreover, haplotypes containing SNPs up to several centimorgans in distance away (several megabases) from each other could potentially contribute to the additive heritability of a trait, since the haplotype will be inherited mostly as an intact unit, even though over past history recombinations have occurred. The same is not true of interactions between SNPs more distant than this—i.e., these interaction effects would not make a significant contribution to the heritability of a trait, except for the most closely related individuals, because they would rarely be passed on to more distant descendants, see Chap. 8 for discussion of GWAS-based heritability analysis.

Recently Hu and Lin [38] have shown in a slightly different setting (SNP rather than haplotype imputation) that when haplotypes involving unmeasured SNPs (i.e., SNPs seen in a reference panel but not genotyped) are to be imputed, the statistical behavior of the ML methods may represent an important improvement over the substitution approach under the alternative hypothesis. That is, the ML estimates of haplotype-specific risk have less bias and likelihood-based confidence intervals for β_h have better coverage properties. Again, however, these benefits are mainly seen when the true magnitudes of β_h are quite large; tests for $\beta_h = 0$ based upon the expectation-substitution approach were observed by Hu and Lin to retain good type I error properties and to be reasonably powerful compared to ML.

Homework

1. Show that if the mean of outcome Y is linear in the count, δ_h, of haplotype h but if δ_h is unmeasured, then the expected value of Y is also linear (with the same slope parameter) in the expected count $E(\delta_h|G)$ where G are the measured genotypes. Assume non-differential errors in estimating δ_h

2. Estimate R_h^2 as the ratio of the observed variance over the expected variance, $2p_h$ $(1 - p_h)$, for all the counts of common and rare haplotypes seen in the CYP17 or CYP19 example. Is there a relationship between haplotype frequency, p_h, and R_h^2 in these data?

3. Using the R function *expected_haplotypes* in *expected_haplotypes.r*, predict haplotype counts separately for cases and controls in the CYP17 example. As described above, this leads to differential error in the estimation. How serious is this error?

    (a) Compared to using all the samples, how different are the haplotype counts for the common haplotypes when cases are imputed separately from controls?

    (b) When the haplotype counts are used in logistic regression, do the results of the analysis appear to be the same as in the text above?

    Note: Follow directions in the *expected_haplotypes.r* file for setting up the call to the program tagSNPs that does the actual imputation.

4. Use a different program, one or more of BEAGLE [39], IMPUTE2 [40], or MACH [41], see links below, to impute haplotype dosage for the same SNPs in the CYP17 or CYP19 example. How do the results of these programs compare to each other and to the output of the *expected_haplotypes* function?

5. Download the program HAPSTAT [42]. This program implements maximum likelihood estimation and correction for haplotype uncertainty in estimation of disease associations. Try this program on the CYP17 example data and compare to the results shown in the text using the expectation-substitution approach.

6. Review the haplotype-based association tests that are implemented in the program PLINK; which tests and analyses described above can be implemented (e.g., logistic or linear regression testing for individual haplotype effects and joint tests for no haplotype effects)? If you have access to the JAPC data, consider haplotype analysis using PLINK of the 8q24 region, a region that has many strong SNP associations. Are any of the haplotype associations stronger than nearby SNP associations?

Links

BEAGLE genetic analysis software program http://faculty.washington.edu/brow ning/beagle/beagle.html

IMPUTE2 Genotype imputation and haplotype phasing program http://mathgen. stats.ox.ac.uk/impute/impute_v2.html

MACH Markov Chain based haplotyper. http://www.sph.umich.edu/csg/abecasis/ MaCH/

HAPSTAT: Software for the statistical analysis of haplotype–disease association. http://dlin.web.unc.edu/software/hapstat/

References

1. Daly, M. J., Rioux, J., Schaffner, S., Hudson, T., & Lander, E. (2001). High-resolution haplotype structure in the human genome. *Nature Genetics, 29*, 229–232.

2. Gabriel, S. B., Schaffner, S. F., Nguyen, H., Moore, J. M., Roy, J., Blumenstiel, B., et al. (2002). The structure of haplotype blocks in the human genome. *Science, 296*, 2225–2229.

3. Barrett, J. C., Fry, B., Maller, J., & Daly, M. J. (2005). Haploview: Analysis and visualization of LD and haplotype maps. *Bioinformatics, 21*, 263–265.

4. Nackley, A. G., Shabalina, S. A., Tchivileva, I. E., Satterfield, K., Korchynskyi, O., Makarov, S. S., et al. (2006). Human catechol-O-methyltransferase haplotypes modulate protein expression by altering mRNA secondary structure. *Science, 314*, 1930–1933.

5. Roten, L. T., Fenstad, M. H., Forsmo, S., Johnson, M. P., Moses, E. K., Austgulen, R., et al. (2011). A low COMT activity haplotype is associated with recurrent preeclampsia in a Norwegian population cohort (HUNT2). *Molecular Human Reproduction, 17*, 439–446.

6. Zhang, J., Chen, Y., Zhang, K., Yang, H., Sun, Y., Fang, Y., et al. (2010). A cis-phase interaction study of genetic variants within the MAOA gene in major depressive disorder. *Biological Psychiatry, 68*, 795–800.

7. Alfadhli, S., AlTamimy, B., AlSaeid, K., & Haider, M. (2011). Endothelial nitric oxide synthase gene haplotype association with systemic lupus erythematosus. *Lupus, 20*, 700–708.

8. Mouaffak, F., Kebir, O., Bellon, A., Gourevitch, R., Tordjman, S., Viala, A., et al. (2011). Association of an UCP4 (SLC25A27) haplotype with ultra-resistant schizophrenia. *Pharmacogenomics, 12*, 185–193.

9. Chen, H. Y., Chan, I. H., Sham, A. L., Leung, V. H., Ma, S. L., Ho, S. C., et al. (2011). Haplotype effect in the IGF1 promoter accounts for the association between microsatellite and serum IGF1 concentration. *Clinical Endocrinology, 74*, 520–527.

10. Lee, Y. J., Huang, C. Y., Ting, W. H., Lee, H. C., Guo, W. L., Chen, W. F., et al. (2011). Association of an IL-4 gene haplotype with Graves disease in children: Experimental study and meta-analysis. *Human Immunology, 72*, 256–261.

11. Cheong, H. S., Park, B. L., Kim, E. M., Park, C. S., Sohn, J. W., Kim, B. J., et al. (2011). Association of RANBP1 haplotype with smooth pursuit eye movement abnormality. *American Journal of Medical Genetics Part B: Neuropsychiatric Genetics, 156B*, 67–71.

12. Stram, D. O., Haiman, C. A., Hirschhorn, J. N., Altshuler, D., Kolonel, L. N., Henderson, B. E., et al. (2003). Choosing haplotype-tagging SNPs based on unphased genotype data from a preliminary sample of unrelated subjects with an example from the Multiethnic Cohort Study. *Human Heredity, 55*.

13. Excoffier, L., & Slatkin, M. (1995). Maximum-likelihood estimation of molecular haplotype frequencies in a diploid population. *Molecular and Biological Evolution, 12*, 921–927.

14. Zaykin, D. V., Westfall, P. H., Young, S. S., Karnoub, M. A., Wagner, M. J., & Ehm, M. G. (2002). Testing association of statistically inferred haplotypes with discrete and continuous traits in samples of unrelated individuals. *Human Heredity, 53*, 79–91.

15. Xie, R., & Stram, D. O. (2005). Asymptotic equivalence between two score tests for haplotype-specific risk in general linear models. *Genetic Epidemiology, 29*, 166–170.

16. Qin, Z. S., Niu, T., & Liu, J. S. (2002). Partition-ligation-expectation-maximization algorithm for haplotype inference with single-nucleotide polymorphisms. *The American Journal of Human Genetics, 71*, 1242–1247.

17. Carroll, R. J., Ruppert, D., Stefanski, L. A., & Crainiceanu, C. (2006). *Measurement error in nonlinear models: A modern perspective* (2nd ed.). New York, NY: Chapman and Hall.

18. Kraft, P., Cox, D. G., Paynter, R. A., Hunter, D., & De Vivo, I. (2005). Accounting for haplotype uncertainty in matched association studies: A comparison of simple and flexible techniques. *Genetic Epidemiology, 28*, 261–272.

19. Rosner, B., Spiegelman, D., & Willett, W. (1992). Correction of logistic relative risk estimates and confidence intervals for random within-person measurement error. *American Journal of Epidemiology, 136*, 1400–1409.

20. Stram, D. O., Pearce, C. L., Bretsky, P., Freedman, M., Hirschhorn, J. N., Altshuler, D., et al. (2003). Modeling and E-M estimation of haplotype-specific relative risks from genotype data for a case–control study of unrelated individuals. *Human Heredity, 55*, 179–190.

21. Lin, D. Y., & Zeng, D. (2006). Likelihood-based inference on haplotype effects in genetic association studies. *Journal of the American Statistical Association, 101*, 89–104.

22. Lin, D. Y., & Huang, B. E. (2007). The use of inferred haplotypes in downstream analyses. *The American Journal of Human Genetics, 80*, 577–579.

23. Scheet, P., & Stephens, M. (2006). A fast and flexible statistical model for large-scale population genotype data: Applications to inferring missing genotypes and haplotypic phase. *The American Journal of Human Genetics, 78*, 629–644.

24. Browning, S. R., & Browning, B. L. (2007). Rapid and accurate haplotype phasing and missing-data inference for whole-genome association studies by use of localized haplotype clustering. *The American Journal of Human Genetics, 81*, 1084–1097.

25. Stephens, M., Smith, N. J., & Donnelly, P. (2001). A new statistical method for haplotype reconstruction from population data. *The American Journal of Human Genetics, 68*, 978–989.

26. Kraft, P., & Stram, D. O. (2007). Re: The use of inferred haplotypes in downstream analysis. *American Journal of Human Genetics, 81*, 863–865. author reply 865–866.

27. Haiman, C. A., Stram, D. O., Pike, M. C., Kolonel, L. N., Burtt, N. P., Altshuler, D., et al. (2003). A comprehensive haplotype analysis of CYP19 and breast cancer risk: The multiethnic cohort study. *Human Molecular Genetics, 12*, 2679–2692.

28. Louis, T. (1982). Finding the observed information matrix when using the EM algorithm. *Journal of the Royal Statistical Society B, 44*(2), 226–233.

29. Spinka, C., Carroll, R. J., & Chatterjee, N. (2005). Analysis of case–control studies of genetic and environmental factors with missing genetic information and haplotype-phase ambiguity. *Genetic Epidemiology, 29*, 108–127.

30. Zhao, L. P., Li, S. S., & Khalid, N. (2003). A method for the assessment of disease associations with single-nucleotide polymorphism haplotypes and environmental variables in case–control studies. *The American Journal of Human Genetics, 72*, 1231–1250.

31. Dudbridge, F. (2006). A note on permutation tests in multistage association scans. *American Journal of Human Genetics, 78*, 1094–1095. author reply 1096.

32. Dudbridge, F., & Koeleman, B. P. (2004). Efficient computation of significance levels for multiple associations in large studies of correlated data, including genomewide association studies. *The American Journal of Human Genetics, 75*, 424–435.

33. Dudbridge, F., & Koeleman, B. P. (2003). Rank truncated product of P-values, with application to genomewide association scans. *Genetic Epidemiology, 25*, 360–366.

34. Lin, D. Y. (2006). Evaluating statistical significance in two-stage genomewide association studies. *The American Journal of Human Genetics, 78*.

35. Marchini, J., Donnelly, P., & Cardon, L. R. (2005). Genome-wide strategies for detecting multiple loci that influence complex diseases. *Nature Genetics, 37*, 413–417.

36. Millstein, J., Conti, D. V., Gilliland, F. D., & Gauderman, W. J. (2006). A testing framework for identifying susceptibility genes in the presence of epistasis. *The American Journal of Human Genetics, 78*, 15–27.

37. Evans, D. M., Marchini, J., Morris, A. P., & Cardon, L. R. (2006). Two-stage two-locus models in genome-wide association. *PLoS Genetics, 2*, e157.

38. Hu, Y., & Lin, D. (2010). Analysis of untyped snps, maximum likelihood and Imputation Methods. *Genetic Epidemiology, 34*, 803–815.

39. Browning, B. L., & Browning, S. R. (2009). A unified approach to genotype imputation and haplotype-phase inference for large data sets of trios and unrelated individuals. *The American Journal of Human Genetics, 84*, 210–223.

40. Howie, B. N., Donnelly, P., & Marchini, J. (2009). Impute2: A flexible and accurate genotype imputation method for the next generation of genome-wide association studies. *PLoS Genetics, 5*, e1000529.

41. Li, Y., Willer, C. J., Ding, J., Scheet, P., & Abecasis, G. R. (2010). MaCH: Using sequence and genotype data to estimate haplotypes and unobserved genotypes. *Genetic Epidemiology, 34*, 816–834.

42. Lin, W. Y., Yi, N., Zhi, D., Zhang, K., Gao, G., Tiwari, H. K., et al. (2012). Haplotype-based methods for detecting uncommon causal variants with common SNPs. *Genetics Epidemiology, 36*(6), 572–82.

Chapter 6
SNP Imputation for Association Studies

Abstract This chapter also (as does Chap. 5) discusses an extension of association analyses to include a larger set of hypotheses beyond just the single markers that have been genotyped in a particular study. Imputed SNP analysis is in certain respects identical to haplotype analysis since the imputed SNPs are on specific haplotypes or haplotype combinations. Testing imputed SNPs as well as genotyped SNPs is thus simply a more focused kind of haplotype analysis and serves to extend the set of hypotheses that are tested to encompass known but ungenotyped variants. Imputed SNP analysis plays a special role during a post-GWAS phase when during *meta-analysis* many studies are combined in efforts to find associations that are too small to be detectable in any one study. Imputation is necessarily relied upon when (as is generally the case) not all studies used the same genotyping platform or chip version.

This chapter discusses the basic statistical method, namely, *Hidden Markov Model* (*HMM*) that is used for fast and very large-scale SNP *imputation* in a number of high-performance programs. A brief introduction to the HMM methods is provided and the basic principles behind estimating the parameters of an HMM are illustrated with *R* code. The basics of a particular algorithm, patterned loosely after that implemented in the program *MACH*, are described.

Since nearly all large-scale SNP imputation methods require that *phased haplotypes* be provided for SNPs to be imputed (or measured for the purpose of imputation), a discussion of the use of *phasing* algorithms is also provided, with the details also modeled after the MACH program.

The use of imputed SNPs as independent variables in regression analysis is introduced with the discussion mostly focused on the same approach (expectation substitution) used in haplotype analysis. Use of imputed SNPs in association analyses for a single study is described, although the use of imputed SNPs in meta-analysis is deferred until Chap. 8.

D.O. Stram, *Design, Analysis, and Interpretation of Genome-Wide Association Scans*, Statistics for Biology and Health, DOI 10.1007/978-1-4614-9443-0_6, © Springer Science+Business Media New York 2014

6.1   The Role of Imputed SNPs in Association Testing

Similar to haplotype analysis, imputed SNPs are used to extend the number of hypotheses that are tested during association analysis. In order to be able to impute unmeasured alleles in an association study, there must first be information available about the LD pattern relating the markers that are genotyped in the association study to those SNPs that are not genotyped directly. For the purposes of discussion here, the set of SNPs or markers that are to be tested in the association study is denoted as the set of *imputation targets*. It is assumed that all the alleles in the *imputation target* are genotyped in a reference panel of individuals but that only a subset of target alleles will actually be genotyped in the association study; these SNPs are termed the *main study genotypes*. Note that the SNPs constituting the imputation target must contain the SNPs genotyped in the main study and hence in any given analysis will include SNPs for which actual genotypes, rather than only imputed genotypes, are available for association testing. At times the imputation target will be referred to as the *reference panel genotypes* when this is clear.

In standard applications, the reference panel participants will be considerably smaller in number than the number of association study members. For many past studies, HapMap phase 2 has served as reference panel, with the specific reference panel chosen to best correspond to the ethnic makeup of the participants in the association study [1]. More recently the *1000 Genomes Project* has become the provider of the "standard" list of target SNPs for imputation with the proviso that as of the writing of this chapter, SNP discovery and validation in this project remains an ongoing process and more samples are being added. Going beyond the 1000 Genomes Project, it is almost certain that with the advent of high-throughput next-generation sequencing, data suitable for use as reference panel genotypes and samples will continue to expand.

For a GWAS, the main study genotypes consist of the SNPs on a specific GWAS chip. In candidate gene or fine-mapping studies, the reference panel genotypes may be focused on specific regions of the genome, and selection of the SNPs to be used for the main study genotypes (rather than using a fixed SNP array) becomes a necessary component of the study.

Here we first go over the basic principles of SNP imputation in a way that is most applicable to smaller studies and then introduce key methods used in large-scale imputation.

6.2   EM Algorithm and SNP Imputation

When haplotype frequency estimates are available for a target set of SNPs but main study genotypes are only available for a subset, it is possible to use those haplotype frequency estimates to estimate the number of copies of the unmeasured SNPs using an algorithm which is identical in spirit to the methods introduced in Chap. 5.

The computation of the expected value of either (1) the number of copies of a given allele for SNP or (2) the probability that the number of copies of that SNP equals 0, 1, or 2 is performed for each subject conditionally on the genotypes that are available. Begin by assuming that haplotype frequencies are known. Then if (following the framework of Chap. 5 for haplotype estimation) $n_A(H)$ counts the number of copies (0, 1, or 2) of allele A for an SNP not genotyped in the main study that is contained in the pair of haplotypes, H, the expected number of copies of allele A (the dosage estimate) is computed as

$$E\left(n_A|G_i\right) = \frac{\displaystyle\sum_{H \sim G_i} n_A(H) p_{h_1} p_{h_2}}{\displaystyle\sum_{H \sim G_i} p_{h_1} p_{h_2}}, \tag{6.1}$$

with the summation over the set of haplotype pairs, H, for the target SNPs which are compatible with the genotypes, G_i, observed for the main study SNPs. These dosage estimates may then be used in the expectation-substitution method for association testing of the ungenotyped SNPs by fitting outcome models like

$$g(E(Y_i)) = \mu + \beta n_{i,A},$$

by replacing the unobserved $n_{i,A}$ with the observed $E(n_A|G_i)$ see below and Chap. 5. If the interest is in fitting codominant rather than additive models, i.e., models of form

$$g(E(Y_i)) = \mu + \beta_1 I(n_A = 1) + \beta_2 I(n_A = 2), \tag{6.2}$$

then it is necessary to estimate the conditional probabilities

$$E\{I(n_A = k)|G_i\} = \frac{\displaystyle\sum_{H \sim G_i} I\left(n_A(H) = k\right) p_{h_1} p_{h_2}}{\displaystyle\sum_{H \sim G_i} p_{h_1} p_{h_2}}, \quad \text{for } k = 1, 2 \tag{6.3}$$

and substitute accordingly into (6.2).

This method of SNP imputation is easily described, but there can be several complications to this procedure. For example, as given above, if the haplotype frequency estimates are obtained for the reference panel completely separate from the calculation of haplotype dosage for the association study, then there occasionally will be subjects whose genotypes, G, are not compatible with any of the pairs of haplotypes that were estimated to have nonzero frequency in the reference panel, i.e., an observed genotype combination seen for one or more individuals in the association study appears to have zero probability of occurrence using the haplotype frequencies estimated in the reference panel. This is not particularly surprising when the number of association study subjects is much greater than those genotyped in the reference panel, since some rare haplotypes seen in the association study will be likely to have been missed in the reference panel. One possible solution to this problem is to include the association subjects as if they were reference panel members (with missing data for all the ungenotyped target SNPs) in the haplotype estimation phase so as to estimate haplotype frequencies and perform (at the convergence of the EM) the SNP predictions simultaneously. Doing this will insure that no observed genotype combination is given zero probability in the EM algorithm; however the large number of subjects with a large amount of missing data being used in the EM algorithm tends to dramatically slow down the estimation of haplotype frequencies.

Another serious impediment to directly using (6.1) is more logistical in nature especially when very large numbers of SNPs have been genotyped. Since it is impossible (even with the PLEM) to run the EM algorithm for very large numbers of SNPs, it is first necessary to decide, for each SNP in the target SET, the set of SNPs in the basis set to actually use in the imputation. This may be done, for example, by setting up windows of nearby SNPs or by dividing all SNPs into haplotype blocks, with only the basis SNPs in the same window or blocks as the target SNPs used in the EM algorithm; however fine-tuning such algorithms can be tricky.

An alternative approach is to use SNP tagging software [2–4] to find, for each SNP in the target set, a short list of basis SNPs that in combination serve as tags for the target. This was done in Haiman et al. [5]. In this large-scale candidate gene study, a total of 2,897 SNPs were successfully genotyped in a special purpose reference panel, and 1,234 SNPs were chosen as the tag SNPs to be genotyped in the association study. The program Tagger [6], as implemented in Haploview [7], identified a maximum of 3 tag SNPs as haplotype predictors of each target SNP, and the list of the predictors for each target SNP was retained for later use. After the association study genotyping had been completed, the data for all subjects genotyped with the tag SNPs (including both the reference panel and the association study members) was run through the program TagSNPs [8] to perform haplotype frequency estimation and SNP imputation using (6.1). The genotypes that were processed by each run of the TagSNPs program included only the single target SNP genotypes plus the genotypes of the tag SNPs that had been identified by Tagger for that target SNP. Therefore for each target SNP, a complete EM algorithm was run (involving from 2 to 4 SNPs) prior to SNP imputation.

Another fairly simple approach to SNP imputation which has been discussed to some degree in the literature [3, 9] is to replace the EM-haplotype frequency-based SNP imputation with linear regressions. That is, SNP genotype in the target set is analyzed by ordinary regression analysis using the main study SNPs as (linear) explanatory variables. As discussed by Stram [3], this method gives similar results to haplotype-based imputation so long as the target SNP and the SNPs used for prediction are in complete linkage disequilibrium (no recombinant haplotypes evident). In general, however, it does not appear to be as effective a method for SNP imputation as the haplotype-based methods described above.

6.3 Phasing Large Numbers of SNPs for the Reference Panel

As we will see in the discussion of more current software, large-scale SNP imputation using current packages generally requires that all target SNPs for the reference panel subjects be initially phased to begin the imputation process. From the discussion of haplotype uncertainty in Chap. 5, it is clear that phasing of large numbers of genotypes for a panel of unrelated individuals must be inherently unreliable. For example, if as few as 7 very common SNPs are in linkage equilibrium, then the estimate of the number of copies (0, 1, or 2) of any given haplotype that are carried is predicted quite poorly (as indicated by R_h^2 in Fig. 5.2). This is overcome to some degree if data from nuclear families is available—for example, if parents and single-child trios are genotyped, then a doubly heterozygous parent has uncertain haplotype counts only if the child's genotypes are also doubly heterozygous and the other parent is heterozygous for at least one of the two SNPs. However uncertainty in haplotype assignment while reduced still remains (see discussion in Chap. 5). Despite this inherent uncertainty, we will see that imputed long-range phased haplotypes for the HapMap data and variants observed in the 1000 Genomes Project are routinely required as a starting point for SNP imputation. The phasing of the SNP data provided by the HapMap and 1000 Genomes Project, especially for those groups (e.g., the Japanese and Chinese HapMap samples) where no family members, specifically no offspring, have been genotyped, should be regarded as "pseudo-phasing" that is only accurate over regions of limited linkage disequilibrium. The empirical success of SNP imputation methods that rely on initial phasing of the reference panel data (phased reference panel data is available for the HapMap and thousand genomes or can be computed using such programs as PHASEII [10], MACH [11], fastPHASE [12], or SHAPEIT [13]) implies that SNP imputation is not very dependent on the strict accuracy of the initial phasing especially over long genomic distances. This is undoubtedly because of the flexibility of the probability models that the HMM-based imputation methods rely upon as seen below.

6.4 Brief Introduction to Hidden Markov Models

An important special case of the EM algorithm is estimation of the parameters (including transition probabilities, initial distribution, most probable path) for a Markov chain when the transitions are not directly observed. Introductions to Hidden Markov Models (HMMs) for certain genetic applications are available from a number of sources (e.g., [14] Chap. 3, [15] Chap. 9). An interesting historical note is that the original papers on the Hidden Markov Model [16–18] describing the updating procedure predated the classic EM paper (Dempster et al. [19]) by a number of years, and indeed the earlier papers proved many of the basic properties of the EM algorithm.

Using the notation of Rabiner 1989 [20], an HMM consists of a *Markov chain* Q_t which takes values, q_t, $t = 1, \ldots, T$ from a set of possible states $S = \{S_1, \ldots, S_N\}$.

In a Markov chain, the complete probability distribution of the sequence of states q_t is defined by the initial distribution $\pi_i = p(q_1 = i)$ and a state transition probability matrix $\mathbf{A} = \{a_{ij}\}$, i.e., the probability of moving from state S_i (at a given time t) to state S_j at time $t+1$ conditional on being in state S_i at time t. This allows the evaluation of the probability of a sequence of states $Q = (q_1, \ldots, q_T)$ given the model parameters $\theta = (\mathbf{A}, \pi)$ as

$$\Pr(Q|\theta) = \pi_{q_1}\left[\prod_{t=2}^{T} a_{S_{t-1}S_t}\right].$$

Now consider the problem of estimating the state transition probabilities

$$p(S_i, S_j) = \Pr(q_{t+1} = S_j | q_t = S_i).$$

In order to simplify the notation for the remainder of this section, we will denote $p(S_i, S_j)$ as a_{ij} and refer the states in S as simply states 1 to N.

Now suppose we wanted to estimate the transition probabilities by observing the Markov chain for a total of T transitions, i.e., we observe the sequence $q_1, \ldots, q_T$, for this purpose.

Clearly the MLE of a_{ij} would be just the observed number of transitions from state i to state j divided by the total number of times that q_t is observed to be in state i for $t = 0, 1, \ldots, T - 1$:

$$\hat{a}_{ij} = \frac{\Sigma_{t=2}^{T} I(q_{t-1} = i \text{ AND } q_t = j)}{\Sigma_{t=2}^{T} I(q_{t-1} = i)}. \tag{6.4}$$

Let us consider now the *Hidden Markov Model* where instead of seeing directly the states, q_t, at each time t, we saw output (called signals) $O = (O_1, O_2, \ldots, O_M)$ at each time, but this output is ambiguous in the sense that the same signals can be generated from more than one state. A Hidden Markov Model is characterized by the following:

1. N the number of states, $S = \{S_1, S_2, \ldots, S_N\}$ in the underlying Markov chain.
2. M the number of distinct observation symbols with the possible signals taking values from the set $V = \{v_1, v_2, \ldots, v_M\}$.
3. The state transition matrix $A = \{a_{ij}\}$ where

$$a_{ij} = P\left[q_{t+1} = S_j | q_t = S_i\right].$$

4. The observation symbol probability distribution in state j

$$B = \{b_j(k)\},$$

where $b_j(k) = P[O_t = v_k | q_t = S_j]$, $1 \leq j \leq N$, $1 \leq k \leq M$.
5. The initial state distribution $\pi = \{\pi_1, \pi_2, \ldots, \pi_N\}$

Given values of N, M, A, B, and π, the HMM can be used as a generator to give an observation sequence $O = O_1 O_2 \ldots O_T$ as follows:

1. Choose an initial state $q_1 = S_i$ according to the initial state distribution π.
2. Set $t = 1$.
3. Choose $O_t = v_k$ according to the symbol probability distribution in state S_i, i.e., $b_i(k)$.
4. Transit to a new state $q_{t+1} = S_j$ according to the state transition probability distribution for state S_i, namely, a_{ij}.
5. Set $t = t + 1$; return to step 3 if $t < T$; otherwise terminate.

There are three basic problems that are posed by an HMM. These are:

Problem 1: Given the observation sequence $O = O_1 O_2 \ldots O_T$ and a model $\lambda = (A, B, \pi)$, how do we efficiently compute the probability, $P(O|\lambda)$, given the model?

Problem 2: Given the observation sequence $O = O_1 O_2 \ldots O_T$, how do we choose a corresponding state sequence $Q = q_1 q_2 \ldots q_T$ which is optimal in some sense?

Problem 3: How do we adjust the model parameters λ to maximize $P(O|\lambda)$?

Problems 1 to 3 involve the *Baum–Welch forward and backward algorithms* (see below) or sometimes the closely related *Viterbi* algorithm (for solving Problem 2). We note that Problem 3 can be solved[1] using the EM algorithm. For example, for estimating the transition probabilities a_{ij} from just the observation sequence O, the EM algorithm requires that we compute estimates of the conditional probabilities of a transition from i to j given the observed data O and initial estimates of the model parameters $\lambda = (\mathbf{A}, \mathbf{B}, \pi)$. Define (using the initial estimates as if they were the true values) the conditional probability of a transition from S_i to S_j at time t as

$$\eta_{ij}(t) = p\left(S_t = i, S_{t+1} = j \middle| O; \theta\right) \tag{6.5}$$

(computing these constitutes the *E*-step) and then (in the *M*-step) update the $\mathbf{A}$ matrix as

$$\hat{a}_{ij} = \frac{\Sigma_{t=1}^{T-1} \eta_{ij}(t)}{\Sigma_{t=1}^{T-1} P(q_t = i)}, \tag{6.6}$$

where $P(q_t = i) = \displaystyle\sum_{j=1}^{N} \eta_{ij}(t)$, i.e., we have computed the expected value of the function of the data, i.e., (6.4), that would be used to estimate the a_{ij} if the q_t were

---

[1] Actually the EM algorithm generally will only find a local maximum; running the EM repeatedly using multiple starting values for the parameters in λ is recommended for assessment of whether a global maximum has been achieved.

observed. Again efficiently computing $\hat{a}_{ij}$ involves the Baum–Welch forward and backward variables (computed by the forward and backward algorithms, respectively). The solution for updating initial estimates of the initial probabilities π is

$$\hat{\pi}_i = \sum_{j=1}^{S} \eta_{ij}(0).$$

In addition we can estimate the probabilities of being in state i at any particular time t as

$$\hat{\pi}_i(t) = \sum_{j=1}^{S} \eta_{ij}(t).$$

6.4.1   The Baum–Welch Algorithm

The Baum–Welch algorithm is essentially a way of quickly computing $\eta_{ij}(t)$ through two sets of recursive calculations, one going forward in time t and the other going backward in t. First consider how the probability of a given observation sequence $O_1 O_2 \ldots O_T$ can be computed. Define the auxiliary variable $\alpha_i(t)$ as

$$\alpha_t(i) = p\big(O_{1:t}, q_t = i | \theta\big).$$

Here we have used the notation $O_{1:t} = (O_1, \ldots, O_t)$.
The algorithm to compute $p(O|\theta)$ is as follows:
Initialization:

$$\alpha_1(i) = b_i(O_1)\pi_i \quad \text{for } 1 \le i \le N.$$

Iteration:

$$\alpha_{t+1}(j) = \left[\sum_{i=1}^{N} \alpha_t(i)a_{ij}\right] b_j(O_{t+1}) \quad \text{for } 1 \le t \le T - 1, \ 1 \le j \le N.$$

Termination:

$$p(O|\lambda) = \sum_{i=1}^{N} \alpha_T(i). \tag{6.7}$$

This computation is called a "forward pass" through the series, and this computation thus gives the solution to Problem 1 above, i.e., we have computed the probability of the observation O given the model parameters. To solve the other two problems, we continue as follows:

Now consider the "backward pass," compute $\beta_t(i) = p(O_{t+1}, O_{t+2}, \ldots O_T | q_t = i, \lambda)$.

This can be done similarly to the forward pass:
Initialization:

$$\beta_T(i) = 1, \quad 1 \leq i \leq N.$$

Iteration:

$$\beta_t(i) = \sum_{j=1}^{N} a_{ij} b_j(O_{t+1}) \beta_{t+1}(j), \quad t = T - 1, T - 2, \ldots, 1, \quad 1 \leq i \leq N.$$

We can now compute the conditional probability of a transition from state i to j at time $t + 1$, i.e.,

$$\eta_{ij}(t) = \frac{1}{Z_t} \alpha_t(i) a_{ij} b_j(O_{t+1}) \beta_{t+1}(j), \tag{6.8}$$

where Z_t is a normalizing constant so that $\sum_{i,j=1}^{S} \eta_{ij}(t) = 1$. Then the M-step for a_{ij} is as in (6.6) above.

For our purposes (of SNP imputation), we focus on solving Problem 2, i.e., giving some sort of optimal estimate for the state sequence since if the state sequence is known, then we will know the genotypes for each SNP that is missing in the main study. The key issue is to estimate the conditional probability distribution of being in state S_i at time t given the observation sequence O and the model parameters; this can be readily computed from the forward and backward variables and using the solution to Problem 1, i.e., the calculated value of $\Pr(O|\lambda)$. Defining $\gamma_t i)$ as $\Pr(q_t = S_i|O, \lambda)$ we have

$$\gamma_t(i) = \frac{\alpha_t(i)\beta_t(i)}{\Pr(O|\lambda)}. \tag{6.9}$$

One relatively easy solution then to estimating the state that is occupied at time t is just as the state with the maximum probability

$$\hat{q}_t = \underset{1 \leq i \leq N}{\operatorname{argmax}} [\gamma_t(i)], \tag{6.10}$$

so that at time, t, the value of the individually most likely state is chosen. Another approach is to attempt to find the state sequence, Q, that maximizes $\Pr(Q|O, t)$, which is not necessarily equivalent to a choice of the sequence of individually most likely values $(\hat{q}_1, \hat{q}_2, \ldots, \hat{q}_T)$ from (6.10). Maximizing $\Pr(Q|O,t)$ is accomplished using a technique known as the *Viterbi* algorithm; however this is tangential to our interests and is not discussed here; see Rabiner [20] for more information. Updating the basic model parameters, i.e., the initial state, the parameters in the transition matrix or the output sequence probabilities from each state all involve the transition probabilities at time t, i.e., $\eta_{ij}(t)$ from (6.8). However, it should be noted that creating identifiable models (for which the observation sequence alone provides sufficient information for estimation) typically involves developing models for the transition matrix and the output signal probabilities that involve a relatively small number of parameters; these parameters, rather than, for example, the entire matrix of transition probabilities, are then estimated from the estimates of $\eta_{ij}(t)$ and the corresponding estimates of the number of transitions into and out of each state, treating these estimated data points as if they had been observed directly. Note that this will correspond to an EM algorithm that uses the expectation of the number of transitions (computed during the E-step) as if it was data actually observed from the underlying Markov chain model.[2]

6.5 Large-Scale Imputation Using HMMs

The problem of imputing target genotypes for members of the study (using basis genotypes) is greatly simplified if we can assume that phase is known for both the reference panel genotypes as well as the main study genotypes. This not only simplifies the imputation algorithm but also corresponds to a recommended approach for imputation of the 1000 Genomes target [13]. Since the 1000 Genomes target is still (as of this writing) subject to significant revisions and extensions (and other extensive datasets are and will continue to become available) and since imputing missing genotypes when phase is known for the main study is much faster than when phase is not known, the following heuristic algorithm is advocated by Delaneau et al. [13] and others [21]:

1. Genotype the main association study, perform quality control, identify the basis genotypes, and finalize the association genotype dataset.
2. Phase the finalized association study genotype data.
3. Download the phased haplotypes for the 1000 Genomes Project version X (reference panel).
4. Impute target genotypes for the main study using results of Steps 2 + 3.
5. Perform association analysis of imputed genotype data.

When the new and improved 1000 Genomes version $X + 1$ is released, increment X and repeat from Step 3.

Step 2 may take many hours of computer time (and may require a cluster of computers) and generally involves first splitting up each chromosome into many partly overlapping pieces of manageable size and then piecing the imputation results

---

[2] In other settings, the EM algorithm requires calculating expectations of sufficient statistics or of log likelihood functions in toto, rather than just the unobserved data; see [19]. It is because the HMM is a model for multinomial data (i.e., number of transitions), and since the log of the likelihood of a multinomial is linear in the observed or unobserved counts, calculating the expectation of unobserved transitions, given observed data (signals), is sufficient for the estimation of model parameters.

back together. Once Step 2 is done then as each version of the 1000 Genomes data is released, only the very much less time-consuming Steps 2 and 3 are to be performed. Therefore rather than discuss here the problem of inferring target genotypes when phased haplotypes are available only for the reference panel, we describe both phasing genotype data (without the benefit of a reference panel) and imputing missing genotypes when both the reference panel and main study are already phased.

Since Step 4 is far less complicated than Step 2, Step 4 is discussed first.

6.6 Using an HMM to Impute Missing Genotype Data when Both the Reference Panel and Study Genotypes Are Phased

One basic approach to applying an HMM to the problem of imputing alleles for the missing markers (i.e., for the ungenotyped SNPs) relies on an assumption that most or all haplotypes in the association study can be regarded as recombinations of the haplotypes for the reference panel members. Suppose that there are N haplotypes in the reference panel and n members of the association study, the problem of imputing missing markers at a given location, i, consists of identifying, for a given association study haplotype, which of the reference panel haplotypes at that location is the most probable given the marker allele information that is available.

To illustrate a basic HMM (in R) as follows with very simple data, we consider that the haplotypes for N individuals at T markers are available for reference panel. For purposes of illustration, we work with 19 markers and 12 reference panel subjects defining the 12×19 matrix H of reference panel haplotypes as (these are data from [22]):

```
> H<-rbind(
>     c(1,4,3,1,2,1,2,4,3,3,1,4,4,4,1,2,3,1,4),
>     c(1,3,3,1,2,1,1,4,3,3,3,4,2,2,3,3,1,1,4),
>     c(1,3,3,4,4,1,1,4,2,2,3,2,2,2,3,3,1,1,4),
>     c(1,4,1,1,2,1,1,4,3,3,4,2,2,2,3,3,1,1,4),
>     c(1,4,3,4,4,3,1,2,3,3,3,2,2,2,3,3,3,1,2),
>     c(1,4,1,4,4,1,1,4,2,2,3,2,2,2,3,3,1,4,4),
>     c(1,4,3,1,2,1,1,4,3,3,3,4,2,2,3,3,1,1,4),
>     c(1,4,3,4,4,1,1,4,2,2,3,2,2,2,3,3,1,4,4),
>     c(1,3,3,1,2,1,1,4,3,3,3,4,2,2,3,3,3,1,2),
>     c(1,4,3,1,2,1,2,4,3,3,1,4,2,4,1,2,3,1,4),
>     c(4,4,3,1,2,1,1,4,3,3,3,4,2,2,3,3,1,1,2),
>     c(1,4,3,4,4,1,1,4,2,2,3,2,2,2,3,3,1,1,4)
>     )
> N<-dim(H)[1]
> Tt<-dim(H)[2]  # Note: use Tt rather than T since T is short for
>                # logical "TRUE" in R
```

The possible states are $S = (1,2, \ldots,N)$ with $q_t = i$ meaning that at location t the association study haplotype corresponds to reference panel haplotype i. There are a total of T diallelic markers in the reference panel.

There are $M = 3$ three possible output symbols, V, consisting of $\{0, 1, \varnothing\}$. The output symbol 1 is produced at state j with probability 1 if the genotype at the current position (t) is equal to 1 and with probability zero if that genotype is 0, and similarly for output symbol zero. The output symbol $\varnothing$ (indicating missing data and coded here as 9) is assumed to be produced with equal probability from any state.

Following the above, we define the emission probabilities (probability of reporting a signal, o, depending on the state, j, and position t (which takes values from 1 to T_t) as:

```
> b<-function(t,j,o) # emission probabilities probability of seeing a
> # signal o from state j -- in this problem this is a function of t
> {
>    if (o!=9) outp<-ifelse(H[j,t]==o,1,0) # 9 means not genotyped
>    else outp<-1/N  # the point here is that it is equally likely for
>                    # any state j to produce missing output(at time t)
>    outp
> }
```

Note that in the above we have not allowed for the possibility of genotyping error in the main study. We could allow a (small) probability that a 1 is produced if the true state has genotype zero and vice versa; this might reduce the number of recombinations that are estimated by the algorithm, but for now we ignore this possibility.

We next define the recombination probability (probability of a crossover between haplotypes) to be a constant value θ here set to be equal to 0.1. This corresponds to an assumption that the genetic distance between every pair of neighboring SNPs is equal. This can be (and is in many programs) modified according to genome map data. This assumption allows us to define the transition probabilities as an R function:

```
> theta<-0.1
> a<-function(i,j) # transition probabilities
>   { if (i==j) tp=1-theta+theta/N
>     else tp=theta/N
>   tp}
```

The definition explicitly allows for (when i and j are the same state) the possibility of a crossover between identical haplotypes which is why the second line of function a includes the θ/N term.

We now define the initial probabilities π_0 as equal as in:

```
> Pi<-rep(1/N,N)
```

To run the algorithm, we observe an observation sequence (i.e., read in a main study haplotype) such as:

```
> O<-c(4,3,3,9,9,3,1,2,3,9,9,2,2,4,1,2,9,1,9)
> # here 9 means not genotyped only main study snps are genotyped
```

For the time being, we consider only the problem of producing a "best" estimate of the state sequence $Q = (q_1, q_2, \ldots, q_{T_i})$ corresponding to the observation sequence, O.

The Baum–Welch algorithm consists of first calculating the forward variable, $\alpha(t, q_t)$, $\Pr(O_{1:t}, q_t = i)$ for $t = 1, \ldots, T$, $i = 1, N$. In order to do this, we work on the log scale (and utilize a helper algorithm, logsum, which computes the log of the sum of very small numbers stored as logarithms) (see *haplo_impute.r* for its definition):

```
> # calculate the forward variable alpha(t,q_t) = Pr(O_{1:t},q_t=i)
> # for t=1,Tt i=1,N
> # work on log scale
> logalpha<-matrix(0,Tt,N)
> # initialize logalpha at time 1
>     for( i in 1:N) logalpha[1,i]<-log(Pi[i])+log(b(1,i,O[1]))
> # iterate to finish logalpha
>     for (t in 1:(Tt-1))
>       for(j in 1:N){
>       sx=rep(0,N)
>       for (i in 1:N)
>       {
>             sx[i]=logalpha[t,i]+log(a(i,j))
>       }
>       logalpha[t+1,j]=logsum(sx)+log(b(t+1,j,O[t+1]))
>     }
```

and we terminate by calculating the probability of the observation sequence, (6.7), as:

```
> logPO <-logsum(logalpha[Tt,]) # log of probability of observation
                                # sequence O
```

After this we calculate the backward variable (again using logs) as:

```
> logbeta<-matrix(0,Tt,N) # logbeta[Tt] is set to zero as required
>   for (t in (Tt-1):1) for (i in 1:N) {
>     sx=rep(0,N)
>     for (j in 1:N)
>           sx[j]=log(a(i,j))+log(b(t+1,j,O[t+1]))+
>           logbeta[t+1,j]
>     logbeta[t,i]=logsum(sx)
>   }
```

From this we can calculate the conditional state probabilities, $\gamma_t i$), (6.9), as:

```
> loggamma=matrix(0,Tt,N)
> for (t in 1:Tt){
>     for (i in 1:N) {
>             loggamma[t,i]=logalpha[t,i]+logbeta[t,i]-logPO
>     }
> }
```

and we can maximize the individual state probabilities to give an individually "best" sequence as:

```
> Qbest<-rep(0,Tt)
> for (t in 1:Tt) Qbest[t]<-which.max((loggamma[t,]))
```

Now we can calculate the alleles of the imputed haplotype as:

```
> iG<-rep(0,Tt)
> for (t in 1:Tt) iG[t]<- H[Qbest[t],t]
```

Finally we display the results observed and imputed haplotypes as well as the "best state" itself:

```
> cbind(O, Qbest, iG)
        O Qbest iG
 [1,]  4    11  4
 [2,]  3     2  3
 [3,]  3     2  3
 [4,]  9     5  4
 [5,]  9     5  4
 [6,]  3     5  3
 [7,]  1     5  1
 [8,]  2     5  2
 [9,]  3     5  3
[10,]  9     5  3
[11,]  9     5  3
[12,]  2     5  2
[13,]  2     5  2
[14,]  4    10  4
[15,]  1    10  1
[16,]  2    10  2
[17,]  9    10  3
[18,]  1    10  1
[19,]  9    10  4
```

Here we see that the state estimate first starts with state 11, which makes sense because the 11th row of table H (the reference panel haplotypes, see above) is the only haplotype with a 4 in the first position. The best state then switches to state 3 for the next two SNPs and then settles on state 5 (which matches the observed haplotype at SNPs 6 through 9 and at SNPs 12 and 13, with SNPs 11 and 12 unobserved) for SNPs 4–13 and finally switches to state 10 which matches the observed haplotypes at all remaining observed positions.

Note that from the discussion in the previous chapter, it is important, for association testing, to allow for the uncertainty in haplotype estimation, by providing the expected genotype count values at each position, where the count will be of the number of copies of a reference allele; for convenience, the reference allele is taken to be the allele contained by the first reference panel haplotype. The expected count can be calculated as follows:

```
> gam<-exp(loggamma) # unlog the probability distribution
> ExpectedG<-rep(0,Tt)
> RefAllele=H[1,] # use the first haplotype to define reference allele
> for (t in 1:Tt)
>     for (i in 1:N)
>         ExpectedG[t]=
>         ExpectedG[t]+as.numeric(H[i,t]==RefAllele[t])*gam[t,i]
```

and the results displayed as:

```
> cbind(O, Qbest, iG,RefAllele, ExpectedG)
        O Qbest iG RefAllele    ExpectedG
 [1,]   4    11  4         1  0.000000000
 [2,]   3     2  3         4  0.000000000
 [3,]   3     2  3         3  1.000000000
 [4,]   9     5  4         1  0.359618753
 [5,]   9     5  4         2  0.187247295
 [6,]   3     5  3         1  0.000000000
 [7,]   1     5  1         2  0.000000000
 [8,]   2     5  2         4  0.000000000
 [9,]   3     5  3         3  1.000000000
[10,]   9     5  3         3  0.962855058
[11,]   9     5  3         1  0.002382856
[12,]   2     5  2         4  0.000000000
[13,]   2     5  2         4  0.000000000
[14,]   4    10  4         4  1.000000000
[15,]   1    10  1         1  1.000000000
[16,]   2    10  2         2  1.000000000
[17,]   9    10  3         3  0.947791165
[18,]   1    10  1         1  1.000000000
[19,]   9    10  4         4  0.930851979
>
```

We see now that in general when there is a missing genotype value in the observed data, there remains some uncertainty about the true genotype. For example, at base position 4, there remains a 36 % probability that the underlying genotype is actually a 3 rather than the "best" prediction of 4, and at position 5, there is a 19 % chance that the true genotype is a "2" rather than a "4." At the other positions where the observed sequence is missing data, the uncertainty is a bit less. As described in the previous chapter, it is the estimated genotype counts that should be used as the genetic "dosage" variable in haplotype association studies.

Note that we have obtained seemingly good results for these data without going through any additional steps, specifically we have not considered the updating of the model parameters (Problem 3 above); here there really only are two parameters that could be updated: one is the recombination probability and the other is the initial probability (probability of state 1, i.e., values for the first SNP). Running the above algorithm (with the same input data) for a range of values of recombination probability, rp, from 0.01 to 0.90 does not change the "best" missing genotype assignments, but does modify the certainty with which the genotypes are assigned, with the larger values of recombination probability leading to larger uncertainties. By considering the values of the log of the observation probability ($\log PO$ which equals -28.9 for $\theta = 0.1$, -34.9 for $\theta = 0.01$, and -30.9 for $\theta = 0.9$ in the R program), we can see that for these data a considerably better fit to the observed data is provided by using the larger (e.g., 0.1 or 0.9) than the smaller $p = 0.01$ crossover probability; this makes sense given that the algorithm was forced to "jump" several times in order that the observed genotypes matched for the reference haplotype of interest.

Note however that we would not actually consider implementing an EM procedure to maximize the likelihood with respect to θ after having seen only one observation sequence (i.e., main study genotype). Maximization over any of the parameters would be done when all the data has been processed. Assuming that the main study genotypes are independent of one another, one would apply the maximization stage of the EM algorithm (solving Problem 3) in order to maximize the product of all observation probabilities, not the probability of each of them; see Section V.B. of Rabiner [20].

Keeping the same basic structure, we could modify aspects of the model; for example, rather than using a fixed recombination probability, one could allow genetic map information to be used to provide an external source of information about how θ varies from position to position, and this is allowed in most programs. Note that the usual genetic maps describes the recombination probability for a single meiosis; here θ corresponds to a population-level observed rate of historical recombination, which might best be modeled as a constant times genetic map distances rather than equal to genetic distance in the traditional sense.

Another parameter that appears in the model is the probability of missing data (an emission of a $\varnothing$, coded as 9 in the R program); varying this parameter from 0.02 to 0.8 has a large effect on $\log PO$ (with larger values more likely than smaller values, since after all 6 out of 19 markers are missing in the observation sequence) but has no effect at all on the estimation of the best state or the uncertainty in the imputed genotype. Another change would be to model main study haplotypes as the result of mutation as well as recombination of the main study haplotypes; this is incorporated by modifying the output function b introducing an "error" parameter ε. As pointed out by Li et al., such a parameter encompasses a number of possibilities including genotyping error, mutation, and gene conversion.

6.7   Using an HMM to Phase Reference or Main Study Genotypes

We now consider the complications that would be involved in modifying the R program so that it would be able to predict haplotype phase for a large number of SNPs and for a large number of panel or study members. Starting from scratch, with no phased data to provide guidance or to build from, naively would involve all 2^T choose 2 possible states where state now refers to the combination of 2 possible haplotypes that an individual could carry. This is not tractable and conceptually more complicated methods are required. We focus upon the methods that are described for the program MACH (Li et al. [11], Appendix). We break the problem into two parts:

1. Given a current set of possible haplotypes for the reference panel or study group, the assignment of a haplotype pair for each individual with genotype data.
2. Initialization and subsequent updating of the current set of possible haplotypes.

Consider now the modifications to the HMM procedure to take account of Problem (1). Let the number of haplotypes currently assigned be equal to h. At each location t, there are a total of $N = h^2$ possible states $S_t = (x_t, y_t)$, where x_t denotes the haplotype for the first chromosome at position t and y_t the haplotype for the second chromosome. The transition probabilities, i.e., $\Pr(S_t | S_{t-1})$, can be defined as

$$
\begin{aligned}
&P\left(S_t | S_{t-1}\right) \\
&= \begin{cases}
\theta^2/h^2, & \text{if } x_t \neq x_{t-1} \text{ and } y_t \neq y_{t-1} \\
(1-\theta)\theta/h + \theta^2/h^2, & \text{if } x_t \neq x_{t-1} \text{ or } y_t \neq y_{t-1} \\
(1-\theta)^2 + 2(1-\theta)\theta/h + \theta^2/h^2 & \text{if } x_t = x_{t-1} \text{ and } y_t = y_{t-1}
\end{cases}
\end{aligned}
\tag{6.11}
$$

Here the probability of one change, i.e., the second line of (6.11), allows for the probability of exactly one crossover to the current state or of two crossovers but in which one of the crossovers was between identical haplotypes, and the third line (probability of no changes) counts the probability of no crossovers plus the probability of one or two crossovers between identical haplotypes. The first line is the probability of two crossovers from state S_{t-1} to reach S_t.

In order to simplify implementation in R, we first convert the table of current haplotypes (we will use those defined above) into a matrix of 0's and 1's so that that the H matrix counts the number of reference genotypes as follows:

```
> # Redo the H table so that H consists of zeros and ones using
> # first column as reference
> refAllele<-H[1,]
> W<-matrix(0,dim(H)[1],dim(H)[2])
> for (i in 1:N)
> W[i,]<-1*(H[i,]==H[1,])
> H<-W
```

We rewrite the function a in R as follows:

```
> a<-function(i,j){ # probability of a transition from
>                   # state S_i to S_j at time t
>                  # state is defined as pair of two haplotypes
>                  # each pair is coded as a single number 1 -- h^2
>    x_i=trunc((i-1)/h)+1  # gives first haplotype
>                   # corresponding to state i
>    y_i=i-(x_i-1)*h    # gives second
>    x_j=trunc((j-1)/h)+1  # gives first haplotype corresponding to
>                   # state j
>    y_j=j-(x_j-1)*h  # gives second
> # Now return the transition probability
>       if ((x_i != x_j) &    (y_i != y_j)) return(theta^2/h^2)
>       if ((x_i != x_j) | (y_i != y_j) )
>            return(theta^2*(1-theta)/h+theta^2/h^2)
>       # otherwise
>       return((1-theta)^2+2*(1-theta)*theta/h+theta^2/h^2)
> }
```

Here, in order to minimize any other needed changes in the program, the single state encodes the two haplotypes (from 1 to $N = h^2$) into a single value so that state 1 corresponds to the haplotype pair $(1, 1)$ and state 2 to pair $(1, 2)$, continuing all the way up to state N which corresponds to haplotype pair (h, h); here the numbers 1 to h refer to haplotype appearing in the rows of the table H. The first few lines of a simply decodes the state information for state i and j into the haplotype pairs (x_i, y_i) and (x_j, y_j).

The emission probabilities $\Pr(G_t|S_t)$ are now defined (including the error probability ε) as [23]

$$P\big(G_t\big|S_t\big) = \begin{cases} (1-\varepsilon)^2 + \varepsilon^2, & \text{if sum}(S_t) = G_t \text{ and } G_t = 1 \\ 2(1-\varepsilon)\varepsilon, & \text{if sum}(S_t) \neq G_t \text{ and } G_t = 1 \\ (1-\varepsilon)^2 & \text{if sum}(S_t) = G_t \text{ and } G_t \in (0, 2) \\ (1-\varepsilon)\varepsilon & \text{if sum}(S_t) = 1 \text{ and } G_t \in (0, 2) \\ \varepsilon^2 & \text{if sum}(S_t) \text{ and } G_t \in (0, 2) \text{ but } S_t \neq G_t \end{cases} \qquad (6.12)$$

For example, the last line of (6.12), where the genotype implied by state S_t, i.e., sum(S_t) and the observed G_t are opposite homozygotes, can only occur if there are two "errors" in the emission of signal from state S_t; this occurs with probability ε^2 assuming independence. These emission probabilities can be implemented in R, and also including possibility of missing genotypes, not considered in (6.12) as follows:

```
> eps<-0.005 # probability of error
> pmiss<-0.2 # (probability of missing genotype from any state)
> b<-function(t,j,G) # emission probabilities:probability of
>                     # seeing a signal G from state j
>                     # (in this problem this is a
>                     #function of location t)
> {
>   if (G==9) return(pmiss)  # 9 means not genotyped:
>                            # all states are equally possible
>   # otherwise
>            # split the state number j (going from 1 to h^2)
>            # into two numbers (indicating
>            # the two haplotypes in the pair)
>   j1=trunc((j-1)/h)+1  # points to first haplotype (row of H)
>                        # corresponding to state j
>   j2=j-(j1-1)*h        # points to second haplotype
>   sumhaps<-H[j1,t]+H[j2,t] # This gives the true genotype that
>                            # corresponds to
>                            # haplotypes j1 and j2 at time t
> # now consider all cases
>   if ((sumhaps==G) & (G==1)) return((1-eps)^2+eps^2)
>   if ((sumhaps!=G) & (G==1)) return(2*(1-eps)*eps)
>   if ((sumhaps==G) & (G %% 2 == 0)) return((1-eps)^2)
>   if ((sumhaps==1) & (G %% 2 == 0)) return((1-eps)*eps)
>   # otherwise
>   return(eps^2)
> }
```

Also we will change to a more realistic recombination probability for these data, namely,

```
> theta<-0.5
```

The same iterations as above can be used to develop the "current" estimate of best state (haplotype pair) corresponding to a given G; see *haplo_impute.r*. For example, consider a genotype $G = (2,0,1,1,2,1,0,1,1,2,0,2,0,1,0,0,1,2,1)$. With these changes in the a and b (transition and emission probabilities), running the same code shown above to perform the forward and backward algorithms (see *haplo_impute.r*) sets the R variable Q_{best} equal to $Q_{best} = (33,33,41,41,41,41,41,$ $41,41,45,45,45,45,45,45,45,45,45,45)$, indicating that the best (current) estimate of the haplotypes that correspond to this genotype is the haplotype pairs $(3, 9)$ in the first two locations, $(4, 5)$ from location 3–9, and $(4, 9)$ thereafter; here 3 refers to row 3 of matrix H that holds the current haplotypes, 4 refers to row 4, etc. Putting this together, the current estimate of the phased haplotype for this observation is displayed using

R code as:

```
>    j=Qbest
>    j1=trunc(((j-1)/h)+1 # points to 1st haplotype
>                         # corresponding to state j at position t=1 to N
>    j2=j-(j1-1)*h        # points to 2nd haplotype at position j for t=1
>                         # to N
>    Hhat=matrix(0,Tt,2)
>    for (t in 1:Tt) {
>       Hhat[t,1:2]=c(H[j1[i],t],H[j2[t],t])
>    }
>    colnames(Hhat)<-c("h1","h2")
>    cbind(j1,j2,Hhat,G)
        j1 j2 h1 h2 G
 [1,]   3  9  1  1  2
 [2,]   3  9  0  0  0
 [3,]   6  9  0  1  1
 [4,]   6  9  0  1  1
 [5,]   4  4  1  1  2
 [6,]   4  5  1  0  1
 [7,]   5  6  0  0  0
 [8,]   5  6  0  1  1
 [9,]   5  6  1  0  1
[10,]   5  9  1  1  2
[11,]   9  9  0  0  0
[12,]   9  9  1  1  2
[13,]   9 10  0  0  0
[14,]   9 10  0  1  1
[15,]   4  9  0  0  0
[16,]   4  9  0  0  0
[17,]   4  9  0  1  1
[18,]   4  9  1  1  2
[19,]   4  9  1  0  1
```

The actual haplotype assignments h1 and h2 are shown as the third and fourth columns of this output, and we see the consistency of the haplotype assignments with the genotype data G. Note, however, that when phasing data without the benefit of an existing reference panel, we are not interested in finding the single best estimate of h1 and h2; instead we need to address the second question of this section, namely, the initialization and updating of the current list of haplotypes.

6.7.1 Initializing and Updating the Current List of Haplotypes

Up to this point, all the imputations have been dependent upon the prior existence of a table of possible haplotypes from which recombinants are formed. All programs that are capable of performing large-scale haplotype imputation rely upon sampling haplotypes from among the set of possible haplotypes that are compatible with a given observed genotype sequence, G. The number of haplotype pairs that are compatible with the sequence G is equal to $2^{N_{hets}}$ where N_{hets} is the number of heterozygous markers in G. One approach to initializing haplotypes (used by MACH) is simply to randomly sample compatible haplotypes. For example, for the observed sequence $G = (2,0,1,1,2,1,0,1,1,2,0,2,0,1,0,0,1,2,1)$ used above, a pair of compatible haplotypes would be simply

$$\left\{ \begin{array}{l} (1,0,x_1,x_2,1,x_3,0,x_4,x_5,1,0,1,0,x_6,0,0,x_7,1,x_8) \\ (1,0,1-x_1,1-x_2,1,1-x_3,0,1-x_4,1-x_5,1,0,1,0,1-x_6,0,0,1-x_7,1,1-x_8) \end{array} \right\},$$

where each of x_i for $i = 1, \ldots, 8$ is sampled as independent Bernoulli draws with frequency 0.5. Thus if we are trying to impute haplotypes for N individuals, then we could initialize the table, H, by adding two sampled haplotype pairs for each individual to H. In R if the matrix G_{table} contains the genotype counts for (here 11) individuals in the panel to be phased:

```
> Gtable
      [,1] [,2] [,3] [,4] [,5] [,6] [,7] [,8] [,9] [,10] [,11] [,12] [,13] [,14] [,15] [,16] [,17] [,18] [,19]
 [1,]   2    2    2    2    2    2    1    2    2    2     1     2     1     2     1     1     1     2     2
 [2,]   2    2    2    2    2    2    2    2    2    2     2     2     2     2     2     2     2     2     2
 [3,]   2    0    2    2    2    2    0    2    2    2     0     2     0     2     0     0     0     2     2
 [4,]   2    2    1    2    2    2    1    2    2    2     1     2     1     2     0     0     0     2     2
 [5,]   2    0    2    2    2    2    0    2    2    2     0     2     0     2     0     0     0     2     2
 [6,]   2    1    2    2    2    2    1    2    2    2     0     2     0     1     1     1     1     2     2
 [7,]   2    0    1    1    2    1    0    1    1    2     0     2     0     1     0     0     1     2     1
 [8,]   2    2    2    2    2    2    2    2    2    2     2     2     2     2     2     2     2     2     2
 [9,]   2    2    1    2    2    1    2    2    2    1     2     1     2     1     1     1     1     2     2
[10,]   2    2    1    2    2    2    1    2    2    2     1     2     1     2     1     1     1     2     2
[11,]   1    2    2    1    1    2    0    2    1    1     0     1     0     2     0     0     0     1     1
```

then the initial estimate of H can be computed as:

```
> H<-matrix(0,2*Nsubj,nSnps)
> for (i in 1:Nsubj){
>     k=(i-1)*2+1
>     L=k+1
>     for (j in 1:nSnps) {
>         if (Gtable[i,j]==0) H[k:L,j]<-0
>         if (Gtable[i,j]==2) H[k:L,j]<-1
>         if (Gtable[i,j]==1) {x<-rbinom(1,1,.5);H[k,j]<-x;H[L,j]<-(1-x)}
>     }
> }
```

This gives (as one possible realization) a table H equal to:

```
> H
      [,1] [,2] [,3] [,4] [,5] [,6] [,7] [,8] [,9] [,10] [,11] [,12] [,13] [,14] [,15] [,16] [,17] [,18] [,19]
 [1,]   1    1    1    1    1    1    0    1    1    1     1     1     0     1     0     1     1     1     1
 [2,]   1    1    1    1    1    1    1    1    1    1     0     1     1     1     0     0     1     1     1
 [3,]   1    1    1    1    1    1    1    1    1    1     1     1     1     1     1     1     1     1     1
 [4,]   1    1    1    1    1    1    1    1    1    1     1     1     1     1     1     1     1     1     1
 [5,]   1    0    1    1    1    1    0    1    1    1     0     1     0     1     0     0     0     1     1
 [6,]   1    0    1    1    1    1    0    1    1    1     0     1     0     1     0     0     0     1     1
 [7,]   1    1    0    1    1    1    1    1    1    1     1     1     0     1     1     0     1     1     1
 [8,]   1    1    1    1    1    1    0    1    1    1     0     1     0     1     0     0     0     1     1
 [9,]   1    1    1    1    1    1    0    1    1    1     0     1     0     1     0     0     0     1     1
[10,]   1    0    1    1    1    1    0    1    1    1     0     1     0     1     0     0     0     1     1
[11,]   1    1    1    1    1    1    1    1    1    1     0     1     0     1     0     1     1     1     1
[12,]   1    0    1    1    1    1    0    1    1    1     0     1     0     1     1     0     0     1     1
[13,]   1    0    1    0    1    0    0    0    1    1     0     1     0     0     0     0     1     1     0
[14,]   1    0    0    1    1    1    0    1    0    1     0     1     0     1     0     0     0     1     1
[15,]   1    1    1    1    1    1    1    1    1    1     1     1     1     1     1     1     1     1     1
[16,]   1    1    1    1    1    1    1    1    1    1     1     1     1     1     1     1     1     1     1
[17,]   1    1    0    1    1    1    1    1    1    1     0     1     1     1     0     0     1     1     1
[18,]   1    1    1    1    1    1    0    1    1    1     1     1     0     1     0     1     1     1     1
[19,]   1    1    1    1    1    1    0    1    1    1     1     1     0     1     0     1     0     1     1
[20,]   1    1    0    1    1    1    1    1    1    1     0     1     1     1     1     0     1     1     1
[21,]   0    1    1    0    0    1    0    1    1    1     0     1     0     1     0     0     0     1     0
[22,]   1    1    1    1    1    1    0    1    0    0     0     0     0     1     0     0     0     0     1
>
```

This table is only used temporarily, however. In particular, after one run through the observed genotype vectors, G, for each individual, new haplotypes will be assigned, and these will replace the current table H.

For example, running the forward and backward algorithm on the first line of G_{table}, i.e., on the observation sequence, $G = (2,2,2,2,2,1,2,2,2,1,2,1,2,1,1,1,2,2)$, using H given above, produces the log probability of all states at location t as the array *loggamma*. Now, however, we are not really interested in the "best" sequence of states that correspond to this observation sequence; instead an update of the current assignment of states is performed by sampling a new state (i.e., new pair of haplotypes) with the sampling at each time point t using the expression for $\gamma_t i$) in (6.9) as the posterior distribution to be sampled from. Doing this for all genotype vectors G in G_{table} produces a new table H to be used in the next round. This procedure is allowed to iterate, typically around 20 times or so as described in Li et al. [11].

We can implement the sampling as follows:

1. First, sample initial state q_1 proportional to $\Pr(Q_1 = S_i | O, \lambda)$, i.e., proportional to *exp(loggamma[1,])* in the R program.
2. Next, use the combination of forward and backward variables to compute the probabilities of a transition from the sampled state q_1 to each of the possible states $j \in \{1, \ldots, N\}$ which from (6.8) is proportional to

$$\alpha_1(q_1)a_{q_1,j}b_j(O_2)\beta_2(j).$$

3. Iterate through the remaining states so that if state q_t is sampled at location t, the sampling probabilities for a transition to state j at time $t + 1$ is proportional to

$$\alpha_t(q_t)a_{q_t,j}b_j(O_{t+1})\beta_{t+1}(j).$$

This sampling can be performed using the R program code as:

```
>    sampledQ<-rep(0,Tt)
>    sampledQ[1]=sample(N,size=1,prob=exp(loggamma[1,]))
> # finish according to Eq (6.8)
>    for (t in 1:(Tt-1)){
>      probs<-rep(0,N)
>      Qt<-sampledQ[t]
>      for (j in 1:N){
>           probs[j]=exp(logalpha[t,Qt])*a(Qt,j)*b(t+1,j,G[t+1])
>                   *exp(logbeta[t+1,j])
>      }
>      probs<-probs/sum(probs)
>      sampledQ[t+1]<-sample(N,size=1,prob=probs)
>    }
```

The replacement pair of haplotypes is provided by decoding *sampleQ* as in:

```
> j=sampledQ
> j1=trunc((j-1)/h)+1   # gives first haplotype corresponding
>                       # to state j
> j2=j-(j1-1)*h # gives second
> Hhat=matrix(0,Tt,2)
> for (i in 1:Tt) {
>       Hhat[i,1:2]=c(H[j1[i],i],H[j2[i],i])
> }
> cbind(j,j1,j2,Hhat,G)
```

which gives something like:

```
        j  j1 j2 h1 h2 G
 [1,]   3   1  3  1  1 2
 [2,]   3   1  3  1  1 2
 [3,]   3   1  3  1  1 2
 [4,]   3   1  3  1  1 2
 [5,]  52   3  8  1  1 2
 [6,]  52   3  8  1  1 2
 [7,]  52   3  8  1  0 1
 [8,]   2   1  2  1  1 2
 [9,]  49   3  5  1  1 2
[10,]  49   3  5  1  1 2
[11,]  49   3  5  1  0 1
[12,]  49   3  5  1  1 2
[13,]  49   3  5  1  0 1
[14,]  49   3  5  1  1 2
[15,]  49   3  5  1  0 1
[16,]  49   3  5  1  0 1
[17,]  49   3  5  1  0 1
[18,]  49   3  5  1  1 2
[19,]  49   3  5  1  1 2
```

Repeating this sampling process for each genotype in turn and over a number of iterations should gradually improve the assignment of haplotypes for each study participant.

6.8   Practical Issues in Large-Scale SNP Imputation

Notice that the main loops above (for the calculation of *logalpha* and *logbeta* using the Baum–Welch algorithm in the above) are linear in the number of SNPs and in the number of samples being phased or imputed but are quadratic in the number of states, i.e., there are two nested *for* loops over the N states in the calculations of *logalpha* and *logbeta* above. The number of states is the square of the number of haplotypes (h^2 in the code above)[3] so that the whole run time would be a polynomial in the 4th power of the number of haplotypes used to define states. Therefore the number of haplotypes being considered must be quite small for any run, so that our above device, of starting with twice the number of haplotypes as genotypes to be phased is not feasible for large reference panels or main studies. An analysis and description of the run times of a number of different algorithms is provided as a part of Delaneau et al.'s [13] description of the program *SHAPEIT*. The success of the modern programs (including *SHAPEIT*) in providing useful phasing information and imputation for very large numbers of SNPs in feasible amounts of time is very impressive; while many important modifications are required to achieve this success, the fundamental ideas of encoding the imputation and phasing problems into an HMM and solving these problems using relatively standard Baum–Welch algorithms are at the heart of all the current high-performance algorithms.

Clearly also (as the reader can judge by running the above code selections, see also *haplo_impute.r*) the time required for the R interpreter to go through the loops described above is far too great for R to serve as a native language for this type of work. Typically, programs are written in C++ and are run simultaneously on multiple computer clusters breaking up the jobs either by chromosome or most often into many smaller segments. The state of knowledge of SNPs and other variants is constantly changing so that available reference panels are a moving target. As described above, it is useful to break up the overall imputation process into two parts, first phasing the main study data in its entirety and then running and rerunning as necessary the much faster haplotype-based imputation methods as reference panels are modified.

6.8.1 Assessing Imputation Accuracy

The most useful statistic for assessing the quality of imputation of an SNP or other allele is the correlation between true genotype count and imputed dosage variable [24]. Of course, except in special experiments, e.g., that of [24], we do not directly observe both genotyped and imputed variables for the main study SNPs being imputed. However we can estimate imputation R^2 in a number of ways. First of all, a formal calculation based on Hardy–Weinberg equilibrium for the imputation accuracy can be performed when haplotype frequencies are known and is similar to the calculation of haplotype imputation accuracy, R_h^2, discussed in Chap. 5. This calculation involves computing the "fraction of variance explained" as ($\text{Var}(E(n_A|G_i))/2p(1-p)$) where n_A is an allele count with frequency p. Since $E(n_A|G_i)$

---

[3] The number of unique states, N, can be reduced to $h(1 + h)/2$ since haplotype order is not being considered here. The R code above becomes slightly less intelligible when mapping the state number j to the pair of haplotypes referred to by j which is why this redundancy has not been removed.

is the imputed allele "dosage," one quasi-empirical estimate of imputation accuracy is simply the observed variance of the computed dosage variable divided by estimated $2\hat{p}(1-\hat{p})$ where $\hat{p}$ is the estimated allele frequency; this can be computed using the dosages as one half the average value of the dosage estimate, i.e., the estimate of $E(n_A|G_i)$. This is termed a quasi-empirical imputation R^2 because its calculation depends upon the correctness of the estimate of $E(n_A|G_i)$ in the first place (if the imputations were completely off base or biased, then the variance of the estimated dosage variables would not be informative). A more direct assessment of overall imputation accuracy is to mask some fraction of either the main study genotypes or the reference panel samples. The former calculation is routinely performed by many or all of the current imputation programs. Typically a few percent of the main study genotypes are "hidden" (treated as ungenotyped) and then imputed; and the sample correlations between the imputations and genotypes are directly calculated. The weakness of this approach is that it does not give an accuracy estimate for the (unmeasured) SNPs where the imputations are of any direct interest. It may be overoptimistic to assume that imputation accuracy for measured but hidden SNPs can be translated to the unmeasured SNPs for a variety of reasons including differences in population structure, minor allele frequency, and LD patterns. The second approach (hiding reference panel samples) is potentially informative but generally requires that a very large reference panel is available, especially if the accuracy of rare SNPs is to be carefully evaluated. Each of these measures, i.e., the *quasi-empirical*, SNP-based, and sample-based R^2 statistics, has been examined in certain publications [11, 24, 25]. Generally for common SNPs, the quasi-empirical and SNP-based R^2 statistics are reasonably consistent with each other; for example, see Fig. 3 of [24].

6.8.2   Imputing Rare SNPs

As is described in more detail in Chap. 8, the target sets of variants of interest for association studies have increasingly included rarer variants and SNPs. Following the logic described in Chap. 2, all variants are expected to have a single origin, and the specific chromosome that the variant arose upon is uniquely identifiable by patterns of marker variants nearby the site of origin. It follows that rare SNPs should be imputable on the basis of rare haplotypes of the common SNPs that are typically present on a GWAS array. Since rare SNPs are (in the absence of selective pressures) almost always of recent origin, it follows that the marker haplotype marking the new variant may still be unaffected by recombination occurring after the origin of the rare variant and thus still be recognizable. This means that the imputation of rare variants may be possible using common SNPs.

One of the crucial questions has to do with the necessary size of the reference panel needed in order to get good imputation quality. The required reference panel size increases as the frequency of the SNPs (or haplotypes in the above discussions) that are being imputed decreases. An analysis by Liu et al. [24] considered imputation of both common and rare SNPs that were genotyped in about 2,000 subjects. They found that with this many individual samples (and withholding genotyped data so that "dosage R^2," i.e., R^2 between imputed dosage variable and true genotype could be directly examined), a reference panel of ~2,000 samples could impute with $R^2 \geq 0.8$ SNPs with minor allele frequency in the range from 1 % to 3 %. Note that alleles with frequency 1 % would be seen an expected 40 times in a reference panel of 2,000 individuals. This is roughly the same number of minor alleles that would be expected to be seen in a reference panel of 40–100 samples (e.g., approximately HapMap sized) for SNPs in frequency range 0.2 to 0.5, and indeed SNPs in this frequency range are generally highly imputable with HapMap data [25]. Naively scaling this to rarer SNPs implies that reference panels of size at least 20,000 samples are required to impute SNPs with minor allele frequencies at 1/10 of 1 % with this same level of imputation accuracy.

In this naïve scaling, however, the issue of haplotype uncertainty as embodied in the R_h^2 calculation of Chap. 5 has been neglected. Without recombination there is a limit on the total number of haplotypes (and hence also a limit on the number of rare haplotypes), so if many rare haplotypes are to be defined by common SNPs, then recombination must be present. If a rare SNP falls on one or more rare haplotypes of common SNPs, it may not be well imputed by the common SNPs since imputation accuracy declines with the amount of recombination as described in the previous chapter.

6.8.3   Use of Cosmopolitan Reference Panels

As of the writing of this chapter, the most widely used reference panel and set of target genotypes for imputation are those available from phase 1 of the 1000 Genomes sequencing project. The 1000 Genomes Project is multiethnic and quite diverse. One important question is whether for a given project it is necessary to pick and choose from reference panels in order to do imputation and specifically whether it is important to match the reference study to the main study according to race/ ethnicity. As illustrated in Chap. 5, haplotype imputations and by implication imputed genotypes are dependent upon which reference group is selected, and it would be very bad to select (to give an extreme example) European or Asian reference panels in order to impute SNPs in a main study with participants of African origin. Two papers have looked at the use of the combined HapMap phase 2 genotypes (YRI, CEU, JPT, and CHB) [4, 26] for tag SNP selection (and by implication for imputation purposes) with the general conclusion that either a weighted or unweighted cosmopolitan panel is an appropriate choice. Here a weighted panel would be a combined panel with the fraction of individuals included in the panel weighted according to approximate admixture fractions (either recent or historical) of the study population. In a recent analysis of diabetes risk in a Singapore Chinese population quite close genetically to the 286 East Asians in the

1000 Genomes Project, Chen et al. [27] used the full set of thousand genomes (1,009 individuals) (rather than only the Asian) samples as a reference panel with evident success, showing that many unmeasured diabetes variants could be imputed and directionally validated in terms of their association with diabetes risk. While further investigation of this topic would seem worthwhile, it seems likely that (as in Chen et al.) all individuals in the 1000 Genomes Project are likely to be included in the reference panel for many projects.

6.9   Estimating Relative Risks for Imputed SNPs

6.9.1   Expectation Substitution

Based on the discussion of haplotype inference given in Chap. 5, expectation substitution of $E(n_A|G_i)$ in place of n_A in association analysis of the trait of interest can be expected to have good type I error probabilities and reasonable power relative to other (e.g., maximum likelihood) methods that jointly estimate risk parameters and haplotype frequencies when fitting models such as

$$g(E(Y_i)) = \alpha + \beta n_A. \tag{6.13}$$

More generally, if the model

$$g(E(Y_i)) = \alpha + \beta_0 I(n_A = 0) + \beta_1 I(n_A = 1) + \beta_2 I(n_A = 2) \tag{6.14}$$

is of interest, the probabilities that n_A equals 0, 1, or 2 given the observed genotype data (i.e., the expected values of the indicator functions) are used as the explanatory variables in (6.14).

More discussion of the behavior of expectation-substitution methods in unmeasured SNP analysis is provided in Chap. 8 (post-GWAS meta-analysis). SNPs that are well imputed may also safely be taken into multi-marker analyses, such as conditional analyses in which the effect of one variant is evaluated after allowing for the effects of another in order to determine if multiple associations seen in a single region are likely coming from the same or independent sources.

6.10   Chapter Summary

SNP imputation is very important in both extending the hypotheses being tested and for combining incompletely overlapping datasets. This chapter has tried to give the flavor of the HMM-based methods that form the basis of today's software. While some authors [28] have stressed the importance of more sophisticated methods, simple expectation substitution is the basic for nearly all association testing using imputed variants and is reasonably reliable at least for testing the effects of single variants. The 1000 Genomes Project as a cosmopolitan reference panel is a good source of information about LD patterns for the imputation of common SNPs, whereas targeting rarer alleles requires larger reference panels. Imputation of rare alleles using only common markers must ultimately be less accurate than imputing common markers, no matter how large the reference panel, based on considerations of haplotype uncertainty in the presence of recombination.

Homework

1. In the first example above (imputing genotypes from phased data for both the reference and main study), there was no allowance for genotyping error (e.g., function b in the R code above, see also *haplo_impute.r*). Modify this so that there is a high probability of genotyping error and rerun the imputation for the same data. What is the effect on the imputation?
2. Try replacing some of the observed data with missing in the first example (i.e., change the vector `O<-c(4,3,3,9,9,3,1,2,3,9,9,2,2,4,1,2,9,1,9)` so that one or two of the non-missing genotypes are set to missing, i.e., set to 9. Run the imputation again and compare the imputed genotypes to their true values. How successful does the imputation seem to be?
3. If not already available, download IMPUTE2 from the IMPUTE2 website (see links below) and install on your computer. Download the HapMap phase 3 phased genotypes (haplotypes) for the CEU and YRI groups for the SNPs on chromosome 22. Download the phased haplotypes for the ASW group and remove 1/2 of the SNPs (i.e., mask them in the analysis). Use the CEU + YRI data as the reference panel and impute the missing SNPs for the ASW group. Compare the imputed SNPs for ASW to the true values by calculating R^2 between the imputed and true SNP allele counts. What is the distribution of R^2? If necessary (for ease in testing the programs and manipulating the data) do the experiment first using only a few hundred SNPs within a short region of the chromosome.
4. IMPUTE2 provides an imputation quality score for each imputed SNP. How does that imputation quality score compare to the R^2 calculated above? For example, plot the quality scores against the R^2 values. Also compute the imputation R^2 as Var(SNP allele dosage)$/(2\hat{p}(1-\hat{p}))$ with $\hat{p}$ the estimated allele frequency for the imputed SNP ($\hat{p}$ is the mean of the dosage divided by 2). Compare the imputation R^2 with the IMPUTE2 quality score and the observed R^2 from the masking experiment. How well do they compare (e.g., are they highly correlated)?
5. If you have access to the JAPC data, try extracting the SNPs in the 8q24 region near the top hits as listed in the Cheng et al. paper (see Chap. 3) and use the HapMap phase 2 data for JPT + CHB samples in the same region as the reference panel and target genotypes. Run either MACH or IMPUTE2 to impute the genotypes in HapMap phase 2 that are not in the JAPC data. Run association tests using either R, SAS, or PLINK, to relate the dosage estimates to prostate cancer risk. Are there any imputed SNPs that appear to have stronger results than the genotyped SNPs?

6.10.1 Links

IMPUTE2, Genotype imputation and haplotype phasing program, http://mathgen. stats.ox.ac.uk/impute/impute_v2.html#download

MACH, Markov Chain based haplotyper. http://www.sph.umich.edu/csg/abecasis/ MACH/index.html

References

1. Howie, B., Marchini, J., & Stephens, M. (2011). Genotype imputation with thousands of genomes. *G3 (Bethesda), 1*, 457–470.
2. Carlson, C. S., Eberle, M. A., Rieder, M. J., Yi, Q., Kruglyak, L., & Nickerson, D. A. (2004). Selecting a maximally informative set of single-nucleotide polymorphisms for association analyses using linkage disequilibrium. *The American Journal of Human Genetics, 74*, 106–120.
3. Stram, D. O. (2004). Tag SNP selection for association studies. *Genetic Epidemiology, 27*, 365–374.
4. de Bakker, P. I., Burtt, N. P., Graham, R. R., Guiducci, C., Yelensky, R., Drake, J. A., et al. (2006). Transferability of tag SNPs in genetic association studies in multiple populations. *Nature Genetics, 38*, 1298–1303.
5. Haiman, C. A., Hsu, C., de Bakker, P., Frasco, M., Sheng, X., Van Den Berg, D., et al. (2007). Comprehensive association testing of common genetic variation in DNA repair pathway genes in relationship with breast cancer risk in multiple populations. *Human Molecular Genetics, 17* (6), 825–834.
6. de Bakker, P. I., Yelensky, R., Pe'er, I., Gabriel, S. B., Daly, M. J., & Altshuler, D. (2005). Efficiency and power in genetic association studies. *Nature Genetics, 37*, 1217–1223.
7. Barrett, J. C., Fry, B., Maller, J., & Daly, M. J. (2005). Haploview: Analysis and visualization of LD and haplotype maps. *Bioinformatics, 21*, 263–265.
8. Stram, D. O., Haiman, C. A., Hirschhorn, J. N., Altshuler, D., Kolonel, L. N., Henderson, B. E., et al. (2003). Choosing haplotype-tagging SNPs based on unphased genotype data from a preliminary sample of unrelated subjects with an example from the Multiethnic Cohort Study. *Human Heredity, 55*(1), 27–36.
9. Chapman, J. M., Cooper, J. D., Todd, J. A., & Clayton, D. G. (2003). Detecting disease associations due to linkage disequilibrium using haplotype tags: A class of tests and the determinants of statistical power. *Human Heredity, 56*, 18–32.
10. Stephens, M., & Donnelly, P. (2003). A comparison of bayesian methods for haplotype reconstruction from population genotype data, *American Journal of Human Genetics*, 73, 1162–1169.
11. Li, Y., Willer, C. J., Ding, J., Scheet, P., & Abecasis, G. R. (2010). MaCH: Using sequence and genotype data to estimate haplotypes and unobserved genotypes. *Genetic Epidemiology, 34*, 816–834.
12. Scheet, P., & Stephens, M. (2006). A fast and flexible statistical model for large-scale population genotype data: applications to inferring missing genotypes and haplotypic phase. *The American Journal of Human Genetics, 78*, 629–644.
13. Delaneau, O., Marchini, J., & Zagury, J.-F. (2011). A linear complexity phasing method for thousands of genomes. *Nature Methods, 9*, 179–181.
14. Durbin, R., Eddy, S., Krogh, A., & Mitchison, G. (1998). *Biological sequence analysis.* Cambridge, UK: Cambridge University Press.
15. Siegmund, D., & Yakir, Y. (2007). *The statistics of gene mapping.* New York, NY: Springer.

16. Baum, L. E., & Eagon, J. A. (1967). An inequality with applications to statistical estimation for probabilistic functions of Markov processes and to a model for ecology. *Bulletein of the American Mathematical Society, 73*, 360–363.

17. Baum, L. E., Petrie, T., Soules, G., & Weiss, N. (1970). A maximization technique occurring in the statistical analysis of probabilistic functions of Markov chains. *The Annals of Mathematical Statistics, 41*, 164–171.

18. Baum, L. E. (1972). An inequality and associated maximization technique in statistical estimation for probabilistic functions of Markov processes. *Inequalities, 3*, 1–8.

19. Dempster, A., Laird, N., & Rubin, D. (1977). Maximum likelihood from incomplete data via the EM algorithm. *JRSS-B, 37*, 1–22.

20. Rabiner, L. R. (1989). A tutorial on hidden Markov models and selected applications in speech recognition. *Proceedings of the IEEE, 77*, 257–286.

21. Howie, B., Fuchsberger, C., Stephens, M., Marchini, J., & Abecasis, G. R. (2012). Fast and accurate genotype imputation in genome-wide association studies through pre-phasing. *Nature Genetics, 44*, 955–959.

22. Haiman, C. A., Stram, D. O., Pike, M. C., Kolonel, L. N., Burtt, N. P., Altshuler, D., et al. (2003). A comprehensive haplotype analysis of CYP19 and breast cancer risk: The multiethnic Cohort study. *Human Molecular Genetics, 12*, 2679–2692.

23. Howie, B. N., Donnelly, P., & Marchini, J. (2009). Impute2: A flexible and accurate genotype imputation method for the next generation of genome-wide association studies. *PLoS Genetics, 5*, e1000529.

24. Liu, E. Y., Buyske, S., Aragaki, A. K., Peters, U., Boerwinkle, E., Carlson, C., et al. (2012). Genotype imputation of Metabochip SNPs using a study-specific reference panel of 4,000 haplotypes in African Americans from the Women's Health initiative. *Genetic Epidemiology, 36*, 107–117.

25. Li, L., Li, Y., Browning, S. R., Browning, B. L., Slater, A. J., Kong, X., et al. (2011). Performance of genotype imputation for rare variants identified in exons and flanking regions of genes. *PLoS One, 6*, e24945.

26. Egyud, M. R., Gajdos, Z. K., Butler, J. L., Tischfield, S., Le Marchand, L., Kolonel, L. N., et al. (2009). Use of weighted reference panels based on empirical estimates of ancestry for capturing untyped variation. *Human Genetics, 125*, 295–303.

27. Chen, Z., Pereira, M. A., Seielstad, M., Koh, W.-P., Tai, E. S., Teo, Y.-Y., et al. (2013). Joint effects of known Type 2 diabetes susceptibility loci in genome-wide association study of Singapore Chinese: The Singapore Chinese health study. *PLOS ONE In Press*

28. Hu, Y. J., & Lin, D. Y. (2010). Analysis of untyped SNPs: Maximum likelihood and imputation methods. *Genetic Epidemiology, 34*, 803–815.

Chapter 7
Design of Large-Scale Genetic Association Studies, Sample Size, and Power

Abstract The subject of this chapter is sample size and power calculations for studies of genetic associations for both case–control studies and prospective studies of a quantitative phenotype or trait. This chapter starts with a comparison of three different methods for calculating power for the simplest single marker studies and then goes on to consider the general statistical approach to power calculations that are embodied in the very widely used QUANTO (Gauderman, W., & Morrison, J. (2006). *QUANTO 1.1: A computer program for power and sample size calculations for genetic-epidemiology studies.* http://hydra.usc.edu/gxe) program for a variety of study designs, including those which are impervious to population stratification, specifically sibling-matched and parent-affected-offspring studies. The chapter then discusses additional considerations affecting sample size and power including (1) control for multiple comparisons, (2) control for population stratification by the principal components methods discussed in Chap. 4, (3) multi-staged genotyping designs, (4) fine-mapping of associations using multi-marker analyses, (5) power calculations for haplotype analysis and imputed marker analysis, and (7) reuse of existing data for new studies.

7.1 Design Considerations

Design considerations include (1) source(s) of samples including cases and controls in retrospective studies, (2) control for population stratification either directly or indirectly, (3) control of multiple comparisons, (4) genotyping plan, and (5) data reuse/meta-analysis plans.

All human genetic studies are inherently observational studies. The goal of a genetic association study is to find results (associations between phenotype and variant) which can be reliably reproduced if not in all human populations (which may be impossible since allele frequencies and LD patterns can vary widely between populations) at least in populations with similar ancestral origins. There are many potential pitfalls in genetic association studies, not the least of which is

D.O. Stram, *Design, Analysis, and Interpretation of Genome-Wide Association Scans*, Statistics for Biology and Health, DOI 10.1007/978-1-4614-9443-0_7, © Springer Science+Business Media New York 2014

the possibility that population structure may introduce bias and/or unexpected correlations between phenotypes into association results. Two well-known designs, sibling-matched designs and affected-offspring (trio) designs, have the advantage of being immune to usual concerns about population structure and confounding, since the ancestry of the parents is completely adjusted for (conditioned out) in the analysis of data from these two designs. However in most settings these designs have important logistical disadvantages compared to studies of "unrelated" subjects. Admixture between groups with varying disease susceptibility was early on [1] recognized as a serious potential problem; one solution, when studying diseases such as diabetes in admixed populations, is to only consider "stratification-proof" designs and accept the limitations that this implies on study size and conduct. Luckily as we have seen, when large amounts of genotype data are available (large-scale SNP data) additional approaches to controlling for admixture and other kinds of population structure open up. Previously justified admonitions to take extreme care in seeking highly homogeneous sources of case and controls [1] to avoid the possibility of hidden stratification or admixture differences are less relevant when admixture can be detected directly and adjusted for in the analysis.

7.2   Sample Size and Power for Studies of Unrelated Subjects

7.2.1   Power for Chi-Square Tests

Many different kinds of tests can be approximated as single or multi-degree of freedom central and non-central chi-square statistics under the null (central chi-square) or alternative (non-central chi-square) hypotheses. To briefly review, a central chi-square random variable with one degree of freedom arises as the square of a standard normal random variable, z, having mean zero and unit variance. A non-central chi-square with one degree of freedom and the non-centrality parameter μ^2 arise as the square of a normal random variable, with mean μ and variance 1. Central chi-squares with more than one degree of freedom, p, arise as the sum of squares of p independent standard normal random variables. A non-central chi-square random variable with p degrees of freedom arises as the sum of normal random variables, z_i, $i = 1, \ldots, p$, each having means μ_i and variance 1. The non-centrality parameter for the distribution is $\lambda^2 = \sum_{i=1}^{p} \mu_i^2$. The non-central chi-square distribution has mean $p + \lambda^2$ and variance $2(p + 2\lambda^2)$.

Consider a one degree of freedom test. Assume that there is a single parameter of interest, β, in a model for the outcome data (which may also involve other nuisance parameters) and that β has an estimator, $\hat{\beta}$, which converges to β and which has a variance estimate $\hat{\mathrm{Var}}(\hat{\beta})$. For most generalized linear models under certain regularity conditions (required to remove pathological cases) we can assume that for large samples $\hat{\beta}$ is distributed as a normal random variable with mean β and that the variance estimate will converge to the true variance $\text{Var}(\hat{\beta})$, of $\hat{\beta}$. Further assume that we are testing the null hypothesis that $\beta = 0$ against the two-sided alternative $\beta \neq 0$. In this case the test statistic $\hat{\beta}^2/\hat{\text{Var}}(\hat{\beta})$, will, for large samples, have a χ_1^2 distribution with non-centrality parameter equal to the true value, β^2, divided by the true variance $\text{Var}(\hat{\beta})$ (For tests of other null hypotheses, i.e., $\beta = \beta_0$ the non-centrality parameter is $(\beta = \beta_0)^2/\text{Var}(\hat{\beta})$). This non-centrality parameter is key to evaluating power of the test. For example, in order to obtain power at least equal to s (i.e., sensitivity, or one minus the type II error rate) to test a null hypothesis $\beta = 0$ using a test with type 1 error rate α then the non-centrality parameter must be at least as large as

$$\left[\Phi^{-1}(1 - \alpha/2)\Phi^{-1}(s)\right]^2,\tag{7.1}$$

where $\Phi^{-1}(x)$ is the inverse of the CDF function for a standard normal random variable, z, i.e., $\text{Pr}(z \leq \Phi^{-1}(x)) = x$ when z is normal with mean 0 and variance 1.

In a simple univariate least squares regression problem, where outcome, Y_i, is a linear function of a predictor, X_i, with both variables observed for $i = 1, \ldots, N$ subjects, the estimate of the slope parameter, β, is equal to $\hat{\beta} = \left(\sum_{i=1}^{N}(X_i - \overline{X})(Y_i - \overline{Y})\right)/\sum_{i=1}^{N}(X_i - \overline{X})^2$. Assuming that the OLS model is correct (i.e., the mean of Y_i is linear in X_i and that the variance of Y_i is equal to a constant σ^2 for all i), then the variance of $\hat{\beta}$ is equal to $\sigma^2/\sum_{i=1}^{N}(X_i - \overline{X})^2$. The non-centrality parameter of the χ^2 test, $\hat{\beta}^2/\text{Var}(\hat{\beta})$, of the null hypothesis that $\beta = 0$ is equal to $\beta^2/\sigma^2 \sum_{i=1}^{N}(X_i - \overline{X})^2$. Note that this non-centrality parameter can be obtained by a method which we term following Longmate 2001 [2] as the *exemplary data substitution approach* as follows. We take the formula for the chi-square statistic

$$\frac{\hat{\beta}^2}{\text{Var}(\hat{\beta})} = \frac{\left(\dfrac{\sum(X_i - \overline{X})(Y_i - \overline{Y})}{(X_i - \overline{X})^2}\right)^2}{\dfrac{\sigma^2}{\sum(X_i - \overline{X})^2}} = \frac{\left(\sum(X_i - \overline{X})(Y_i - \overline{Y})\right)^2}{\sigma^2 \sum(X_i - \overline{X})^2}\tag{7.2}$$

and replace Y_i and $\overline{Y}$ with their expected values $\mu + \beta X_i$ and $\mu + \beta\overline{X}$, respectively so that the RHS of (7.2) becomes $\left(\sum(X_i - \overline{X})(\beta X_i - \beta\overline{X})\right)^2/\sigma^2 \sum(X_i - \overline{X})^2 = (\beta^2/\sigma^2)\sum(X_i - \overline{X})^2$, which is the non-centrality parameter. It turns out that for ordinary least squares regression this substitution approach can be utilized to determine the non-centrality parameter for a great number of tests, both single and multi-degree of freedom. In general the chi-square statistics relevant to linear regression can all be written as $Y'AY/\sigma^2$ where A is a symmetric projection matrix with rank equal to the number of hypotheses, p, being simultaneously tested. It is easy to show that the expected value of this statistic is equal to

$$\text{rank}(A) + E(Y)'AE(Y)/\sigma^2 = p + E(Y)'AE(Y)/\sigma^2,$$

so that the non-centrality parameter λ^2 is obtained by substitution of the vector $Y = (Y_i, Y_2, \ldots, Y_N)'$ with its expected value, $E(Y) = (E(Y_i), E(Y_2), \ldots, E(Y_N))'$, into the formula for the statistic itself; i.e., to obtain the non-centrality parameter we *analyze* $E(Y)$ in the same way we would analyze the actual observed data Y. This idea is expanded upon in the next sections. Note that $(\beta^2/\sigma^2)\sum (X_i - \overline{X})^2$ increases linearly with the sum of squares term, $\sum_{i=1}^{N} (X_i - \overline{X})^2$. Typically the sum of squares can be assumed to increase linearly with the number of subjects (if for example the sampled X_i are representative of an underlying population of possible values so that each individual brings on average the same amount of information to the study). This is also generally true for the non-centrality parameter, $E(Y)'AE(Y)/\sigma^2$, for multiple degrees of freedom test.

As usually described, tests of null hypotheses in ordinary linear regression utilize F, rather than chi-square, statistics to perform hypothesis testing. The F tests, by taking into account the variability of the estimate of σ^2 ($\hat{\sigma}^2$, equal to the sum of the square of the residuals divided by the residual degrees of freedom), are exact for any sample size when, in addition to being linear in X_i and homogeneous in variance, the Y_i are normally distributed. The chi-square statistics described above form the numerator and denominator of these F tests (after division by the number of degrees of freedom, p), and the non-centrality parameter for the F is equal to the non-centrality parameters for the numerator. As the number of degrees of freedom for the residual error estimate, $\hat{\sigma}^2$, increases, the conclusions of the F test (i.e., the p-values obtained from the test) approach those of the chi-square statistic.

Once the non-centrality parameter for a single or multi-degree of freedom test is computed it is very simple to obtain the power of a chi-square test using the R code functions *pchisq* and *qchisq*, which give (respectively) the CDF and inverse CDF functions of the chi-square distributions. The function *Power_chisq* defined below takes arguments equal to the number of degrees of freedom and non-centrality parameter as well as the test size α used to determine significance:

```
> # power function for chi-square tests
> Power_chisq<-function(ndf, ncp, alpha){
>     crit=qchisq(1-alpha,ndf) # critical value for central chi-square
>     1-pchisq(crit,ndf,ncp) # prob of exceeding this critical value
>                            # for noncentral chi-square
> }
```

The power function for F tests is a function also of the same ncp and alpha parameters, but includes both the numerator and denominator (residual) degrees of freedom in the calculations. R code for this function is:

```
> # power function for f tests
> Power_f<-function(ndf1,ndf2, ncp, alpha){
>    crit=qf(1-alpha,ndf1,ndf2)
>    1-pf(crit,ndf1,ndf2,ncp)
> }
```

Finding the non-centrality parameter that corresponds to a fixed value of power is easy for 1 degree of freedom chi-square tests using (7.1). For multiple degrees of freedom tests a simple search can be used to solve for the ncp value that satisfies a given power requirement. When the non-centrality parameter can be assumed to be linear in sample size, finding the non-centrality parameter also finds the sample size needed to meet specific study requirements on power and type I error rate α.

The *exemplary data approach* to power calculation applies this substitution method to tests which can be assumed to have an asymptotic chi-square distribution; our main focus will be upon likelihood ratio tests for generalized linear regression. While the underlying statistical justification of this approach can be quite complex it is an extremely useful and relatively simple approximation technique [2–4].

As described in previous chapters there is more than one way to analyze genetic associations in case–control data (here we concentrate on diallelic variants), for example, we may

1. Perform tests for allele frequency differences (allele A versus allele a) between cases and controls, using standard binomial statistics.
2. Use the Armitage test NR^2 to test for correlation between case–control status, D, and the count, $n(A)$, of the number of copies of allele A.
3. Perform logistic regression relating individual case–control status, D_i, to $n_i(A)$ by fitting the logistic model.

$$\log[E(D_i) - \log[1 - E(D_i)] = \mu + \beta_0 G_{i0} + \beta_1 G_{i1} + \beta_2 G_{i2}, \qquad (7.3)$$

with G_{ik} equal to the indicator variable $I[n_i(A) = k]$ for $k = 0, 1, 2$.

We now consider power calculations for all three of these. Consider several possible constraints on the β_k parameters in model (7.3).

1. The *dominant* model constrains $\beta_0 = 0$ and $\beta_1 = \beta_2$.
2. The *recessive* model constrains $\beta_0 = \beta_1 = 0$.
3. The *log additive* model constrains $\beta_0 = 0$ and $\beta_2 = 2\beta_1$.

In addition μ is a free parameter that will play a role as well in the following. Of course in a case–control study the estimated value of μ is mainly reflective of matching frequency ratios and not of background rates of disease in a population.

7.2.2 Calculation of Non-centrality Parameters for Chi-Square Tests in Generalized Linear Models

We begin our analysis of power by computing the expected genotype probabilities $\Pr(n_i(A) = k|D_i)$ conditional on case–control status ($D_i = 0$ or $D_i = 1$) assuming (1) that the frequencies of alleles a and A are in Hardy–Weinberg equilibrium in the source population for the case–control study with allele A having frequency p and (2) that model (7.3) applies. We use Bayes' Rule to compute

$$\Pr\big(n_i(A) = k\big|D_i\big) = \frac{\Pr\big(D_i\big|n_i(A) = k\big)\Pr(n_i(A) = k)}{\sum_{l=0}^{2}\Pr\big(D_i\big|n_i(A) = l\big)\Pr(n_i(A) = l)}. \tag{7.4}$$

Illustrative values coming from the calculations are displayed in Table 7.2. Here we focus on an example involving a rare disease ($\mu = 10^{-5}$ in the population) and a modest log odds ratio parameter $\beta = \log(1.3)$ for a common variant having frequency equal to $p = 0.1$.

R code to compute the second line of Table 7.1 is given below; note that this uses the built-in R function *dbinom* which gives the probability function for the binomial distribution; the first argument for *dbinom* is the number of successes, the second is the index (number of trials), and the third the frequency parameter p

```
> # case_control_power.r
> logit<-function(x) log(x)-log(1-x) # logistic link function
> expit<-function(x)exp(x)/(1+exp(x)) # inverse of logit function > >
> log(x/(1-x))
> # joint distribution function for n and D
> p_d_n<-function(n,D,mu,beta0,beta1,beta2,p) {
>    Pr1=expit(mu+beta0*(n==0) + beta1*(n==1)+beta2*(n==2))
>    # probability that D=1
>    dbinom(D,1,Pr1)*dbinom(n,2,p)
> }
> # conditional distribution of n given D
> p_n_given_d<-function(n,D,mu,beta0,beta1,beta2,p){
>    pr=0; # sum to get marginal prob that status=D
>    for (nn in 0:2) pr=pr+p_d_n(nn,D,mu,beta0,beta1,beta2,p)
>    p_d_n(n,D,mu,beta0,beta1,beta2,p)/pr
> }
> # Now compute line2 of Table 7.1
> #additive model
> mu=logit(1e-5);beta0=0;beta1=log(1.3);beta2=2*beta1;p=.1

> pc_case=
> c(p_n_given_d(0,1,mu,beta0,beta1,beta2,p),
>    p_n_given_d(1,1,mu,beta0,beta1,beta2,p),
>    p_n_given_d(2,1,mu,beta0,beta1,beta2,p)
> )
> pc_control=
> c(p_n_given_d(0,0,mu,beta0,beta1,beta2,p),
>    p_n_given_d(1,0,mu,beta0,beta1,beta2,p),
>    p_n_given_d(2,0,mu,beta0,beta1,beta2,p)
>)

>round(c(pc_case,pc_control),4)
```

Table 7.1 Illustrative values of $\Pr(n(A)|D)$

Model	$D = 1$			$D = 0$		
	$\Pr(n_i(A) = 0)$	$\Pr(n_i(A) = 1)$	$\Pr(n_i(A) = 2)$	$\Pr(n_i(A) = 0)$	$\Pr(n_i(A) = 1)$	$\Pr(n_i(A) = 2)$
$\mu = \mathrm{logit}(10^{-5})$, null, $\beta = 0$, $p = 0.1$	0.81	0.18	0.01	0.81	0.18	0.01
$\mu = \mathrm{logit}(10^{-5})$, additive, $\beta = \log(1.3)$, $p = 0.1$	0.7635	0.2206	0.0159	0.8100	0.1800	0.0100
$\mu = \mathrm{logit}(10^{-5})$, dominant, $\beta = \log(1.3)$, $p = 0.1$	0.7663	0.2214	0.0123	0.8100	0.1800	0.0100
$\mu = \mathrm{logit}(10^{-5})$, recessive, $\beta = \log(1.3)$, $p = 0.1$	0.808	0.179	0.013	0.810	0.180	0.010
$\mu = \mathrm{logit}(0.5)$, additive, $\beta = \log(1.3)$, $p = 0.1$	0.7894	0.1983	0.0122	0.8317	0.1607	0.0076

The other lines are computed by altering the parameters, p, μ, and the βs accordingly.

With Table 7.1 in hand consider power calculations for each of the tests above.

The binomial test assumes that each of the genotype count variables for cases and controls is distributed as a binomial random variable with number of trials equal to 2 and tests for a frequency difference between the two groups. A standard asymptotic χ_1^2 test statistic is

$$\frac{(\hat{p}_1 - \hat{p}_0)^2}{\hat{\text{Var}}(\hat{p}_1 - \hat{p}_0)}. \tag{7.5}$$

The variance estimator is

$$\left(\frac{\hat{p}_1(1 - \hat{p}_1)}{2n_1} + \frac{\hat{p}_0(1 - \hat{p}_0)}{2n_0} \right),$$

where $\hat{p}_1$ and $\hat{p}_0$ are the sampled frequencies of allele A in the cases and controls respectively and $\hat{p}$ is the frequency in the combined sample (cases and controls). The non-centrality parameter for test (7.5) is

$$\frac{(p_1 - p_0)^2}{\text{Var}(\hat{p}_1 - \hat{p}_0)}, \tag{7.6}$$

with $\text{Var}(\hat{p}_1 - \hat{p}_0)$ equal to $(p_1(1 - p_1)/2n_1) + (p_0(1 - p_0)/2n_0)$. Consider now the power of testing for allele frequency differences in a scenario in which the population allele frequency, p, equals 10 %; the model for disease given allele count $n(A)$ is log additive with $\beta_1 = \log(1.3)$ (and $\beta_2 = 2\log(1.3)$) in a study which samples 500 cases and 500 controls from a population with background disease frequency specified by $\mu = \text{logit}(10^{-5})$. From Table 7.1 we see that in this scenario the genotype count probabilities for the cases are $\Pr(n(A) = 0) = 0.7635$, $\Pr(n(A) = 1) = 0.2206$, and $\Pr(n(A) = 2) = 0.0159$. Therefore the true A allele frequency is $P_1 = (0.2206 + 2 \times 0.0159)/2 = 0.1262$ for the cases. For the controls $\Pr(n(A) = 0) = 0.81$, $\Pr(n(A) = 1) = 0.18$, and $\Pr(n(A) = 2) = 0.01$, with mean frequency 10 % as in the population. Upon substitution the non-centrality parameter is equal to

$$\lambda^2 = 1,000 \frac{0.0262^2}{0.1262(1 - 0.1262) + 0.10(1 - 0.10)} = 3.4275.$$

Substituting this into the *Power_chisq* function above:

```
>Power_chisq (1,3.4275,.05)
```

gives a power of 0.4568 under the alternative hypothesis.

Table 7.2 Expected distribution of case–control status and genotype computed in a case–control study with 500 cases and 500 controls for the above example

$n(A)$	D	$\Pr(n(A),D)$	$E(N_{n(A),D})$
0	0	0.4050	405
1	0	0.0900	90
2	0	0.0050	5
0	1	0.38175	381.75
1	1	0.1103	110.3
2	1	0.0080	7.95

Each value $E(N_{n(A),D})$ is the expected number of subjects and is computed as 1,000 times $\Pr(n(A),D)$ which equals $\Pr(n(A)|D)\pi(D)$ for $n(A) = 0, 1, 2$ and $D = 0, 1$. Here $\pi(D)$ is the fraction of sampled subjects with disease state D. In this 1:1 matching $\pi(D)$ equals ½ for both $D = 0$ and $D = 1$

For the Armitage trend test (computed as NR^2 where N is the total number of subjects and R^2 is the squared correlation between case–control status and genotype count) we can compute the correlation between case–control status and genotype count for this example. The joint probability distribution of genotypes and case–control status for a 1:1 frequency-matched study will be as shown in Table 7.2 which is computed using the R function $p\_n\_given\_d$ defined above.

Analyzing these data as if they are observed data can be done (approximately) as follows:

```
> Expected_gc<-c(rep(0,405),rep(1,90),rep(2,5),
  rep(0,382),rep(1,110),rep(2,8))
> Expected_D <-c(rep(0,500),rep(1,500))
> 1000*cor(Expected_gc,Expected_D)^2 # the NCP
```

which gives 3.364 as the non-centrality parameter.

For a more precise answer we can use the *cov.wt* function in R which allows for weights and analyze Table 7.2 directly as

```
> D<-c(0,0,0,1,1,1)
> G<-c(0,1,2,0,1,2)
> wgts<-1000*c(.4050,.0900,.0050, .38175, .1103, .00795)
> x<-matrix(c(G,D),6,2)
> 1000*cov2cor(cov.wt(x,wgts)$cov)[1,2]^2 # the NCP
```

which gives 3.4163 as the non-centrality parameter (here the *cov2cor* function is used to compute a correlation matrix from an input covariance matrix which is computed using *cov.wt*). Using the latter in function *Power_chisq* gives power = 0.5745, close to the power determined from the test of binomial frequencies above.

Table 7.3 Non-centrality parameters calculated for the parameter values given in Table 7.1

	Allele counting	Armitage test	Logistic regression exemplary data
$\mu = \text{logit}(10^{-5})$, additive, $\beta = \log(1.3)$, $p = 0.1$	3.4275	3.4163	3.4260
$\mu = \text{logit}(10^{-5})$, dominant, $\beta = \log(1.3)$, $p = 0.1$	2.6735	2.5739	2.5907
$\mu = \text{logit}(10^{-5})$, recessive, $\beta = \log(1.3)$, $p = 0.1$	0.0343	0.0064	0.0065
$\mu = \text{logit}(0.5)$, additive, $\beta = \log(1.3)$, $p = 0.1$	3.1664	3.0160	3.0224

Finally we can use Table 7.2 to approximate the power for a likelihood ratio test of no association between disease, D, and outcome. We fit a logistic regression model to the data in Table 7.2 either approximately as in:

```
# ncp for LR test
> fit_glm<-glm(Expected_D~Expected_gc,family=binomial())
              # save model fit
> anova(fit_glm)
```

which returns ncp $= 3.37395$ or directly (using a weight function in the call to the *glm* function) as:

```
> # ncp for LR test use definition of D, G, and wgts, from above
> fit_glm2<-glm(D~G,family=binomial(),weights=wgts) # save model fit
> anova(fit_glm2)
```

which gives ncp $= 3.426016$.

All of these non-centrality parameters give similar estimated study power of 45.7–45.9 %.

Table 7.3 gives non-centrality parameters for the three tests (allele counting, Armitage, and Logistic regression) corresponding to all the parameter choices given in Table 7.1.

Notice that the non-centrality parameters are far smaller for the recessive model than for the dominant or additive models (which is expected since the risk genotype, the AA, is very rare). Also notice that the non-centrality parameter computed for the allele counting method for the recessive model is noticeably larger than for either the Armitage test or for logistic regression. This needs to be interpreted carefully; in this case the a priori assumption, used by the allele counting method, of Hardy–Weinberg equilibrium of genotypes in both the cases and controls is not valid. Compared to a binomial distribution with the same mean the distribution among the cases has too many homozygotes (*aa* or *AA*) and too few heterozygotes. This means that the allele counting test underestimates the variance of $\hat{p}_1$ and therefore of the test statistic, $(\hat{p}_1 - \hat{p}_0)$; hence this test may not control the false-positive rate at the required type I error level. The dominant model (second line of Table 7.3) also shows a small discrepancy between the distribution of genotypes in the cases and that expected with the binomial distribution with the same mean. In this case the discrepancy again leads to a slight overestimation of the power for the allele counting test. The same appears to be true for a log additive model (last line of Table 7.3) in which the disease is assumed to be common (background frequency of 0.5). In general the allele counting test is only fully appropriate for an additive logistic model when the disease is rare, since only then does the distribution of $n(A)$ in both the cases and the controls follow HWE (see Homework).

The exemplary data method is a very flexible method for approximating non-centrality parameters for case–control studies [2]: it can be extended to the computation of power for tests of gene $\times$ environment and gene $\times$ gene interactions using standard logistic regression analysis (i.e., unconditional analysis), conditional logistic regression [3], and case-only analysis (for interactions), etc. For each choice of parameters in Table 7.2 models for the distribution of disease, given genetic variants and covariates, (including interactions with covariates), are combined with models for the distribution of genetic variants and covariates in the population as a whole to produce the expected numbers given in the table.

A fairly complicated example of the exemplary data method is given in Longmate [2] who describes power calculations for a gene–environment interaction, in this case between smoking and a candidate gene for lung cancer. In order to compute power for such a study it is necessary to specify (1) the risk allele frequency in the population, (2) the frequency of smoking in the population, (3) the relationship between smoking and probability of disease, and (4) how this smoking risk depends upon the number of risk alleles, $n(A)$, that an individual carries. It was assumed in Longmate 2001 that smoking is independent of $n(A)$ in the population as a whole, that the population frequency of never smoking was 34 % (coded as Smoking = 1), 44 % for former smoking (Smoking = 2), and 22 % for current smoking (Smoking = 3), and that the frequency of the risk allele A was 80 %. Next it was assumed that for individuals in which $n(A) = 0$ (noncarriers) smoking multiplied the risk of lung cancer by a factor of 2 and 4 for former and current smokers compared to never smokers, respectively; for $n(A) = 1$ disease risk was assumed to be increased by a factor of 4 and 8 for former and current smokers, and $n(A) = 2$ further increased the relative risk of disease to 5 and 10 for former and current smokers. No main effects were attributed to $n(A)$, i.e., the risk allele count had no effect on lung cancer risk among never-smokers. Finally it was assumed that in the case–control design there was an oversampling of nonsmoking cases (15 % of the total sample) with 50 % of subjects being controls, not sampled on the basis of smoking and the remaining 35 % either former or current smokers. Based on all this information the expected data distribution was calculated and summarized in Table 2 of that paper.

Table 2 of that paper can be reexpressed (for a study of 2,000 total cases and controls) as Table 7.4.

Here the stratum variable (dependent on smoking and disease) takes the value 1 for controls, 2 for nonsmoking cases, and 3 for former or current smoking cases.

Table 7.4 Exemplary data for example from Longmate 2001 [2]

Disease	$n(A)$	Smoking	Stratum	$w = \text{Pr}(n(A)|\text{Smoking, Disease}) \times \pi(\text{stratum})$	$E(N_{D,n(A),S})$
0	2	1	1	0.1088	217.6
0	2	2	1	0.1408	281.6
0	2	3	1	0.0704	140.8
0	1	1	1	0.0544	108.8
0	1	2	1	0.0704	140.8
0	1	3	1	0.0352	70.4
0	0	1	1	0.0068	13.6
0	0	2	1	0.0088	17.6
0	0	3	1	0.0044	8.8
1	2	1	2	0.0960	192
1	2	2	3	0.1228	245.6
1	2	3	3	0.1228	245.6
1	1	1	2	0.0480	96
1	1	2	3	0.0491	98.2
1	1	3	3	0.0491	98.2
1	0	1	2	0.0060	12
1	0	2	3	0.0031	6.2
1	0	3	3	0.0031	6.2

Summing over the elements composing the stratum we have $\sum_{\text{stratum}=1} w = 0.5$, $\sum_{\text{stratum}=2} w = 0.15$, and $\sum_{\text{stratum}=3} w = 0.35$ as planned for the study.

These data can be used to calculate non-centrality parameters for each of the effects, smoking, allele count, and the interaction between smoking and allele count using the *glm* function and display them in an analysis of deviance table using anova as follows:

```
> D=c(rep(0,9),rep(1,9))
> S=factor(rep(1:3,6))
> G<-factor(rep(c(2,2,2,1,1,1,0,0,0),2))
> wgts=c(108.8,140.8,70.4,54.4,70.4,35.2,6.8,8.8,4.4,9.6,122.8,
>     122.8,48,49.1,49.1,6,3.1,3.1)
> anova(glm(D~S+G+S*G,family=binomial(),weights=wgts))
```

which returns:

```
      Df Deviance Resid. Df Resid. Dev
NULL                    17    2772.59
S      2    42.69        15    2729.90
G      2     5.88        13    2724.02
S:G    4     3.56         9    2720.46
```

Finally power is computed using the *Power_chisq* function, using the changes in deviance as the non-centrality parameter in each case. The power of this study is computed as equal to *Power_chisq(2,42.69,.05)* = 99.99 % for the smoking effect,

Power_chisq(2,5.88,.05) = 57 % for the marginal effect of genotype count, G, and
Power_chisq(4,3.56,.05) = 29 % for the smoking by gene interaction.

7.3 QUANTO

The widely used QUANTO program authored by Gauderman and Morrison [5] is a
power calculator that computes power for detection of effects on phenotype mean
or case–control status, for gene, environment, and gene × environment or gene ×
gene interactions using a modification of the exemplary data method. It allows
many types of study designs and outcome analyses including (1) ordinary least
squares regression analysis, (2) 1:M frequency-matched designs using unconditional analysis, (3) 1:1 individual-matched data including sibling-matched designs,
(4) the parent-affected-offspring (trio) design, and (5) the case-only approach for
testing of G × G and G × E interactions.

As described in two papers [6, 7] Gauderman and coworkers implement a
modification of the exemplary data method in order to compute power for complex
case–control designs. This method is a bit more complex than that described above.
Rather than using the expected counts (i.e., the last column of Tables 7.1 or 7.3)
directly as observed data, they are used instead to compute the maximum value of
the expected log likelihoods for both the null and alternative hypothesis, when
fitting parameters in the models of interest. It is worthwhile going through the
calculations for the example in Table 7.2. Table 7.5 adds two additional (the fourth
and fifth) rows to Table 7.2, which is the log likelihood contribution for each cell.

The expected log likelihood for the null hypothesis (calculated using the
$E(N_{n(A),D}$ above), which is computed using the parameter values under the alternative hypothesis), is

$$(381.75 + 110.3 + 7.95)$$
$$\alpha - (381.75 + 110.3 + 7.95 + 405 + 90 + 5)\log(1 + e^{\alpha})$$
$$= 500\alpha - 1,000\log(1 + e^{\alpha}).$$

This easily shows that the maximum of this function is achieved when $\alpha = 0$ and
maximum value is $- 1,000 \log(2) = - 693.1472$. Under the alternative hypothesis the expected log likelihood is

$$-786.75\log(1 + \exp(\alpha)) - 200.3\log(1 + \exp(\alpha + \beta))$$
$$-12.95\log(1 + \exp(\alpha + 2\beta)) + 500.00\alpha + 126.20\beta.$$

This expression can be maximized with respect to α and β with the following
R code which uses a multidimensional search program, *optim*, for optimization, that
is, provided by R:

Table 7.5 Expected distribution of case–control status and genotype computed in a case–control study with 500 cases and 500 controls for the above example as in Table 7.2

$n(A)$	D	$\Pr(n(A),D)$	Contribution to null log likelihood	Contribution to alternative log likelihood	$E(N_{n(A),D})$
0	0	0.4050	$-\log(1 + e^{\alpha})$	$-\log(1 + e^{\alpha})$	405
1	0	0.0900	$-\log(1 + e^{\alpha})$	$-\log(1 + e^{\alpha+\beta})$	90
2	0	0.0050	$-\log(1 + e^{\alpha})$	$-\log(1 + e^{\alpha+2\beta})$	5
0	1	0.3818	$\alpha - \log(1 + e^{\alpha})$	$\alpha - \log(1 + e^{\alpha})$	381.75
1	1	0.1103	$\alpha - \log(1 + e^{\alpha})$	$\alpha + \beta - \log(1 + e^{\alpha+\beta})$	110.3
2	1	0.0080	$\alpha - \log(1 + e^{\alpha})$	$\alpha + 2\beta - \log(1 + e^{\alpha+2\beta})$	7.95

Disease	$n(A)$	Smoking	Stratum	$w = \Pr(n(A)\vert\text{Smoking}, \text{Disease}) \times \pi(\text{stratum})$	$E(N_{D,n(A),S})$
0	2	1	1	0.1088	217.6
0	2	2	1	0.1408	281.6
0	2	3	1	0.0704	140.8
0	1	1	1	0.0544	108.8
0	1	2	1	0.0704	140.8
0	1	3	1	0.0352	70.4
0	0	1	1	0.0068	13.6
0	0	2	1	0.0088	17.6
0	0	3	1	0.0044	8.8
1	2	1	2	0.0960	192
1	2	2	3	0.1228	245.6
1	2	3	3	0.1228	245.6
1	1	1	2	0.0480	96
1	1	2	3	0.0491	98.2
1	1	3	3	0.0491	98.2
1	0	1	2	0.0060	12
1	0	2	3	0.0031	6.2
1	0	3	3	0.0031	6.2

The contribution to the log likelihood of each cell under the null and alternative hypothesis is added to the table

```
> f<-function(par){   # set up function to be maximized
>    a=par[1] # mu
>    b=par[2] # beta
>    -786.75*log(1+exp(a))-200.3*log(1+exp(a+b))-
>    12.95*log(1+exp(a+2*b))+500.00*a+126.20*b
> }
> par=c(0,log(1.3)) # starting values
> m_e_like_alt<-optim(par,f,control=list(fnscale=-1)) # perform the
>                                    # maximization using optim
> m_e_like_alt # display the results
```

This gives results showing $par (the maximized values of the parameters) $value (the maximized value of f) and other information:

```
$par
[1]  -0.05906569    0.26240039

$value
[1]  -691.4342

$message
NULL
```

We can now compute the non-centrality parameter as the expected change in deviance (twice the change in log likelihood) as:

```
> m_e_like_null=-1000*log(2)# maximized value of
>                          # expected null likelihood
> ncp=-2*(m_e_like_alt$value  -  m_e_like_null)
```

which returns ncp equal to 3.426014 which is indistinguishable from the NCP calculated using the exemplary data method (3.426016) as given in the previous section. Power is therefore estimated to be Power_chisq(1,3.4260,0.05) = 45.7 %.

The expected change in likelihood method can also be extended to more complicated tests as for example in Table 7.4. If the null hypothesis includes the presence of an effect of G and S but not of $G \times S$ term then we specify initial values for five parameters in the null model

$$\log\left(\Pr(D = 1)/(1 - \Pr(D))\right) = \mu + \beta_{S2}S_2 + \beta_{S3}S_3 + \beta_{G1}G_1 + \beta_{G2}G_2$$

(here the S and G variables are appropriate indicator functions for smoking and gene count, $n(A)$ respectively, with μ representing the odds of disease for nonsmokers with $n(A) = 0$). We then calculate the log of the likelihood, $l_{\text{null},k}$, for each data configuration given in Table 7.4 ($k = 1,\ldots,18$, with k indexing the rows of Table 7.4). For example, for the configuration $D = 0$, $n(A) = 2$, $S = 0$ (row 8 of Table 7.4) the log likelihood will be equal to $l(\mu^0,\beta^0)_{\text{null},8} = \log(1 - (\exp(\mu^0 + \beta_{G2}^0))/(1 + \exp(\mu^0 + \beta_{G2}^0)))$ and for configuration given $D = 1$, $n(A) = 1$, $S = 2$ (the 14th row) the log likelihood will be equal to $l(\mu^0,\beta^0)_{\text{null},14} = \log(\exp(\mu^0 + \beta_{S2}^0 + \beta_{G1}^0)/1 + \exp(\mu^0 + \beta_{S2}^0 + \beta_{G1}^0))$. We calculate the expected value as $E\{(l_{\text{null}}(\mu^0, \beta^0)\} = \sum_{k=1,\ldots18}^{18} = w_k l(\mu^0\beta^0)_{\text{null},k}$ then we must search for parameter values, $(\mu, \beta_{S2}, \beta_{S3}, \beta_{G1}, \beta_{G2})$, which maximize this expectation, i.e., find we find arg $\max[E\{(l_{\text{null}}(\mu, \beta))\}]$ and save the corresponding maximized value as $l_{\text{null}}^{\max}$. This computes the first step of the power calculation.

The next step is to perform the same procedure again this time using the likelihood under the alternative hypothesis, i.e., the likelihood function that includes the four interaction terms $\beta_{G1,S2}G_1S_2$, $\beta_{G1,S3}G_1S_3$, $\beta_{G2,S2}G_2S_2$, and $\beta_{G2,S3}G_2S_3$ in the model and perform a maximization (including the added parameters) to find the maximized value, $l^{\text{max}}_{\text{alternative}}$, of the expected log likelihood including the two interaction parameters, using the same weights as before. Finally the non-centrality parameter for the test (here a 4 degree of freedom test) is computed as $2(l^{\text{max}}_{\text{alternative}} - l^{\text{max}}_{\text{null}})$.

Coding this all in *R* and using the *optim* function twice (see the accompanying file *power_functions.R*) give a non-centrality parameter of 2.80 (power = 23 %) compared to 3.56 (power = 28 %) using the exemplary data method; thus in more complex models these two methods are likely to diverge to some degree.

7.3.1 Use of QUANTO to Compute Power to Detect Main Effects of Genetic Variants in Case–Control Studies

QUANTO is available at the URL http://hydra.usc.edu/gxe/. On start-up (after installation) an initial screen appears showing default values. Normally a user will begin by clicking on the "Wizards" menu item and then choosing "New," this being a series of input screens which specify the choice of study design as well as (for main effects analysis) allele frequency and range of genetic effects of interest. In addition (for case–control studies) the baseline probability of disease in the population is required (as discussed above) in order to compute the expected data configurations. For the example given in the first line of Table 7.3 (see Fig. 7.1), choose "Unmatched Case–Control Study" with frequency matching of 1 case to 1 control from the Outcome/Design section and choose "Gene Only" from the Hypothesis section. On the next screen set the allele frequency to 0.10 and the Inheritance Mode to "Log Additive". On the third screen set the Baseline Risk to 0.00001 and the Genetic Effect to 1.3. On the last screen specify the sample size as 1,000 and the type I error rate as 0.05. Finally choose "Finish" and click the calculator icon on the main menu. This gives the output

Parameter	Power	Null	Full
Gene	0.4570	$\beta_G = 0$	β_G

The power reported is in agreement with the 45.7 % power found above for the same example.

7.4 Alternative Designs

As described in previous chapters control for population stratification is an important issue in genetic association studies. This is especially true of small scale studies in which too few markers can be genotyped in order to allow for the methods of correction described in Chap. 4, i.e., the principal components or

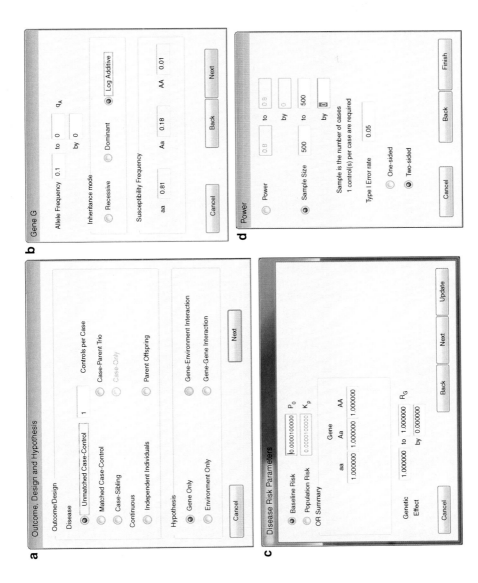

Fig. 7.1 Quanto input screens for example in Table 7.3

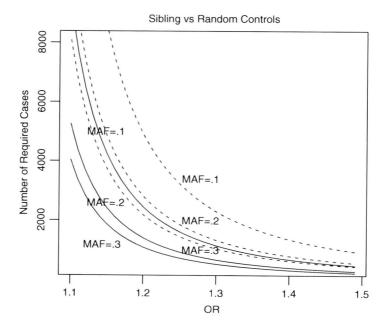

Fig. 7.2 Sample sizes plotted against odds ratios. Sample sizes computed in QUANTO are those required to maintain power of 80 % for detecting the effects of variants with specified ORs and allele frequencies from 10 to 30 % for sibling (*solid lines*) versus random (*dotted lines*) controls

mixed model methods. Control for the effects of population stratification by study design has been discussed extensively in the statistical genetics literature. Here we discuss the two types of such designs that QUANTO can calculate power for, namely, the use of sibling controls in case–control studies and the parent-affected-offspring designs.

7.4.1 Sibling Controls

Studies in which cases are matched to controls selected from among their biological full siblings offer complete control for population stratification because each full sibling has exactly the same ancestry. The analysis of sibling-matched controls must be performed using conditional logistic regression and power calculations for this design must take account of the fact that siblings are more likely to share the genotype of an allele of interest than are randomly selected controls. Figure 7.2 shows sample sizes (number of required cases) computed using QUANTO that are required for the detection of odds ratios ranging from 1.1 to

2.0 for allele frequencies 10–30 % under the log additive model for both the sibling (1:1) matched design and a 1:1 matched case–control design using randomly selected controls. For all the combinations of odds ratios and allele frequencies shown QUANTO finds that it takes almost exactly twice the number of sibling control matched cases to detect (with type I error rate 5 % and power 80 %) the effect of a given variant than using random controls. The loss of effective sample size when sibling controls are used is due to the correlation between the genotypes of the siblings. From Chap. 2 we recall that this correlation is $r = 0.50$. It is because of this strong correlation there are many more non-informative case–control sets (i.e., case–control sets where both the cases and controls have the same genotypes) than there would be if random controls were selected.

The loss of effective sample size for detecting the main effects of genes is a significant detriment to this study design; in modern-day studies where large numbers of markers are genotyped protection against population stratification can be achieved using other methods, for example, by control for principal components. However, as shown below utilization of these methods also causes a loss in effective sample size, although this varies by the degree of differentiation of each marker, so that we need to be careful in concluding that random controls are "always" better than sibling controls

7.4.2 Power for Interactions

As illustrated above a full analysis of power for testing interactions is necessarily quite complicated since power and required sample size depends upon many "nuisance" factors, including, (1) the frequency of the exposure, (2) genotype frequency, (3) marginal effects of exposure on risk, (4) marginal effects of genotypes on risk, (5) the background risk of disease, (6) the correlation of exposure among case–control sets, etc.

Extensive comparisons of the power of tests for gene by environment interactions using sibling controls versus random controls are given in Gauderman et al. [6]. In most cases it turns out the use of sibling controls is somewhat *more powerful* than using random controls, so long as the environmental exposures between the two siblings are not correlated. Once the exposures are correlated within sibship the (generally modest) power advantage of the sibling control design degrades. Intuition is provided for this last result by considering that when both exposures and (necessarily) the SNP genotypes are correlated within sibships, the probability of obtaining pairs that have the same values for both genes and exposures (and hence are non-informative for gene × exposure interactions) becomes larger than for randomly paired cases and controls.

7.4.3 Parent-Affected-Offspring Trios

The parents-affected-offspring design (trio design) also provides full protection against the confounding effects of population stratification. As described in Chap. 3 (Sect. 3.6.2) there are several ways to analyze data from the trio design, QUANTO calculates the maximized expected likelihoods for this design using conditional logistic regression. For main effects analysis the transmission disequilibrium test is a score test for this likelihood. When the model for disease status is log-linear in the number, $n(A)$, of copies of the allele of interest, then the parent–offspring design requires virtually the same number of cases (and hence 3/2 times as many subjects genotyped) as does the unmatched case–control design. For other penetrance models (i.e., dominant or recessive) the parent–offspring design requires somewhat fewer cases than does the unmatched case–control design.

For the study of gene × environment interactions the parent–offspring design is somewhat more powerful than the unmatched case–control design, especially for dominant or recessive penetrance models and this design can be considerably more powerful for the study of gene × gene interactions. As mentioned above the particulars for power calculations for gene × environment (or gene × gene) interactions become complicated, since they depend on a large number of nuisance parameters, the interested reader is directed to the papers by Gauderman and others.

7.4.4 Power for Case-Only Analysis of Interactions

As described by many authors [7, 8], and as seen in Chap. 3 (Sect. 3.7.2), testing for gene by environment or even gene by gene interactions can be much more powerful, for a rare disease, if only the cases are used in an analysis. Such an analysis gains power by reliance on an assumption that in the population as a whole, genetic variants of interest are distributed independently with respect to the exposures of interest and of the other genes (when testing gene × gene interactions). The case-only analysis of interactions essentially tests for dependence, among the cases, between the allele count, $n(A)$, of interest and the particular exposure being studied. If such dependence is noted among the cases in a case–control study, and if independence in the population as a whole is assumed then dependence among cases can be interpreted as being due to interactions between gene and environment. Under the independence assumption, for a rare disease, it takes approximately ½ as many cases to give the same power that a case–control study has for detecting the same effect. For example consider again the data from Longmate. Using only the data for the cases (rows 10–18 of Table 7.4), we form a 3 × 3 table of expected counts as:

```
> cases<-10:18
> etab<-matrix(wgts[cases],3,3)
> colnames(etab)<-c("G=2","G=1","G=0")
> rownames(etab)<-c("S=1","S=2","S=3")
> etab
        G=2   G=1   G=0
S=1 192.0  96.0  12.0
S=2 245.6  98.2   6.2
S=3 245.6  98.2   6.2
```

Next we use the *chisq.test* function in R to test for association between the rows and columns of this matrix:

```
> chisq.test(etab)

          Pearson's Chi-squared test

data:   etab
X-squared = 6.5617, df = 4, p-value = 0.1609
```

We use the test value (6.5617) as the non-centrality parameter, to calculate the power of the test:

```
> Power_chisq(4,6.5617,.05)
[1] 0.5099578
```

This indicates that the case-only test for interaction, with power 51 %, is more powerful than the value calculated for the case–control analysis (29 % power for the test for interaction) using the exemplary data technique above. The power gain for the case–control analysis arises by exploiting the independence assumption (between genes and environment) that was used in calculating the weights for the case–control analysis, but which was not explicitly incorporated into the analysis.

To understand what is going on consider that if there is an interaction between genes and environment then those combinations of genes and environment that lead to especially high risk will be over-represented in the cases so the probability of a case carrying those combinations will be greater than predicted based on the marginal frequency of either of the two among cases. If we assume that there is no relationship between genes and environment in the population as a whole the interaction analysis is simplified to test for independence of genes and environment among cases, a test which is (for rare disease) inherently more direct and powerful than the test for interaction in the cases-control analysis. As described in Chap. 3 (Sect. 3.7.2) the standard case–control analysis of interactions can in fact be thought of as a test for whether the relationship between genes and environment is the same in cases as in the controls. For a rare disease, where the controls represent the population and so G, E independence can be assumed it takes twice as many cases (plus one control per case) to test for interactions in the 1:1 frequency-matched case–control data as does as it does to test for association between genes and environment using the case-only analysis.

7.5   Control for Multiple Comparisons

7.5.1   Single Marker Associations

Large-scale, "agnostic" genetic studies involve the testing of an extremely large number of hypotheses. Testing of single marker associations (main effects) has to date been the main focus of almost all GWAS analyses, often with the inclusion of *imputed* variants as well as the SNPs directly genotyped among the hypotheses to be tested. As described in Chap. 3 (Sect. 3.11) the Bonferroni approach to the correction for multiple hypothesis testing in assignment of the experiment-wise significance of a result from large-scale genetic studies is a reasonable approximation except when the correlations between "nearby" tests is very high. Direct application of the Bonferroni criteria would assign different criteria for significance to different platforms/marker sets. This is somewhat of an inconvenience and does not take into account the use of imputation (Chap. 6) to further extend the number of single marker hypotheses being tested. For common variants (e.g., those above 5–10 % frequency) a general rule of thumb [9] is that there are approximately one million independent hypotheses that "could" be tested using common SNPs (with frequency 5 % or greater) so that a criteria of $0.5/10^6 = 5 \times 10^{-8}$ for global significance of a given association (for either a genotyped or imputed SNP) is an often relied upon guide. It may be justifiable also to use somewhat stricter criteria than this in studies of the older populations, for example, African or African-derived, where the number of common variants is larger and the LD patterns weaker. The effect on power of using a 2.5×10^{-8} vs. 5×10^{-8} significance threshold (allowing for twice as many tests in these populations) can typically be made up for by an increase in sample size of approximately 3 % for a study which is designed to have 80 % power.

7.5.2   More Complex Marker Associations

Figure 7.3 slows a plot of required sample size (obtained from QUANTO) versus number of markers to be tested for a study with 80 % power to reject the null hypothesis in favor of a specific alternative. In the figure the sample size is expressed as the ratio of the number of subjects that are required for testing M hypotheses compared to testing only 1 hypothesis, which allows the plot to be free of the actual alternative value of the odds ratio parameter that is being used in the calculation. This plot is extremely linear in the log of the number of markers. For example a study that is to test $M = 10$ million hypotheses at false-positive error rate, $\alpha = 0.05/M$, must be approximately six times as large as a study that only tests 1 hypothesis at $\alpha = 0.05$. Using this log linear relationship, we can calculate sample size requirements for studies involving a truly forbidding number of hypotheses being tested; consider for example the testing of all two-way

Fig. 7.3 The required sample size for a study with 80 % power to reject a hypothesis at $\alpha = 0.5/M$, where M is the number of markers genotyped. The sample size is plotted relative to the sample size required for testing 1 marker requirements

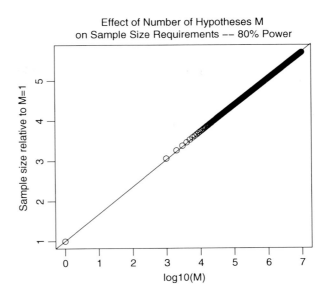

Effect of Number of Hypotheses M on Sample Size Requirements -- 80% Power

interactions between all one million SNPs on a hypothetical GWAS array. We have one million choose two or approximately 500 billion tests being performed, which gives a Bonferroni criteria of 1×10^{-13}. This value is smaller than the (currently) permitted minimum value in QUANTO for the type 1 error criteria. However simple extrapolation, based on the log linearity of Fig. 7.3 readily shows that it would require approximately nine times as many subjects for a study to have 80 % power while controlling for 500 billion tests of gene by gene interactions at a global false-positive error rate of 0.05, compared with a study that has 80 % power to detect an effect of a single gene $\times$ gene interaction. (Here we are assuming that the gene frequencies, as well as the marginal and joint effects on risk of the pairs of variants considered are similar in both studies.)

This discussion has emphasized the simplest but arguably an overly conservative method for control of the false-positive rates when performing multiple comparisons, i.e., the Bonferroni criteria. We have already argued (Chap. 4) that when each association test is only correlated with a limited number of nearby tests that the Bonferroni method performs quite well in comparison to more complex approximations based on theoretical behavior of the Ornstein–Uhlenbeck process. In testing gene by gene interactions the dependence structure between tests is surely more complicated, and it may be worthwhile to consider other methods of assessing significance when such a study is actually conducted; however the point being made here is mainly about the power of having large studies; in an era of large-scale meta-analyses it may (soon) be possible to indeed put together combinations of studies of common diseases that are large enough to effectively control for 500 billion associations using the Bonferroni criteria, moving what can now, with today's sample sizes, mainly be exploratory analysis into the realm of the reliable and reproducible.

7.5.3   *Reliability of Very Small* p-*Values*

Chapter 3 (Sect. 3.12) described briefly some of the considerations involved in evaluating whether asymptotic approximations used to calculate *p*-values, etc. are reliable enough to ensure that the small *p*-values needed to control for experiment-wide single variant tests (e.g., $\sim 5 \times 10^{-8}$) are reliable. It is of course even more difficult to evaluate the reliability of *p*-values smaller than 10^{-13} or so needed to control for hypotheses concerning all pairwise G $\times$ G interactions using the Bonferroni approach. One intuitive approach is motivated by Fig. 7.3. Consider a sample size that is sufficient to reject one hypothesis of interest at the customary 0.05 type I error level reliably, i.e., enough data is available so that the asymptotic approximations are reliable at this rejection rate. Then raise the sample size requirement according to the log linear relationship depicted in Fig. 7.3. Of course determining whether this simple approach is adequate requires additional analysis.

7.6   Two-Staged Genotyping Designs

Many genome-wide association studies have used some form of multistage sampling design [10] because of the considerable savings in genotyping costs this approach offers. Two-stage sampling for GWAS studies is described in detail in Wang [11] based on genotyping part of the sample using a commercial high density panel (typically 500,000 to a million SNPs) and then genotyping the most promising SNPs using a customized panel on the remainder of the sample. A final analysis combining the information from both samples is more powerful than treating the design as a hypothesis generation followed by independent replication [12] because it exploits the additional information about how significant the first-stage associations were, not just the fact that they exceeded some threshold. Formally, two-stage designs can be conceptualized as a family of group sequential tests (one per SNP) with allowance for early stopping for "futility" [13].

Despite the dramatic cost reductions for genotyping of the GWAS era, cost is still a limiting factor in conducting genome-wide association studies and currently there are several potentially important reasons for adopting a multistage genotyping strategy. First, it has been shown [14] that considerable cost savings result by adopting multistage approach to genotyping in a large-scale association study without sacrificing very much power [15]. With the multistage approach, all SNPs are genotyped in the first stage in a fraction of samples, and a liberal significance level threshold is used to identify a subset of SNPs with putative associations. In later stages, these putative associations are retested in a separate sample. This design eliminates waste of resources on noncausal markers and substantially increases power per dollar spent when the principal constraint is the total cost [16]. Another reason for conducting two-stage genotyping studies is that potential data quality concerns, such as heterozygote dropout, or case/control differential call/error rate, may create false positives that are rare in general, but abundant among positive associations detected using a genome-wide technology. Since these artifacts are usually technology specific, genotyping the SNPs selected in stage I on a different platform in later stages may greatly alleviate this practical problem.

Wang et al. [17] focused upon the first of these two problems, by updating these earlier analyses to take account of a number of characteristics of GWAS genotyping. First, in genome-wide scans the total number of SNPs being considered far exceeds those considered in earlier papers and the number of SNPs has an impact upon the optimal sample sizes in the two stages and the threshold for significance in stage I. Second, the per-genotype costs in the first stage and the second stage are dramatically different in a genome-wide scan. Recently cost ratios appear to be in the range of 15 to 20, comparing per-genotype costs using the SNP array in stage I versus the high throughput genotyping platforms generally being considered in stage II. While the costs of both stage I and stage II genotyping technologies have continued to drop rapidly, it seems likely that a large cost differential will remain for the foreseeable future. Third, in the previous work, there has been no consideration of attempting to expand the marker set at promising regions in the second stage.

7.6.1 *Measured SNP Association Tests*

We first assume that the only SNPs of interest are those that actually appear on the SNP chip, so that no imputation of unmeasured SNPs is performed and no increase in marker density is made in stage II. Here we assume a population-based case–control study is used for the genome scan, i.e., all cases and controls are unrelated. In the first stage, the full set of m markers (SNPs) is genotyped on n_1 subjects. A stage I test of association is performed on all markers at a significance level α_1. The significant markers are then genotyped for an additional n_2 subjects, and the stage II statistics based on all $(n_1 + n_2)$ subjects are evaluated at a significance level α_2. Generally α_2 is slightly larger than the overall type I error, α, reflecting the necessity that a marker must be significant in both stages to be significant overall.

Let p denote the population allele frequency and assume Hardy–Weinberg equilibrium. Here the allele of interest is the one that increases disease risk, not necessarily the minor allele. Let δ denote the number of risk alleles a subject carries (allele dosage), $\delta = 0$, 1, or 2. We assume a multiplicative genetic risk model, and let ψ be the increased relative risk (odds ratio, OR) of carrying each additional copy of the disease allele. Details of the optimization method are provided in the Appendix to Wang et al. Briefly, in stage I choose as a test statistic S_1 the difference in average risk allele dosages between cases and controls, and compare this statistic against its asymptotic normal distribution. In the second stage, the test statistic S is based on the combination of data from both samples and the vector (S_1, S) is distributed as bivariate normal with means and covariance given in Appendix. These allow us to compute the power and type I error rate as a function of the sample sizes (n_1, n_2), model parameters (p, β), and critical values (α_1, α_2) at stages I and II respectively. The cost function involves the ratio t_1/t_2 of per-genotype costs at stages I and II, as well as the sample sizes and expected number of markers tested in stage II (determined by the type I error and power for stage I and the number of true causal genes). The optimal design is found by numerically minimizing the total cost for a combination of sample sizes and critical values that yield the desired overall type I error and power. We use a function written in R, see file "2-stage power.R", to perform the searches.

7.6.1.1 Power Calculations for a Specific Two-Stage Design

Before giving results from the optimization procedure it is worthwhile obtaining some basic familiarity with a utility function (called in the optimization) that, for a fixed set of the parameters above, computes power for both the stated two-stage design, as well as a one-stage design in which all subjects are genotyped with the GWAS array. The header for this function is shown below:

```
> twostagePower<-
> function(CC=1,OR=1.4,P0=0.0001,p=0.2,side=2,m=5e5,n1=2000,n2=2000,alpha1=0.0033,
> ALPHA=0.05)
> {
>      #CC                 # number of controls per case
>      #OR                 # Log-additive only, OR of each additional risk allele
>      #P0                 # baseline risk,i.e. Pr(D=1|G=0)
>      #p;                 # causal allele frequency
>      #side               # side=(1,2) for 1- or 2-side test
>      #m;                 # No. of total markers in the first stage
>      #n1;                # number of cases genotyped in stage 1
>      #n2;                # number of cases genotyped in stage 2
>      #ALPHA              # overall false positive rate
>      #alpha1             # type I error of stage I (2-sided)
...
> }
```

Here CC is the number of controls per case in each stage, the OR is the odds ratio as hypothesized under the alternate hypothesis, P_0 is the baseline risk of disease in the population being sampled, p is the hypothesized causal allele frequency, n_1 is the number of cases ($+n_1 \times$ CC controls) genotyped in stage 1, n_2 is the number of cases genotyped in stage 2, m is the total number of markers on the GWAS chip used in the first stage, $ALPHA$ is the desired type I error rate with a default value of 5 %, and finally a_1 is the criteria for significance for moving markers from stages 1 to 2. Consider the use of this function for calculating the power for a one-to-one matched case/control study with 5,000 cases and 5,000 controls in which one million markers are tested initially, and in which various fractions, $n_1/(n_1 + n_2)$, of subjects are genotyped in stage I, and for which the criteria for significance in the

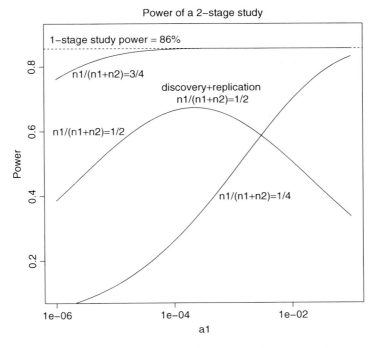

Fig. 7.4 Power of a two stage study to detect an odds ratio of 1.25 for a 20 % allele, according to the fraction of subjects genotyped in stage 1 and the first stage type I error level. Odds ratio is assumed to be equal to 1.25, and frequency 0.2; 5,000 cases and 5,000 controls genotyped. Also shown (*dotted line*) is the power of a "discovery + replication" design with $n_1/(n_1 + n_2) = 1/2$

first stage, α_1, is varied from 10^{-6} to 0.1. We choose OR $= 1.25, p = 0.2$ and keep P_0 and CC at the default values of 0.00001, and 1 respectively. Figure 7.4 plots the results of running the *twostagePower* function (see file "*2-stage power.R*") repeatedly for several choices of the fraction $n_1/(n_1 + n_2)$ in stage 1 and the threshold criteria. For studies in which n_1 and n_2 are equal, nearly full power (i.e., the power of the single-stage design with 5,000 cases and controls) is obtained by setting the criteria, α_1, for significance in the first stage, to 1 % or so. For a study in which the first stage is three times as large as the second stage, close to full power is achieved with a first-stage alpha level of 10^{-4}, and in contrast, when only one fourth of the subjects are genotyped in stage 1 a first-stage alpha level of over 0.1 is required for close to full power.

Figure 7.4 also illustrates (dotted non-monotonic curve) the power of a *discovery + replication* based approach to discover new markers, compared to the use of combined analysis. Here the power of the discover + replication-based method is the product of (1) the power in the first stage that the first-stage test exceeds the significance level α_1 for given markers and (2) the power of the second stage after performing a Bonferroni correction for the number of markers that reach stage

2. Assuming that the number of truly associated markers is small compared to the number of SNPs genotyped in stage 1 we can assume that approximately $\alpha_1 M$ markers will be genotyped in stage 2 (i.e., will meet the criteria for advancement) so that the Bonferroni correction is approximately $\alpha/(\alpha_1 M)$. The R function *onestagePower* can be used as below:

```
> a1=1e-4 # for example
> onestagePower(OR=1.25,p=0.2,m=1e6,n=2500,a=a1,Bonf=0)*
> onestagePower(OR=1.25,p=.2,m=1e6*a1,n=2500,Bonf=1)
```

Which returns 0.663 compared to the power:

```
> twostagePower(OR=1.25,p=0.2,m=1e6,n1=2500,n2=2500,a1=a1)
```

which returns 0.731. This illustrates the results of Skol et al. [12] who found that a proper two-stage analysis is always more powerful than discovery + replication.

7.6.2   Optimal Two-Stage Case–Control Designs

Wang et al. [17] numerically solved the problem of finding the optimal values of n_1, n_2, c_1, c_2 which, for fixed values of the parameters (p, P_0, and ψ) in the risk model satisfied the type I and type II error constraints that $\alpha = \Pr(S_1 > c_1, \ S > c_2|H_0)$ and $\Pr(S_1 > c_1, \ S > c_2|H_A) = 1 - \beta$, while minimizing an expected cost function of form $t_1 n_1 m + t_2 n_2 E(m_2)$ where the expected number of markers, $E(m_2)$ genotyped in the second stage is approximated as $[(m - T)\alpha_1 + T(1 - \beta_1)]$ where T is the number of markers which meet the requirements of the alternative hypothesis (the number of "true" associations), and all other associations are assumed to be null. Generally we would anticipate that T is very small compared to $\alpha_1 m$ and for simplification, we can approximate the expectation of the cost as simply $2(t_1 n_1 m + t_2 n_2 \ \alpha_1 m)$, only a slight underestimate unless there are a huge number of true-positive associations. Here α_1 is defined as $\Pr(S_1 > c_1|H_0)$ and α_2 as $\Pr(S > c_2|H_0)$. Figures 7.5 and 7.6 show (as a function of the number of markers tested, M, and the cost ratio t_2/t_1) the optimal fraction of subjects, $n_1/(n_1 + n_2)$, to genotype in stage 1 (Fig. 7.5) and the optimal fraction of markers, α_1, to genotype in stage 2 (Fig. 7.6), for a study that is designed to achieve 90 % power to detect a variant with a given odds ratio, OR, and frequency, p. While the total number of subjects needed in the study is highly dependent on the assumed value of OR and p, the optimal fractions, $n_1/(n_1 + n_2)$ and α_1, are independent of both quantities. For studies genotyping a large number (0.5 to 1 million) of SNPs in stage 1 where the cost ratio is high ($t_2/t_1 = 20$) then study designs that include about 30 % of subjects in the initial GWAS genotyping and move approximately 1/3 of one percent of markers ($\alpha_1 \sim 0.003$) into stage 2 are optimal in terms of study power.

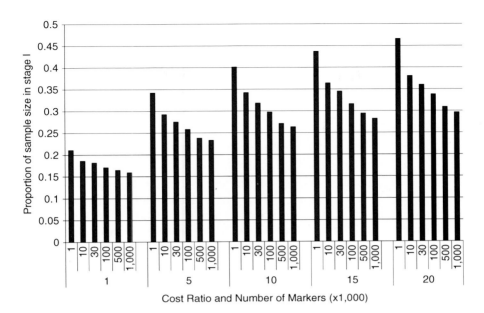

Fig. 7.5 The proportion, $n_1/(n_1 + n_2)$, of sample size allocated to stage I in the optimal design plotted as a function of the cost ratio t_2/t_1 and the number of SNPs, m, genotyped in stage I, for a study with 90 % power to detect an effect with type I error equal to $0.05/m$

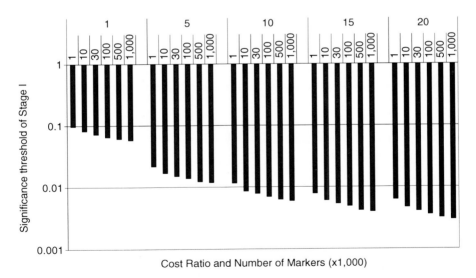

Fig. 7.6 The significance threshold α_1 for promoting a SNP from stages I to II in the optimal design plotted as a function of the cost ratio t_2/t_1 and the number of SNPs, m, genotyped in stage I for a study with 90 % power to detect an effect with type 1 error equal to $0.05/m$

Very often it is not only the constraints on costs that limit the power of a study; the availability of cases for a case–control study may impose limits as well. In this setting studies that are a little bit more expensive, but which retain nearly all the power of a study in which all subjects are genotyped for all markers, can be attractive. For example, when $M = 1$ million and $t_2/t_1 = 20$ then the optimal design would place 32 % of subjects into stage 1 and genotype 0.32 % of markers (Table 3 of Wang et al.). The drawback to this study design can be seen by running:

```
> f1=.32;a1=0.0032;n=5000;twostagePower(m=1e6,p=0.2, OR=1.3,n1=f1*n,
> n2=n-f1*n, a1=a1)
```

The output from this command indicates that this (optimal) design would have 91.2 % power to detect an OR of 1.3 per copy of an allele with 20 % frequency. If the genotyping cost in stage 1 is 0.05 cents per genotype (500 dollars per sample) and 1 cent per genotype in stage 2 then the cost of this study will be about 1.8 million dollars. The drawback to this design is the power loss in comparison to a (much more expensive) study (5 million dollars) that genotypes all subjects in stage 1, since a single-stage study would achieve 98.8 % power. Relaxing the criteria a bit so that 44 % of subjects are in stage 1 and 0.44 % of markers are moved to stage 2 as in:

```
> f1=.44;a1=0.0044;n=5000;twostagePower(m=1e6,p=0.2, OR=1.3,n1=f1*n,
> n2=n-f1*n, a1=a1)
```

gives a study design with almost full power compared to the 1 stage design (97.9 vs. 98.8) and which still saves 2.54 million dollars compared to the 1-stage design (although it costs 37 % more than does the optimal study). Using this same design but with total number of cases equal to 4,000 rather than 5,000 would achieve 92 % power at a cost of 2.0 million dollars. The advantage of this study is that there is little loss of power compared to a one-stage study with this many cases (92 vs. 93.5 % power) and the cost it is still within about 11 % of the optimal study (with 33 % of the 5,000 cases genotyped in the first stage) and remains much less than the single-stage study.

7.7 Control of Population Stratification: Effects on Study Power

Chapter 3 (Sect. 3.6) described two alternative designs (case-sibling and parent-affected offspring) which control completely for population stratification in estimation of genetic main effects and interactions. Both designs have implementation and cost issues and have only relatively rarely been employed in GWAS studies. The use of the correction methods described in Chap. 4 such as principal components and mixed models are generally more feasible and cost-effective than these special designs. It is important to realize that control for population stratification using the genotype data is not cost free either; for testing a marker with the same allele frequency and effect sizes in two populations, one structured and one not, the study without hidden structure will always be more powerful than a study involving hidden structure after correction for the hidden structure. In this section we consider the effect on study power that is a result of having to control for population stratification using the principal components and related methods, in a study of nominally unrelated individuals. We first consider the simplest method, genomic control.

7.7.1   Genomic Inflation and Study Power

Genomic control as originally described [18] involves the division of a given chi-square statistic (e.g., the Armitage test, T^2, for a single SNP association) by a genomic control parameter, λ, prior to the calculation of the corresponding p-value for the statistic. The value of λ is estimated from a large number of similar chi-square statistics, T_k^2, (e.g., one for each SNP, k) as $\hat{\lambda} = \text{median}(T_1^2, \ T_2^2, \ldots, T_M^2)/0.455$. This genomic control procedure can be (as seen in Chap. 4) can be effective method of adjusting for hidden relatedness in which study subjects are related to a number of other individuals but the fraction of individuals that a given subject is related to does not increase with study size. For large-scale hidden stratification or admixture (where the number of other individuals related to a given subject tends to increases linearly with sample size) it is generally less effective than principal components at preserving power while reducing false-positive rates. Consider the impact on the non-centrality parameter for the adjusted test $T^2/\hat{\lambda}$. When there is large-scale population stratification each random variable T_k^2 will be distributed as a χ_1^2 with some (nonzero) non-centrality parameter ncp_k. If we assume that all possible study participants come from the same underlying (infinite sized) stratified population, then all the non-centrality parameters, ncp_k, will increase linearly with sample size N. This implies that that $\hat{\lambda} - 1$ increases proportionately with the number of individuals N for such a study because in this case the non-centrality parameter for each T_k^2 statistic will be increasing linearly with N. The simulation study below illustrates the behavior of $\hat{\lambda} - 1$ with sample size:

```
> # Simulate the behavior of the genomic control parameter lambda
> # with increasing sample size N
> nsims=10
> M=100000 # number of markers used to estimate lambda
> lambda_hat=rep(0,nsims)
> ncp1<-runif(M,0,0.1) # starting noncentrality parameter a random
>                       # sample uniform 0-0.1
>                       # gives a starting lambda of ~ 1.05
> for (n in 1:nsims){ #  n is proportional to population size N
>     T2<-rchisq(M,1,n*ncp1) # non centrality parameter for each
> # statistic increases proportional to sample size
>     lambda_hat[n]=median(T2)/.455
> }
> plot(1:nsims,lambda_hat-1)# linear
```

If $\hat{\lambda} - 1$ is linear in sample size it follows that the non-centrality parameter, $\mathrm{ncp}_k(N)$, for the T^2 statistic for a genuinely casual variant after division by of T^2 lambda, for sample size N will be equal to

$$\mathrm{ncp}_k(N) = \frac{\frac{N}{n}\mathrm{ncp}_k(n)}{1 + \frac{N}{n}(\lambda_n - 1)}, \tag{7.7}$$

where λ_n is the genomic control parameter when sample size equals some initial value n and $\mathrm{ncp}_k(n)$ is the non-centrality parameter for the causal variant also at sample size n. This implies that the non-centrality parameter can get no larger than $\mathrm{ncp}_k(n)/(\lambda_n - 1)$ no matter how large we increase the sample size. For example, if for a given (initial study size) n the genomic control parameter is 1.5 then no study of this population that uses genomic control to control for population stratification can increase the non-centrality parameter for the causal allele by more than twofold, no matter how many-fold the sample size is increased.

As described in Chap. 4, the behavior of the genomic control parameter as sample size increases depends on the specifics of the setting. If there are many clusters of related individuals and if as the sample size increases the number of clusters increase but the size of each cluster does not, then the genomic control parameter will tend to a constant rather than increase linearly; in this case then the genomic control-adjusted non-centrality parameter for the causal allele and hence power to detect the causal allele will continue to increase with sample size.

7.7.2   Correction for Admixture and Hidden Structure by Principal Components

As shown in Chap. 4, when the relationship matrix $\mathbf{K}$ imposed by hidden structure or admixture has only a few leading eigenvalues (and the rest of them are close to 1 in value) then false-positive associations are expected when the covariates (i.e., SNPs) of interest load on the leading eigenvectors of $\mathbf{K}$. The principal components method of Price et al. [19] adjusts for the leading principal components by including them as regression variables in the analysis. Consider the effect on power of having to control for leading principal components compared to not having to, in a given analysis. Let $\mathbf{n}$ be a vector of SNP allele counts of interest, and let $\mathbf{n}^*$ be the vector of residuals of $\mathbf{n}$ after regression of $\mathbf{n}$ on the leading principal components. The non-centrality parameter for the analysis of the continuous trait using $\mathbf{n}^*$ will be equal to

$$\frac{\beta^2}{\sigma_{Y^*}^2} \sum_{i=1}^{N} \left(n_i^* - \overline{n^*}\right)^2 = \frac{\beta^2}{\sigma_{Y^*}^2} N \mathrm{Var}(n^*), \tag{7.8}$$

where β is the regression parameter relating $E(Y)$ to $\mathbf{n}$,* and σ_{Y*}^2 is the variance of the adjusted value of Y, adjusted for the same principal components of $\mathbf{K}$ that were used to adjust the SNP allele counts $\mathbf{n}$. Note that the relationship between Var $(\mathbf{n}^*)$ and Var(n) is that Var$(\mathbf{n}^*) = (1 - R_{n,pc}^2)Var(\mathbf{n})$ where $R_{n,pc}^2$ is the squared multiple correlation between $\mathbf{n}$ and the leading principal components. Also σ_{Y*}^2 is equal to $(1 - R_{Y,pc}^2)$Var(Y). We see that there are two countervailing effects upon the non-centrality parameter for a fixed β. The first is that the numerator of (7.8) decreases compared to NVar$(\mathbf{n})$, thereby decreasing the NCP and hence power, while the denominator also decreases thereby increasing the NCP (although the latter generally has a smaller effect than the former). Since the change in Var(Y) due to the adjustment does not depend upon which SNP count variable is being considered our attention is mainly on the numerator. In cases of recent admixture between formally widely separated groups or of gross population stratification all SNPs are differentiated to some degree between ancestral groups, i.e., they all tend to have the same correlation structure matrix $2p(1 - p)\mathbf{K}$ with the pairwise elements of $\mathbf{K}$ reflecting the ancestral similarities of each pair of study members. This does not mean however that each SNP will all have the same observed correlation with the eigenvectors of $\mathbf{K}$, rather, due to chance some will be more associated with the leading eigenvectors of $\mathbf{K}$ and others will be less associated. Since the leading eigenvectors either closely mirror admixture fraction in admixed samples or act as dummy variables for ancestral origin when there are two or more non-mixing groups, the degree of differentiation of the allele frequency between the ancestral groups determines the sample correlations $R_{n,pc}$ and hence the power reduction. Therefore we would expect that more differentiated SNPs pay a greater penalty for incomplete admixture or hidden structure than do non-differentiated SNPs.

There is a subtlety however to this issue, which can be seen in the case of admixed populations. If SNPs are highly differentiated by ancestral population, i.e., an allele has frequency near 0 in one population and frequency near 1 in the other, then a study in an admixed group will be far more powerful than an equally sized study in either population separately even if global ancestry is adjusted for using principal components. In fact, power is increased over a fairly wide range of allele frequency differences in an admixed compared to non-admixed study. However, studies of a recently admixed population, with little time for recombination to take place, pay a greater price for control of global ancestry than do studies of a less recently admixed population, since more SNPs will align with the ancestry indicators in a recent than an older admixed population. More discussion of this phenomenon is provided in Chap. 8 when adjusting for local, as well as global, ancestry is addressed.

7.7.3   A Retrospective Analysis of Study Power

While we could use (7.7) to compute power of a study in some instances, it is rare for today's studies to depend entirely on genomic control to provide test statistics. The methods described in Chap. 4, Sect. 4.2.5 give one approach to understanding the power characteristics of a study that is required to account for population structure. To review, the retrospective approach to analysis of case–control data (e.g., the Bourgain test [20]) models the genotype counts $\mathbf{n} = (n_1, n_2, \ldots, n_N)$ for an allele of interest as having mean equal to

$$E(\mathbf{n}) = \mu + \mathbf{c}\beta, \tag{7.9}$$

where $\mathbf{c}$ is a vector of zeros and ones indicating case–control status for each study participant so that the mean genotype counts are modeled as $\mu + \beta$ and μ for the cases and controls respectively, for a rare disease μ will correspond to twice the population frequency, p of the allele. The variance–covariance matrix of $\mathbf{n}$ is assumed to be equal to

$$\mathrm{Var}(\mathbf{n}) = 2p(1 - p)\mathbf{K}, \tag{7.10}$$

with $\mathbf{K}$ being equal to twice the kinship matrix (Chap. 2, Sect. 2.1.4). In this model μ, β, and p all depend on the particular marker being considered, while $\mathbf{K}$ is constant for all markers. In the original test described by Bourgain et al. [20], it was assumed that $\mathbf{K}$ was calculated from known pedigree relationships between participants, while in the empirical versions of the test [21–23] $\mathbf{K}$ is estimated from large-scale genotyping data (e.g., GWAS data), for example, using the method of moments approach described in Chap. 2 (Sect. 2.5). The parameters μ and β are estimated using generalized least squares and the non-centrality parameter (if $\mathbf{K}$ is treated as known), for the test of the null hypothesis that $\beta = 0$ is equal to $\left(\beta^2 / \mathrm{Var}(\hat{\beta})\right)$ where $\mathrm{Var}(\hat{\beta})$ is equal to the $(2, 2)$ element of $2p(1 - p)(\mathbf{C}'\mathbf{K}^{-1}\mathbf{C})^{-1}$ with the $2 \times N$ matrix $\mathbf{C}$ having its first column equal to a vector of 1's and the second column equal to the case–control status indicator $\mathbf{c}$ above. When $\mathbf{K}$ is estimated as in Chap. 2 (Sect. 2.5), it is necessary to replace matrix inverses with generalized inverses (since $\hat{\mathbf{K}}$ as given in Sect. 2.5 is not invertible) in order to actually perform the test, but this is ignored for the purposes of power calculations here.

7.7.3.1 Non-Centrality Parameter for the Bourgain Test in the Case of Isolated Populations

We use the Balding–Nichols model (Chap. 2) for allele frequency differences between isolated populations. In this model allele frequencies for an SNP in modern data populations are distributed according to a beta distribution $B(((1 - F)/F) p, ((1 - F)/F)(1 - p)))$ with p the ancestral allele frequency of that SNP. In this model the variance of the modern-day allele frequency is $Fp(1 - p)$, thus F is a parameter specifying the degree of separation between the modern-day and ancestral population. As described in Chap. 4 if genotypes are obtained for randomly sampled individual from two modern-day isolated populations using this model and the separation of each modern-day population from the ancestral population equals F_k (for $k = 1, 2$) statistic then the covariance matrix, $\sigma_j^2 \mathbf{K}$ between subjects for the jth SNP will have diagonal terms equal to $2p_j(1 - p_j)(1 + F_1)$ for members of the first population, diagonal terms equal to $2p_j(1 - p_j)(1 + F_2)$ for members of the second, off diagonal terms of $4p_j(1 - p_j)F_1$, $4p_j(1 - p_j)F_2$, or zero for pairs of individuals who are either both from the first population, both from the second population or from different populations respectively. Here p_j is the frequency in the ancestral population of SNP j.

Consider a case–control study of these two populations in which one population contributes proportionately more cases to the study than the other population, in order to (for example) save on genotyping costs by reusing existing control data.[1] The worst-case example i.e., a study in which all cases come from one isolated population and all controls from another is discussed first. Note that for such a study the use of principal components as fixed effects in the analysis to control for population stratification would not be helpful since with enough markers in play a leading principal component would completely capture population membership so that case–control status would be completely confounded with this component. On the other hand, genomic control (as discussed above) would retain some power to find disease-associated alleles so long as the two study populations were not too different. We analyze this more fully below by computing the non-centrality parameter for the Bourgain test in this situation.

Assume for simplicity that $F_1 = F_2 = F$ (both populations have the same degree of separation from their ancestral source) and that the number of cases and controls are both equal to N so that total sample size is $2N$ (the calculations below can be readily altered for different matching fractions if necessary). Thus we can write the variance of the estimator of the case–control difference for SNP j as

$$\text{Var}(\hat{\beta}_j) = \sigma_j^2 (\mathbf{C}^T \mathbf{K}^{-1} \mathbf{C})^{-1}, \tag{7.11}$$

with the first column of $\mathbf{C}$ being a vector of 1's and the second column of $\mathbf{C}$ a vector of 1's and 0's indicating case–control (and population) status. Using a readily derived formula for the inverse of an $N \times N$ matrix of compound symmetric form

---

[1] For example, the Wellcome Trust Case Control Consortium (WTCCC) study used controls from two sources (the 1958 British Birth Cohort study and a sample of British blood donors) in studies of a total of seven common diseases with cases coming from a variety of different studies. While the studies contributing cases to the WTCCC study were all from the UK one could imagine further reuse of these controls in studies (e.g., of rarer diseases) involving many cases from outside the UK.

$$\begin{bmatrix} a & b & \dots & b \\ b & a & \dots & b \\ \vdots & \vdots & \ddots & \vdots \\ b & b & \dots & a \end{bmatrix}^{-1} = \frac{1}{a^2 + (N-2)ab - (N-1)b^2} \begin{bmatrix} a+(N-2)b & -b & \dots & -b \\ -b & a+(N-2)b & \dots & -b \\ \vdots & \vdots & \ddots & \vdots \\ -b & -b & \dots & a+(N-2)b \end{bmatrix},$$

we can easily write

$$\mathrm{Var}\left(\hat{\beta}_{2j}\right) = 2p_j(1-p_j)\frac{4(N-2)F+2}{N}. \tag{7.12}$$

Thus the non-centrality parameter, $\lambda^2 = \beta_{2j}^2/\mathrm{Var}(\hat{\beta}_{2j})$, of a test of association does not increase linearly in N, but rather is bounded above by the value $(\beta_{2j}^2)/8Fp_j(1-p_j)$. This can impose severe limitations on the power of any study in which there are such differences. To put this in perspective, consider two isolated populations which are each separated from their ancestral population with an F value of 0.0005, and consider an allele that exhibits 40 % frequency in the ancestral population. The variance of the difference between the two isolated modern-day populations in the frequency of this allele is equal to $2p_j(1-p_j)F$ so that we would expect by chance that there is a about a 1.5 % difference in allele frequencies between cases and controls for such an allele. Consider now the detection, in a study of 5,000 cases and 5,000 controls, of a disease-causing allele of the same frequency associated with a 10 % difference in allele frequencies between cases and controls ($\beta_{2j} = 2$). The difference in allele frequencies is approximately six times larger than expected due to population differences, and can be seen to correspond to an odds ratio for disease, under a multiplicative risk model, of 1.5 per copy of the risk allele. From (7.12) the non-centrality parameter $\beta_{2j}^2/\mathrm{Var}(\hat{\beta}_{2j})$ will be equal to 34.73 in this case; on the other hand if F between cases and controls is 0 the non-centrality parameter will equal 208.33. Thus a study that would, given no differences between cases and controls in population of origin, have overwhelming power (>0.9999) to reject the null hypothesis at a genome-wide level significance ($p < 10^{-8}$) is, under this alternative, reduced to having power of only 56 % after correcting for the differences in origins of cases and controls. The survey of European populations by Nelis et al. [24] estimates fixation indices, F_{st}, between populations in SNP allele frequencies which range from less than 0.001 between neighboring populations to 0.023 for Southern Italy versus parts of Finland. Because our F values as defined above are between present-day and ancestral populations the fixation indices calculated between present-day populations by Nelis et al. need to be multiplied by approximately ½ to be consistent with our definition of F (see Chap. 2, Sect. 2.4.1.1). Thus the example we have given ($F=.0005$) corresponds only to the nearest neighbor populations in Europe, even though the value of F is not large, the presence of stratification has a large effect on the power of a test after stratification is considered.

Less extreme situations can be analyzed using this approach by brute force calculation of (7.11). Figure 7.7 shows the non-centrality parameter for the test

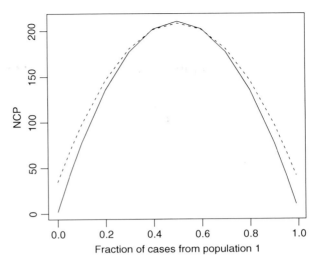

Fig. 7.7 Noncentrality parameter for Bourgain test according to fraction of cases from population 1 and the assumed separation (F_{st}) between populations and ancestral source. The *solid line* is for $F_{st} = 0.01$, and the *dotted* for $F_{st} = 0.0005$. Other parameters are set as described in the text

for two values of F (0.0005 and 0.01) roughly corresponding to nearby and relatively distant European populations, according to the fraction of cases that come from population 1. Here (as above) it is assumed that the two populations contribute equally to the total number of cases and controls. Once there is a fair amount of overlap in ancestry between the cases and controls (with 25–75 % or more of cases coming from population 1) then a considerable fraction of the power is regained.

This general discussion is relevant to the control of simple population stratification by either principal components or genomic control as well as the retrospective methods described here. Using estimated leading principal components as adjustment variables in a fixed effects analysis is not possible when all cases come from a single isolated population and all controls come from another, although in this case genomic control still retains some power, as does the test used here, for detection of strong genetic effects. Once there is some overlap in ancestry between the cases and controls then controlling for ancestry differences by either the fixed effects method or the retrospective approach will regain power, and either will generally be more effective than genomic control in adjusting for simple population structure [19, 25, 26]. Only rarely will a study which collects its own controls in a reasonable fashion suffer a severe loss of power by having to control for the rather minor degree of residual population stratification typical in such settings. Studies that seek to use existing control data while only collecting samples from cases are inherently more susceptible to population stratification and careful analysis of power should be undertaken. Chen et al. [25] give an example of such an analysis focused on the problem of correcting for admixture differences in hypothesized studies of African Americans that reuse existing control data available from a large study of prostate cancer and conclude that such reuse of data is feasible.

7.8   Power of Multi-SNP Conditional Tests

So far we have restricted attention to power in single SNP associations, and simple $G \times E$ interactions, perhaps after having had to adjust for population stratification or admixture. Another important problem, relevant to such topics as fine-mapping (see Chap. 8) around GWAS hits, is assessing the power to detect whether one marker shows either a stronger, or an independent signal than does another marker. For example, if we write a two-SNP model as

$$g(E(Y_i)) = \mu + \beta_1 G_{i1} + \beta_2 G_{i2}, \tag{7.13}$$

then our interest may be in determining whether conditional on a known GWAS association with G_1 the association with a nearby SNP G_2 remains significant. Power to detect the effect of G_2 will depend not only on the size of β_2 and the frequency of G_2 but also on the correlation between G_1 and G_2. Under the assumption that neither G_1 or G_2 explains a large amount of the variance of Y we can approximate the sample size N^* needed to reject the hypothesis $\beta_2 = 0$ at a given type I error rate and power as $N/\left(1 - R^2_{G_1,G_2}\right)$ where N is the sample size needed when only G_2 is in the model, and $R^2_{G_1,G_2}$ is the squared correlation between G_1 and G_2. This follows in an argument similar to that given in Sect. 7.7.2 because the variance of G_2 conditional on G_1 is equal to $\mathrm{Var}(G_2)\left(1 - R^2_{G_1,G_2}\right)$. This implies that we can estimate the sample size N needed to reject $\beta_2 = 0$ conditionally on G_1 being in the model by performing the calculations above (or running Quanto) ignoring G_1 and then adjusting the sample size upward by dividing N by the hypothesized value of $\left(1 - R^2_{G_1,G_2}\right)$. Of course power for testing $\beta_2 = 0$ for model (7.13) can be approached directly using the exemplary data or expected likelihood approach.

7.9   Chapter Summary

This chapter has aimed to give a working knowledge of the standard approaches used to calculate sample size and power for linear and logistic regression, for tests of main effects and interactions, with extensions to other generalized linear models following easily. The chapter introduces the so-called exemplary data method to assessing power in generalized linear models and also describes the generalization of this approach as used in the very popular QUANTO program.

   In addition to standard approaches some unique problems and issues for GWAS studies are addressed with attention devoted to the problem of assessing power after correction for population stratification, reuse of control data, design of two-stage genotyping designs, and large-scale multiple comparisons requirements.

Homework

1. Consider the logistic regression model (7.3) with $\mu = \text{logit}(10^{-4})$, $\beta_0 = 0$, $\beta_1 = \log(3)$, $\beta_2 = \log(9)$, $p = 0.001$.

   (a) Calculate the probabilities $\Pr(n(A)|D)$, for $n(A) = 0, 1, 2$; $D = 0, 1$ that correspond to the columns of Table 7.1 for this configuration.
   (b) For a study of 500 cases and 1,000 controls calculate the joint probabilities $\Pr(n(A), D)$ and the expectations $E(N)$ as given in Table 7.2.
   (c) Using the exemplary data method, calculate the non-centrality parameter for rejecting using logistic regression, the null hypothesis $\beta_1 = \beta_2 = 0$, at type 1 error 0.05 in favor of the (linear in genotype count) alternative that $\beta_2 = 2\beta_1 \neq 0$, what is the power for rejecting the null hypothesis?
   (d) What is the power using the Armitage test to reject this same hypothesis?
   (e) What is the non-centrality parameter for rejecting the hypothesis that $\beta_2 = \beta_1$ using logistic regression?
   (f) What is the power for rejecting the null hypothesis that $\beta_1 = \beta_2 = 0$ against the general alternative that at least one of β_1 and β_2 are nonzero?

2. If $\mathbf{X_1}$ is a $n \times p$ design matrix, of rank p, and $\mathbf{X_2}$ is an $(n) \times (p + r)$ design matrix, of rank $p + r$ that includes the columns of $\mathbf{X_1}$ as well as additional columns for the r new covariates to be tested then

$$\mathbf{A} = \mathbf{X_2}\left(\mathbf{X'_2 X_2}\right)^{-1}\mathbf{X'_2} - \mathbf{X_1}\left(\mathbf{X'_1 X_1}\right)^{-1}\mathbf{X'_1}$$

is used for testing whether the effect of the additional variables contribute significantly to a regression of continuous outcome Y on $\mathbf{X_2}$.

   (a) Special case: What is the A matrix that provides

   (i) The regression sum of squares in univariate linear regression.
   (ii) The residual sum of squares.

   (b) Show that $\mathbf{A}$ is a projection matrix, i.e., that $\mathbf{AA} = \mathbf{A}$. Hint: $\mathbf{X_2}(\mathbf{X'_2 X_2})^{-1} \mathbf{X'_2 X_1}$ is the predicted value of the regression of the columns of $\mathbf{X_1}$ onto the columns of $\mathbf{X_2}$ therefore it must equal $\mathbf{X_1}$.
   (c) What is the rank of A?
   (d) Give an argument that $Y A Y / \sigma^2$ is indeed a chi-square random variable.

3. Show for logistic regression that when the background rate of disease is small and the model is log additive in $n(A)$ that HWE is preserved in both cases and controls. Hint, approximate the logistic as an exponential in this case.

4. Consider the model for continuous outcome Y

$$Y = \mu + \beta_0 G_{i0} + \beta_1 G_{i1} + \beta_2 G_{i2} + e_i,$$

with e_i normal with mean 0 and variance σ^2. Suppose that the true values of the parameters are $\mu = 10$, $\beta_0 = 0$, $\beta_1 = 0.2$, $\beta_2 = 1$ and $\sigma^2 = 0.7$. Consider a study of 100 individuals and an SNP with minor allele frequency equal to 0.2.

(a) If we assume HWE what is the expected number of individuals with 0, 1, and 2 genotypes?

(b) What are the expected values of Y for each of these genotype categories?

(c) Use (7.2) with $E(Y)$ substituted for Y to compute the non-centrality parameter for rejecting the null that $\beta_1 = 0$, $\beta_2 = 0$ in favor of the linear hypothesis that $\beta_2 = 2\beta_1 \neq 0$. What is the power for rejecting this hypothesis (using an F test)?

(d) In R compute (as in problem 2) the **A** matrix for testing the linear hypothesis, verify that the non-centrality parameter $E(Y)' \, \mathbf{A}E(Y)/\sigma^2$ is the same as above. Hint in R matrix the multiplication operator is %*% and transpose is t($\cdot$), inversion is done using solve($\cdot$).

(e) Compute (in R) the **A** matrix for testing the linear hypothesis (that $\beta_2 = 2\beta_1$) against the general hypothesis that either or both of β_1 or β_2 is not equal to zero. What is the non-centrality parameter and power for this test?

5. Power for gene environment interactions. Suppose that X_i denotes the presence or absence of an environmental exposure. Consider the model

$$\text{logit}(\Pr(D = 1)) = \mu + \beta_1(G_{i1} + 2G_{i2}) + \beta_2 X_i + \beta_3 X_i(G_{i1} + 2G_{i2}),$$

with the parameter values $\mu = \text{logit}(10^{-4})$, $\beta_1 = \log(1.3)$, $\beta_2 = \log(1.9)$, $\beta_3 = \log(0.5)$, $p = 0.3$ and $\Pr(X = 1) = 0.5$. Here p is the frequency of the allele of interest:

(i) Make up a table (as in Table 7.4) the probabilities, $\Pr(n(A)|\text{Disease, Exposure})$. Assume that exposure is independent of genotype of interest.

(ii) Assume that 1,000 cases and 1,000 controls will be selected and calculate exemplary data from this model.

(iii) Compute non-centrality parameters for the series of hypotheses $\beta_1 = 0$, $\beta_2 = 0$, and $\beta_3 = 0$ using the *glm* and *anova* procedures in R. Calculate power based on these non-centrality parameters.

(iv) Compare power for each of these hypotheses to the output from QUANTO.

6. Power for conditional analyses. Below is a table of genotype probabilities for minor allele counts of two SNPs in the same region containing GWAS hits.

		SNP2		
		0	1	2
SNP2	0	0.2239	0.1200	0.0161
	1	0.0254	0.3600	0.0946
	2	0.0007	0.0200	0.1393

(a) What is the minor allele frequency of SNP1?

(b) What is the minor allele frequency of SNP2?

(c) What is the squared correlation, R^2, between the counts of the minor alleles of SNP1 and SNP2?

(d) Assume that disease, D, follows a logistic model

$$\text{logit}(\Pr(D = 1)) = \mu + \beta_1 n_1 + \beta_2 n_2$$

with n_1 and n_2 denoting the count of the minor alleles of SNP1 and SNP2, respectively

Suppose that $\mu = \log(10^{-4})$, $\beta_1 = \log(1.3)$, $\beta_2 = \log(1.2)$.

Calculate exemplary data from this model for a study with 500 cases and 500 controls. Use these data to calculate non-centrality parameters and the power for testing:

H1. The null hypothesis that $\beta_1 = 0$ and $\beta_2 = 0$ against the alternative that $\beta_2 \neq 0$.

H2. The null hypothesis that $\beta_1 \neq 0$ and $\beta_2 = 0$ against the hypothesis that $\beta_1 \neq 0$ and $\beta_2 \neq 0$.

How close is the NCP for hypothesis H2 to $(1 - R^2)$(NCP for test H1) as predicted in Sect. 7.8?

References

1. Knowler, W. C., Williams, R. C., Pettitt, D. J., & Steinberg, A. G. (1988). Gm3;5,13,14 and type 2 diabetes mellitus: An association in american indians with genetic admixture. *American Journal of Human Genetics, 43*, 520–526.
2. Longmate, J. A. (2001). Complexity and power in case-control association studies. *American Journal of Human Genetics, 68*, 1229–1237.
3. Self, S. G., Mauritsen, R. H., & Ohara, J. (1992). Power calculations for likelihood ratio tests in generalized linear models. *Biometrics, 48*, 31–39.
4. Brown, B. W., Lovato, J., & Russell, K. (1999). Asymptotic power calculations: Description, examples, computer code. *Statistics in Medicine, 18*, 3137–3151.
5. Gauderman, W., & Morrison, J. (2006). QUANTO 1.1: A computer program for power and sample size calculations for genetic-epidemiology studies. http://hydra.usc.edu/gxe
6. Gauderman, W. J. (2002). Sample size calculations for matched case-control studies of gene-environment interaction. *Statistics in Medicine, 21*, 35–50.
7. Gauderman, W. J. (2002). Sample size requirements for association studies of gene-gene interaction. *American Journal of Epidemiology, 155*, 478–484.
8. Piegorsch, W. W., Weinberg, C. R., & Taylor, J. A. (1994). Non-hierarchical logistic models and case-only designs for assessing susceptibility in population-based case-control studies. *Statistics in Medicine, 13*, 153–162.
9. Pe'er, I., Yelensky, R., Altshuler, D., & Daly, M. J. (2008). Estimation of the multiple testing burden for genomewide association studies of nearly all common variants. *Genetic Epidemiology, 32*, 381–385.
10. Satagopan, J. M., Verbel, D. A., Venkatraman, E. S., Offit, K. E., & Begg, C. B. (2002). Two-stage designs for gene-disease association studies. *Biometrics, 58*, 163–170.
11. Wang, H. (2006). *Staged genotyping and population stratification in genetic association studies*. Department of Preventive Medicine, University of Southern California: Los Angeles, CA.

12. Skol, A. D., Scott, L. J., Abecasis, G. R., & Boehnke, M. (2006). Joint analysis is more efficient than replication-based analysis for two-stage genome-wide association studies. *Nature Genetics, 38*, 209–213.
13. Jennison, C., & Turnbull, B. W. (2000). *Group sequential methods with applications to clinical trials* (Vol. xviii). Boca Raton, FL: Chapman and Hall.
14. Satagopan, J. M., & Elston, R. C. (2003). Optimal two-stage genotyping in population-based association studies. *Genetic Epidemiology, 25*, 149–157.
15. Hirschhorn, J. N., & Daly, M. J. (2005). Genome-wide association studies for common diseases and complex traits. *Nature Reviews Genetics, 6*, 95–108.
16. Ohashi, J., & Clark, A. G. (2005). Application of the stepwise focusing method to optimize the cost-effectiveness of genome-wide association studies with limited research budgets for genotyping and phenotyping. *Annals of Human Genetics, 69*, 323–328.
17. Wang, H., Thomas, D. C., Pe'er, I., & Stram, D. O. (2006). Optimal two-stage genotyping designs for genome-wide association scans. *Genetic Epidemiology, 30*, 356–368.
18. Devlin, B., & Roeder, K. (1999). Genomic control for association studies. *Biometrics, 55*, 997–1004.
19. Price, A. L., Patterson, N. J., Plenge, R. M., Weinblatt, M. E., Shadick, N. A., & Reich, D. (2006). Principal components analysis corrects for stratification in genome-wide association studies. *Nature Genetics, 38*, 904–909.
20. Bourgain, C., Hoffjan, S., Nicolae, R., Newman, D., Steiner, L., Walker, K., et al. (2003). Novel case-control test in a founder population identifies P-selectin as an atopy-susceptibility locus. *American Journal of Human Genetics, 73*, 612–626.
21. Rakovski, C. S., & Stram, D. O. (2009). A kinship-based modification of the armitage trend test to address hidden population structure and small differential genotyping errors. *PLoS One, 4*, e5825.
22. Astle, W., & Balding, D. J. (2009). Population structure and cryptic relatedness in genetic association studies. *Statistical Science, 24*, 451–471.
23. Thornton, T., & McPeek, M. S. (2010). ROADTRIPS: Case-control association testing with partially or completely unknown population and pedigree structure. *American Journal of Human Genetics, 86*, 172–184.
24. Nelis, M., Esko, T., Magi, R., Zimprich, F., Zimprich, A., Toncheva, D., et al. (2009). Genetic structure of Europeans: A view from the North-East. *PLoS One, 4*, e5472.
25. Chen, G. K., Millikan, R. C., John, E. M., Ambrosone, C. B., Bernstein, L., Zheng, W., et al. (2010). The potential for enhancing the power of genetic association studies in African Americans through the reuse of existing genotype data. *PLoS Genetics, 6*, e101096.
26. Price, A. L., Tandon, A., Patterson, N., Barnes, K. C., Rafaels, N., Ruczinski, I., et al. (2009). Sensitive detection of chromosomal segments of distinct ancestry in admixed populations. *PLoS Genetics, 5*, e1000519.

Chapter 8
Post-GWAS Analyses

Abstract The term post-GWAS analyses here refers to two somewhat distinct general topics; first are a compendium of analyses that are typically performed after one or more GWAS studies of a particular disease have been completed. These analyses include pooled or *meta-analysis* used in order to combine results of two or more studies, typically with the help of the of large-scale SNP imputation as discussed in Chap. 6. Additional analyses include replication of results often found first in Europeans, in studies of other racial/ethnic groups. Discussion of this topic is broadened to include what has been called *multiethnic fine mapping*. Adjustment for *local ancestry* in studies of admixed groups, as an aid to fine mapping within a single group is discussed as well. *Heritability* estimation using GWAS data is also considered.

A second set of topics are termed post-GWAS because they relate to issues raised by a new technology, namely, next-generation *whole genome sequencing* (WGS), which is currently being evaluated for large-scale association studies. The main raison d'être for WGS is to allow for interrogation of rare variation that cannot be measured on GWAS SNP arrays used to date. This chapter covers some of statistical topics related to the assessment of the role of rare variation, especially composite groups of rare variation related to each other through their mode of actions, pathway membership, physical location in or between genes, etc.

8.1 Meta-analysis

Meta-analysis is a phrase that has a number of related meanings; most fundamentally meta-analysis refers to the conduct of comprehensive, objective, and quantitative surveys of the state of current knowledge concerning a specific topic, which may involve only published summary data or can involve assembly of raw data from primary sources for combined analysis. Meta-analysis of published data was proposed in the 1970s and 1980s [1–3] in an effort to enhance the scientific credibility of literature reviews, by replacing selective discussion of specific results with more broadly objective and "reproducible" techniques. The scope of meta-analysis in this sense may be very broad, with almost any question that is amenable to experimental, quasi-experimental, or epidemiological investigation a candidate for such analysis. A review of meta-analysis procedures in this broad sense would necessarily include discussion of methods for identifying studies or other sources of information about specific topics, as well as normalization or standardization techniques needed to produce analyzable data that is not simply a collection of "apples and oranges."

More restrictively, the term meta-analysis refers to the statistical techniques that are used in order to summarize data from disparate studies while taking account of sampling variability. Beyond the issue of sampling variability alone, testing for between-study heterogeneity in results is often an important part of meta-analysis. The ability of the meta-analysis to draw conclusions in the presence of heterogeneity is somewhat controversial; however, the estimation of overall or average treatment effects has been considered by many authors [3–6]. This issue closely parallels the interpretation of main effects estimates in a two-way analysis of variance design when it is found that there is an interaction between the two treatments. The usual test of the main effects of treatment A in a two-way design asks whether, when averaged over the levels of B, there is a tendency for the levels of A to be different from each other. In fixed effects analysis, where both A and B are regarded as fixed treatments (and not sampled randomly from a hypothetical population of treatments), the introduction of an interaction between A and B can greatly complicate the conclusions about the efficacy of treatment A. Much of this complication has to do with clarifying whether in future application of treatment A (say when a new drug is released for marketing) factor B will continue to play a role and if so whether that role will be similar to the role that it played in the experimental period. A test for the effects of A when both A and B are regarded as fixed and when there is an interaction is really a test for an effect of A in the presence of B with B being in the same proportions as in the clinical trial. On the other hand, B may by design be regarded as a random effect, with the sampling of factor B that took place in the study being representative of the distribution of factor B (typical examples being plots, animal litters, individuals in repeated measures analysis, etc.) in the underlying population in which A will be used. In this case the main effect of A is clearly meaningful because the concept of averaging over the effects of B is meaningful in both the study sample and in the underlying population. The presence of an interaction between A and B does not change the interpretation of the main effects of A; however, it will change the specific test that is used to test for the effects of A. Referring to the classic decomposition of the total sums of squares (for a balanced design) into effects for A, B, A * B, and error (with mean square errors MS_A, MS_B, MS_{AB}, and MS_E, respectively), the test for an effect of A when B is fixed, with or without the interaction term is based on $F_A = \frac{MS_A}{MS_E}$. However, if B is random and an interaction is present, the test for the main effects of A is to be based on $F_A = \frac{MS_A}{MS_{AB}}$; if the interaction is not present, then the test reverts to $F_A = \frac{MS_A}{MS_E}$.

Fundamentally, the issue is about interpretability. If B is not random and an interaction is present, then the test for A is interpreted as applying to the given assignment of B; that is (speaking somewhat loosely), $F_A = \frac{MS_A}{MS_E}$ tests whether we can expect to see an effect of A averaged over B if we were to run the whole experiment repeatedly with the basic same layout (fraction of subjects assigned to each level of A and B) used each time. If instead the chosen levels of B represent a sample from a population of effects, then the presence of an interaction A*B reduces study power (since MS_{AB} has a larger expectation and fewer degrees of freedom than does MS_E) but does not complicate the interpretation of the main effects of treatment A.

As we see, these same issues arise when interpreting the results of meta-analysis of large-scale SNP data; in this case, factor B could refer to study, while factor A could refer to the allele counts of a particular SNP of interest. Of course, in real studies, things get more complicated, as adjustment variables (for age, sex, race, or principal components to correct for population structure or admixture), etc., are introduced into actual models; nevertheless, the issues remain quite similar.

8.2   Meta-analysis of Linear or Logistic Regression Estimates

The basic model that underlies most meta-analyses in practice corresponds to modeling a two-stage procedure in which there are a number, L, of studies each contributing independent estimates of the effect of a particular variable of interest (typically a SNP count n_A). For a number of reasons, it may not be considered practical to pool all data together in order to estimate the overall effect of n_A. Consider initially, however, a full pooled analysis. This can be written as

$$g\left(E\left(Y_{ij}\right)\right) = \alpha'_j X_{ij} + \beta_j n_{Aij}. \tag{8.1}$$

Here we have complicated the notation used previously so that the index i for subject is nested within study j for $j = 1, \ldots, L$. Here each X_{ij} constitutes a vector of adjustment variables for subject i within study j that may include factors such as age, sex, race, and principal components. The dependency of the parameter vector α_j on the index j simply allows these adjustment variables to have different effects in each study and also allows studies to not necessarily correct for all the same variables, i.e., there may be no need to correct for sex in one study that happened to be all males or for admixture in one study of a homogeneous group, whereas sex or admixture correction may be important in other studies. In any event, the variables in X are not the variables of interest, and further modeling of their effects is not of primary concern here. The dependency of the parameter of interest β on study

j allows for study to study heterogeneity. In particular we consider three possible models:

$$\beta_j = \beta \text{ fixed and equal for all } j, \tag{8.2}$$

$$\beta_j = \beta + \varepsilon_j, \text{ i.e., a random effects analysis,} \tag{8.3}$$

$$\beta_j \text{ heterogeneous but fixed.} \tag{8.4}$$

Model (8.2) imposes a constraint that each β_j in (8.1) be identical; model (8.3) relaxes this by allowing for mean zero random study to study heterogeneity in the true value of β_j, as well as sampling error in the estimate of β_j; the difference between model (8.3) and model (8.4) is that in the former, β has meaning as the expected effect for all studies while allowing for heterogeneity between studies. Model (8.4) simply posits heterogeneity between the studies in the effect of n_A with no attempt to generalize the results to other possible studies. With pooled data, both model (8.2) and model (8.4) are estimable with standard generalized linear model software, and model (8.3) is also available in procedures such as the R function *lme* [7] or the SAS procedure GLIMMIX, under the assumption that ε_j is distributed as a normal random variable with mean 0. A test for heterogeneity (i.e., a test for SNP by study interactions) which tests model (8.2) against either alternative model (8.3) or model (8.4) can be formed as a likelihood ratio test which compares the likelihood of model (8.1) with all β_j equal to the likelihood of the full model with at least one β_j different than the remainder, by fitting model (8.4). Direct tests of the hypothesis that $\text{Var}(\varepsilon_i) = 0$ in model (8.3) can also be performed. These may be expected to provide similar inference as the fixed effects test for heterogeneity in most cases; this holds exactly in two-way (balanced) analysis of variance where the F statistics used to test for the existence of an A*B interaction does not depend upon whether either A or B or both are treated as fixed or random effects.

For any number of reasons, it may be inconvenient to assemble the data required to fit model (8.1) directly in one pooled analysis. In this case meta-analyses will fall back on techniques developed for the analysis of published data such as those discussed by DerSimonian and Laird [3] and many others [4–6]. The DerSimonian and Laird approach starts with an assumption that each study produces an estimate $\hat{\beta}_j$ and an estimate V_j of the variance, i.e., by fitting model (8.1) and reporting the estimate of beta and (the square of) its standard error. A simple model for the $\hat{\beta}_j$ is that

$$\hat{\beta}_j = \beta_j + \zeta_j, \tag{8.5}$$

where it is assumed that the sampling errors, ζ_j, are independent normally distributed with mean zero and variance V_j and are also independently of the values of β_j. This essentially is assuming that the sample size in each study is large enough so that the central limit theorem applies and that the variability in the estimate of V_j can be ignored. If all the β_j are assumed to be equal, then the *best linear unbiased estimate* BLUE, $\hat{\beta}_{\text{BLUE}}$ of the underlying parameter β, is obtained as a weighted mean of the estimates $\hat{\beta}_j$ with the weights being inversely proportional to the variance estimates V_j so that

$$\hat{\beta}_{\text{BLUE}} = \frac{\sum_{j=1}^{L} \frac{1}{V_j} \hat{\beta}_j}{\sum_{j=1}^{L} \frac{1}{V_j}}. \tag{8.6}$$

The variance of the weighted BLUE estimate can be easily shown to reduce to

$$\frac{1}{\sum_{j=1}^{L} \frac{1}{V_i}}, \tag{8.7}$$

so that a test for whether the parameter β is equal to zero is just

$$\left(\hat{\beta}_{\text{BLUE}}\right)^2 \sum_{j=1}^{L} \frac{1}{V_i}. \tag{8.8}$$

Confidence intervals are also readily constructed using the variance (8.7). Assuming that the behavior of the $\hat{\beta}_i$ is adequately described as Gaussian, then this test has a chi-square 1 distribution with a noncentrality parameter equal to the plug-in estimate (see Chap. 7) of $\left(\beta^2 \sum_{j=1}^{L} \frac{1}{V_i}\right)$

A test for heterogeneity, i.e., whether $\beta_j = \beta$, $\forall\, j$ is formed by fitting the model

$$\hat{\beta}_j = \beta + \beta_j + \zeta_j, \tag{8.9}$$

either as a fixed effects model, in which case a constraint on β_j must be imposed, such as $\sum \beta_j = 0$ (as in traditional ANOVA) or $\beta_1 = 0$ (as in glm in R), or as a random effects model with β_j random with mean zero. The fixed effects test for heterogeneity is derived as an $L-1$ degree of freedom contrast test. Starting with the model for the means and variances

$$E \begin{bmatrix} \hat{\beta}_1 \\ \hat{\beta}_2 \\ \vdots \\ \hat{\beta}_L \end{bmatrix} = \begin{bmatrix} \beta_1 \\ \beta_2 \\ \vdots \\ \beta_L \end{bmatrix},$$

with

$$\text{Var}\left(\begin{bmatrix} \hat{\beta}_1 \\ \hat{\beta}_2 \\ \vdots \\ \hat{\beta}_L \end{bmatrix}\right) = \begin{bmatrix} V_1 & 0 & \cdots & 0 \\ 0 & V_2 & 0 & 0 \\ 0 & 0 & \ddots & \\ 0 & 0 & 0 & V_L \end{bmatrix} = \mathbf{\Sigma}.$$

The hypothesis that elements of the parameter vector $\mathbf{\beta}$ are equal to each other can be written as the contrast $\mathbf{C\beta} = 0$ with $\mathbf{C}$ the $L - 1 \times L$ matrix

$$\begin{bmatrix} 1 & -1 & 0 & \cdots & 0 \\ 0 & 1 & -1 & \cdots & 0 \\ 0 & 0 & \cdots & 1 & -1 \end{bmatrix}.$$

The estimated value of this contrast $\mathbf{C\hat{\beta}}$ has variance–covariance matrix $\mathbf{C\Sigma C}'$ so that the Wald test of the null hypothesis that this contrast is zero is

$$\hat{\mathbf{\beta}}'\mathbf{C}'(\mathbf{C\Sigma C}')^{-1}\mathbf{C\hat{\beta}}, \tag{8.10}$$

with some algebra this reduces to $Q = \sum_{j=1}^{L} \dfrac{1}{V_j}(\hat{\beta}_j - \hat{\beta}_{\text{BLUE}})^2$.

Under the null hypothesis that all β_j are equal, Q has a central chi-squared distribution with $L - 1$ degrees of freedom.

8.2.1   Random Effects Models

As described above in the context of analysis of variance, the interpretation of the results of a fixed effects analysis is complicated when there is strong evidence of heterogeneity. If one is willing to think of the studies as having been sampled "randomly" from a population of possible studies, adopting a random effects analysis does three things:

1. It reevaluates the weights in the model.
2. It produces a new "best" estimate, $\hat{\beta}_{\text{RE}}$, of the average, β, of the β_j that underlay the observed $\hat{\beta}_j$.
3. It forms modified tests and confidence intervals regarding the underlying parameter β.

Treating the β_j in model (8.5) as a random effect with mean zero and variance σ_β^2, the total variance of β_j is now $V_j + \sigma_\beta^2$ so that the BLUE estimate will become

$$\hat{\beta}_{\text{RE}} = \frac{\sum_{j=1}^{L} \frac{1}{V_J + \sigma_\beta^2} \hat{\beta}_j}{\sum_{j=1}^{L} \frac{1}{V_J + \sigma_\beta^2}},$$

with variance equal to

$$\text{Var}\left(\hat{\beta}_{\text{RE}}\right) = \sum_{j=1}^{L} \frac{1}{V_J + \sigma_\beta^2}.$$

Estimation of σ_β^2 can be approached either using the method of moments or using maximum likelihood or restricted maximum likelihood. A simple non-iterative method of moments estimator [3] is

$$\hat{\sigma}_\beta 2 = \max\left\{0, \{Q - (L-1)\}/\left[\sum_j w_j - \left(\sum_j w_j^2 / \sum_j w_j\right)\right]\right\},$$

with $w_j = 1/V_j$.

Note that the noncentrality parameter for the test that β is zero is now $\beta^2 \sum_{j=1}^{L} \frac{1}{V_j + \sigma_\beta^2}$ which will be smaller than the NCP for the fixed effects test (unless σ_β^2 is zero).

A more general random effects model for the observed $\hat{\beta}_j$ based on (8.5) is

$$\hat{\beta}_j = \mathbf{X}_j \alpha + \beta_j + \zeta_j. \tag{8.11}$$

The fixed effects term $\mathbf{X}_j \alpha$ is introduced to allow for study-level covariates which may explain some of the heterogeneity between studies; see Stram et al. [4] for an extended discussion.

8.3   Meta-analysis for the GWAS Setting

In the general exposition of meta-analysis (e.g., Borenstein et al. [8]), a good deal of discussion is provided on such topics as the identification of studies to be used in meta-analysis and the potential for biases due to poor selection strategies or due to publication bias (a tendency to only publish positive results). While these problems remain germane here [9] especially for candidate gene studies which have had inconsistent reliability, e.g., [10, 11], GWAS studies generally face a somewhat different set of issues; see, for example, reference [12]. Meta-analysis methods originally designed for published summaries (e.g., counts, effect estimates) have been used even when the studies to be considered are all being conducted by a group of collaborating investigators (e.g., the GENEVA Consortium [13], PAGE collaboration [14]), GAME-ON consortium, who may indeed each have individual access to at least their own data if not all collaborators data. The reason that meta-analysis (e.g., analysis of summary statistics computed for each study) rather than full pooled analysis may be performed is primarily a matter of convenience and sometimes of administrative necessity (due to restrictions on data sharing, patient confidentiality, etc.).

An issue that can be frustrating to deal with in either pooled or summary analysis is the need to rectify any allele/strand differences that may crop up between studies either when genotyping SNPs or when imputing ungenotyped SNPs. Consider, for example, an SNP that when genotyped on the plus strand (see Chap. 1) is an C/T SNP. One study may be using as the risk variable in logistic regression the (observed or expected) number of copies of the allele T for this SNP whereas another study may be counting the number of copies of C; clearly if the SNP allele T is truly a risk factor for the outcome of interest, then the first study will tend to find positive risk associations when the second study will tend to find negative (protective) associations. A third study may be genotyping the same SNP on the minus strand (where it is a G/A SNP) and counting the number of copies of the A allele (the risk allele), while a fourth study may be counting the number of copies of the (protective) G allele on the same strand. The confusion described in this particular example can be easily rectified by simply having each study report the allele that is being counted, A, G, C, or T, in the risk analysis. The meta-analysis can go forward after appropriate reversal of signs of the effect estimates (e.g., linear regression parameters or log odds ratios) so that all studies contribute to the same effect, e.g., the effect of the A allele on the plus strand. As noted in Chap. 1, the problem of rectifying allele/strand differences is a bit trickier for the ambiguous A/T or C/G SNPs (where strand reversal does not change the alleles that are reported). If ambiguous SNPs cannot be avoided altogether, then using the BLAT program (genome.ucsc.edu; see Chap. 1) to match the probes used by each platform to determine strand positivity and then performing appropriate allele "flipping" to resolve complementarities (forcing strand positivity and allele choice for all studies) may be the only really effective measure to avoid nonsense results when the data are combined.

8.3.1   Meta-analysis and Imputation

One of the most unusual aspects of meta-analysis of GWAS data (relative to typical uses of meta-analysis for review purposes) is the large-scale use of imputed geno-types. Since each study to be combined may use different genotyping arrays, or different versions of the same genotyping array, the list of successfully genotyped SNPs can differ for each study to be combined. Rather than dropping whole studies in the analysis of individual SNPs, SNP imputation methods (see Chap. 6) are used so that inference can include all SNPs genotyped by any study or even all SNPs known from either the HapMap [15], 1000 Genomes Project [16], or other source [17] when used as a reference panel for imputation. As stressed in Chap. 6, it is important that the individual studies (e.g., those contributing to the meta-analysis) use the expected indicator or dosage variables when fitting models such as

$$g(E(Y_i)) = \alpha + \beta n_A, \tag{8.12}$$

or 2 df models

$$g(E(Y_i)) = \alpha + \beta_1 I(n_A = 1) + \beta_2 I(n_A = 2), \tag{8.13}$$

for an allele A.

One question frequently asked in this context (e.g., [12]) is whether studies in which allele A is either genotyped or very well imputed should be given more weight in the meta-analysis of the effects of allele A than do studies in which A is less well genotyped. While it may be a good idea to drop very poorly imputed genotypes from analysis, it is helpful to realize that when fitting (for example) model (8.12) using $E(n_A|G)$ (where G is the data used for imputation), less well-imputed genotypes (as measured by the R^2 criteria) are implicitly being down-weighted automatically. This is because the contribution that a specific study will make to the meta-analysis will depend on the variance of the explanatory variable (here, n_A when A is genotyped and $E(n_A)$ when it is not) in that study. If R^2 for a given study is low, then the variance of the predictor, $E(n_A)$, is also low and so the contribution of that study is low, because R^2 can be defined here as $\frac{\text{Var}(E(n_A))}{\text{Var}(n_A)}$. Note that the R^2 values output by such imputation programs as MACH is equal to this expression with the numerator equal to the observed (sample) variance of the expected dosage variable $E(n_A)$ and the denominator replaced by its value under HWE, $2p(1 - p)$, where p is the allele frequency of A. Thus, the use of the expected dosages (or expected indicator variables for 2 degrees of freedom models) already accounts for uncertainty in SNP imputation by implicitly down-weighting the contribution of studies for which SNPs are less well imputed. The calculation of this R^2 of course assumes that the relevant haplotype frequencies have been reasonably well estimated and therefore is model based rather than empirical. See the discussion of other estimates of imputation reliability described in Chap. 6.

8.4 Efficiency of Meta-analysis Versus Pooled Analysis

Pooled analysis refers to the combined analysis of individual data for each study. It is possible to come up with examples in which meta-analysis of study-level results (e.g., log odds ratios and their standard errors) is much less efficient than a pooled analysis. To give an illustrative example, consider an artificial situation in which there are two case–control studies for which effect estimates are to be combined but that one of the studies utilizes a (frequency) matching of 10 controls to each of n cases and the other study matches 10 cases to each of n controls! In a simple comparison of the mean genotype frequency between cases and controls for each study (i.e., using an allele counting test to compare genotype frequencies), the variance (for simplicity evaluated under the null hypothesis of no true difference) of the estimate of the effect (e.g., the difference, d, in allele frequency) is $\mathrm{Var}(\hat{d}_i)$ $= 2p(1-p)[(1/n)+(1/10n)]$ in each study $i = 1, 2$, where p is the population frequency of the allele of interest. Combining the estimates from the two studies, under the assumption that both $\hat{d}_i$ estimate the same quantity, gives $\mathrm{Var}(\text{overall } \hat{d} \text{ from meta-analysis}) = p(1-p)[(1/n)+(1/10n)]$. Pooled analysis of the data from the two studies would give a single study with $11n$ cases and $11n$ controls so that the variance of the difference estimate would be $\mathrm{Var}(\text{overall } \hat{d} \text{ from pooled analysis}) = 2p(1-p)[(1/11n)+(1/11n)]$. Therefore, the pooled analysis has a variance which is less than $1/3$ as large (more precisely $40/121$ times as large) as the meta-analysis. This discussion assumes that there would be no need to adjust for study in the pooled analysis; as soon as a study variable is introduced into the pooled analysis, then the effect estimates for the two situations become essentially indistinguishable. This can be seen by running the R code (with arbitrarily picked parameters):

```
> set.seed(2011)   # so we get the same results each time for
illustration
> p=.2; # allele frequency of allele being tested
> n=100; # number case or controls as above
> v_meta<-p*(1-p)*(1/n+1/(10*n)) # variance under null of the meta
                                 # analysis difference, d
> v_pooled<-2*p*(1-p)*(1/(11*n)+1/(11*n)); # variance under null of d
                                 # in the pooled analysis
> study<-factor(c(rep(1,11*n),rep(2,11*n)))          # study indicator
> cc<-c(rep(1,n),rep(0,10*n),rep(1,10*n),rep(0,n)) # case control
status 0 or 1
> s<-c(rbinom(n,2,p),rbinom(10*n,2,p),rbinom(10*n,2,p),rbinom(n,2,p));
# simulated SNPs
# for cases and controls in each study
> reg1<- lm(s~cc) # simple pooled analysis
> reg2<- lm(s~cc+study) # pooled analysis correcting for study
> sqrt(v_pooled) # gives similar results as reg1
[1] 0.02412091
> summary(reg1)
Coefficients:
            Estimate Std. Error t value Pr(>|t|)
(Intercept)  0.40909    0.01704  24.008   <2e-16 ***
cc          -0.01727    0.02410  -0.717    0.474
---
> sqrt(v_meta) # gives similar results as reg2
0.04195235
> summary(lm(reg2))
Coefficients:
            Estimate Std. Error t value Pr(>|t|)
(Intercept)  0.40695    0.01746  23.303   <2e-16 ***
cc          -0.03650    0.04192  -0.871    0.384
study2       0.02350    0.04192   0.561    0.575
---
```

Note how similar the standard error estimates from the study-corrected pooled regression analysis (0.04195) and the meta-analysis (0.04192) are, as well as from the uncorrected regression (0.02419) and pooled (0.02412). While this is far from a complete analysis, it is illustrative of the fact that when the models being used are comparable, the results from the meta-analytic methods should be similar to the results from pooled analyses, especially when sample sizes are large enough that normality of effect estimates can be safely assumed. Note that all of the analyses above assume that there is no interaction between study and the effect of treatment. If we include a study*cc effect in the regression model as in

```
>summary(lm(s~cc+study+study*cc)
```

then the standard error of the main effects estimate increases further (to 0.05929 in this example). Here, of course we do not need the interaction term (because it is not present in the simulated data). If the interaction was significant, then this would raise issues about the meaning of the main effect parameter. While we have summarized the data as differences in allele frequencies by case–control status rather than as odds ratios, we expect that the same general results (e.g., regarding the relative variances of overall effect estimates) will hold when (log) ORs are computed separately by study and then combined (in a meta-analysis) or when the data are pooled.

8.5 Sources of Heterogeneity in Meta-analysis of GWAS Data

Differences in LD, exposure differences, and gene × gene interactions can all be sources of between-study heterogeneity in meta-analysis results.

8.5.1 LD Differences

As described in Chap. 2, different racial/ethnic groups have different patterns of linkage disequilibrium so that if the same SNP is measured in different groups, it may be in strong LD with a causal allele in one population but not another. It could be, for example, that the causal allele is not present (or is much rarer) in the second population than the first or that the causal allele is in LD with a different set of SNPs in the second population than the first one. A variation on the first possibility (the synthetic association hypothesis [18]) is that the causal allele is very highly penetrant but very rare. Under this scenario LD between the causal allele and common markers such as those typed in GWAS studies would be low, but since the underlying signal is very large, common SNPs with D' equal to 1 with the rare causal allele would still show modest, "synthetic" associations with the outcome of interest. One implication of the synthetic association hypothesis is that the association signal may be spread over long genetic distances since high LD (measured by D', see Chap. 2) between rare and common alleles tends to be more extended than LD between common alleles. In addition since rare alleles are generally more recent in origin than common alleles, rare causal alleles are much more likely to be population-specific so that associations seen in one population are less likely to be replicable in other populations with different genetic ancestry.

8.5.2 Exposure Differences

Populations can and do have different exposures to disease-causing nongenetic factors, and susceptibility to different exposures may well be modified by different SNPs. Even within very similar populations, exposures may change with time or with geographic location; while most examples are fairly hypothetical at this stage, exposure differences clearly are possible sources of heterogeneity in a meta-analysis.

8.5.3 Gene × Gene Interactions

Interactions between alleles complicate the search for causal variants and the role of gene × gene interactions in heritability (see discussion of missing heritability below) of many traits is of considerable past and current interest [19, 20].

When the measured alleles being considered in a meta-analysis (or the causal alleles in linkage disequilibrium with the measured alleles) are interacting with other alleles (or a polygene) which vary greatly in frequency between populations, then the main effects of the alleles of interest can also vary greatly between populations.

Note that a comprehensive identification of interactions is much harder than identifying main effects in GWAS studies (consider, e.g., performing a brute force search of all possible pairwise interactions for one million SNPs, a total of 5×10^{11} tests); Bonferroni correction for 5×10^{11} comparisons requires approximately a ninefold increase in sample size to preserve similar power compared to a single test at $\alpha = 0.05$ (see Chap. 7). Ultimately therefore as sample sizes increase for the most common diseases, it may be possible to perform such agnostic tests, at least for common variants. More focused semi-agnostic tests are already currently possible, for example, to check whether any common variant interacts with one of the known variants.

Homogeneity of effects between most or all populations (especially after LD differences have been dealt with as in multiethnic fine mapping, see below) is an argument against the domination of trait variance by gene by gene interactions. It is interesting, indeed, to note that the analysis of human height by Lango Allen [21] found almost no direct evidence of gene × gene interactions between hundreds of replicated common variants. However, since only single-SNP analyses were used to identify these height variants, it is possible that these are simply the most "additive" variants in the first place and that interactions are not expected with such variants. More extensive analyses will be needed as sample sizes continue to increase.

8.6 Meta-analysis Based on Effect sizes, Z-scores, and *P*-Values

In the analysis above, it is assumed that each estimate, $\hat{\beta}_i$, from each study is estimating fundamentally the same quantity (measured on the same scale), e.g., the increase in phenotype mean, or (log) odds for disease, with the number of risk alleles carried. Historically, however, much work on meta-analysis was in settings [22], where many different measurement instruments existed, which, while considered to be related on a fundamental level, had different scales of measurement and population distributions. A typical example in education research could be student performance on different standardized tests used before and after an intervention or in relation to some sort of predictor variable; class size, for example, has been studied in observational and some experimental studies using a number of different standardized tests [23]. In a study comparing an intervention (such as a reduction in class size) on outcome (test performance), the *effect size* is often defined as the difference between means divided by the standard deviation for the individuals in the control group. Meta-analysis of effect-size estimates in a combined analysis over many schools, etc., can be discussed as above, so long as each effect-size estimate is also given an appropriate variance estimate. Note that distinctions between random and fixed effects models may be less clear when using effect sizes of different instruments because of the inherent dependence of the effect size on the standard deviation in the populations considered. Typically only fixed effects methods seem to be used in these instances; leaving aside this question, however, we consider below some of the well-known methods.

8.6.1 Z-Score Analysis

The test, equation (8.8), of nonzero β can rewritten in terms of Z-scores from each study, i.e., in terms of $Z_i = \hat{\beta}_i / \sqrt{V_i}$ as

$$\frac{\left(\sum_{i=1}^{L} \frac{1}{\sqrt{V_i}} Z_i\right)^2}{\sum_{i=1}^{L} \frac{1}{V_i}}. \tag{8.14}$$

Based at least in part upon the identity between (8.14) and (8.8), weighting
Z-scores by weights that are proportional to the inverse of the standard error of the
effect estimate, or (which often gives similar results) by weights that are proportional to the square root of the sample size of each study, is a popular method for
providing a summary test even when there is no underlying single effect β being
estimated, i.e., when different, but related, instruments are being utilized. It is worth
noting that when there is no underlying single parameter to be estimated, an
"optimal" weighting would intuitively give larger weights to the Z-scores from
the studies with the most power to reject the null hypothesis [24]. Doing so,
however, requires that the effect sizes (or at least their relative sizes) as well as
the sample sizes be known, which is typically more information than is available
[25] when no underlying single effect is being tested.

8.6.2 Fisher's Method of Combining P-Values

Fisher [26] examined the distribution of the product $p_1 p_2 \ldots p_L$ of independent p-
values (each testing different and independent hypotheses) as an overall summary
statistic for the significance of a series of studies. We assume that by construction,
p-values under the null hypothesis are distributed as uniform continuous random
variables. (This not always the case since the underlying test statistics may have not
been uniformly distributed because of either small sample sizes, model misspeci-
fication, or the nature of the hypotheses being tested; for example, the asymptotic
distribution of likelihood ratio tests in maximum likelihood estimation depends on
the parameter space geometry [27].) Applying $-\log(x)$ to a uniform random variable, x, produces an exponential random variable, and doubling an exponential
gives a chi-square with two degrees of freedom. It follows that if each of a set of
L different p_i is from independent tests, all computed under the null, then
$2\sum_{i}^{L} -\log(p_i)$ is a central chi-square with $2L$ degrees of freedom. Comparing the
observed value of this statistic to the critical value from the χ_{2L}^2 distribution forms
an omnibus test of the joint null hypothesis against the alternative that at least one of
the null hypotheses are false. Note that there is no direction implied by this test
(each test specifies a two-sided alternative with no credit for having effects all in the
same direction) and that no weighting of p-values is performed, i.e., a small p-value
from the smallest study is just as influential as from the largest. Because of this, a
number of authors have provided weighted directional versions [25, 28]. One
general approach is to compute a Z-score from a (one-sided) p-value as $Z_i = \Phi^{-1}$
(p_i) with Φ the cumulative standard normal distribution (two-sided tests are first
converted to one-sized tests by dividing each p-value by two and inserting the
direction of each test). With this transformation the methods described above are
then utilized. Another well-known treatment is the Lancaster method [29] which

calculates the statistic $T = \sum_{i}^{L} \left[\chi^2_{(n_i)}\right]^{-1}(1 - p_i)$ having the distribution $T \sim \chi^2_{(\Sigma n_i)}$ under the global null hypothesis. Zaykin 2011 [24] found that this statistic behaves similarly to the Z-score method above with weights proportional either to $\sqrt{n_i}$ or to $1/\sqrt{(V_i)}$ although it should be noted that Lancaster's method, like Fisher's, gives no credit for having individual studies agree on the direction of effect.

8.6.3 Meta-analysis of Score Tests

In some cases (as in the discussion of rare SNPs given below), it may be important to use scores tests rather than Wald tests as the summary statistics. As described in Chap. 3, the score test is a test of the null hypothesis that (univariate) $\beta = 0$ of form $i^{\beta\beta}U\left(\beta = 0, \hat{\lambda}, Y\right)^2$, where $i^{\beta\beta}$ is the element of the inverse of the information matrix evaluated at $\beta = 0$ and at the maximum likelihood value (computed under the null) of the nuisance parameters, here λ, that are also in the model and $U\left(\beta = 0, \hat{\lambda}, Y\right)$ is the component of the score that corresponds to β (also evaluated at zero for β and at $\hat{\lambda}$). Now consider the score statistics for the same risk allele calculated for each of $k = 1, \ldots, L$ studies summarized over each study assuming that the studies each provide independent information regarding the effect of the allele of interest. Since the score test is fundamentally a ratio of the squared score value for β to its variance (which is here $1/i^{\beta\beta}$), we compute a combined score test using all study data as

$$\left[\sum_{k=1}^{L} 1/i_k^{\beta\beta}\right]^{-1}\left[\sum_{k=1}^{L} U_k\left(\beta = 0, \hat{\lambda}, Y\right)\right]^2, \qquad (8.15)$$

where $i_k^{\beta\beta}$ is the appropriate element of the inverse information matrix (evaluated at $\beta = 0$) for the kth study and likewise for $U_k\left(\beta = 0, \hat{\lambda}, Y\right)$. This is a ratio of the square of the total score (combined over all studies) to its estimated variance under the null hypothesis. See Homework for further discussion of the practical significance of this formulation. Note that this test does not actually require that the same set of nuisance parameters λ be used in every study analysis.

8.7 Multiethnic Analyses

Although there have been some improvements in diversifying GWAS studies, as well as pooled or meta-analyses [30–33], GWAS studies using participants from other ethnic groups remain far less common than GWAS studies in Europeans. A primary reason for this is undoubtedly lack of preexisting research infrastructure, i.e., the relative paucity, for other groups, of large-scale case–control and cohort studies with biological samples. Another reason however [34] is the persistence of a general view that homogeneity is required in order for genetic association studies to produce reliable results.

The use of multiple ethnic groups GWAS studies in either pooled analyses or meta-analysis of summary data is useful for at least three reasons:

1. Discovery of additional risk variants
2. Better localization of causal associations and improvement of risk score behavior
3. Enhancement of general knowledge about trait heritability

While alleles that are common in any one large-scale population are generally present in most other such populations, allele frequencies vary considerably between population, and since frequency is a determinant of power (Chap. 7), large-scale ethnically homogeneous but non-European discovery samples have the potential for determining additional risk- or phenotype-associated alleles that are relatively infrequent in Europeans, c.f. [30, 31].

Localization of causal alleles in association studies can be enhanced by use of additional ethnic groups beyond those in which the association was first discovered. Typically when viewing association data for a single population, linkage disequilibrium at the fine scale level ultimately interferes with localization, i.e., there are many similarly performing associated alleles spread out over tens or even hundreds of kilo bases of DNA sequence. If data for other ethnic groups is available then it is possible to rule out a fraction of the similarly performing associated alleles by their behavior in the multiethnic population. Utilization of this approach has been successful in further localizing breast cancer risk in the FGFR2 region [35] and has been attempted in several other studies [32] *other references*. In one specific example, Chen et al. [32] constructed a risk score consisting of the unweighted counts of 19 common genetic variants that had been discovered and reliably shown to be related to breast cancer risk in European or Asian populations. They showed that this score was not reproducible in a large African ancestry study, i.e., the score was not significantly associated with risk in 3,016 cases and 2,745 controls of African ancestry. Chen et al. found however that fine mapping in the 250 kb regions containing the reported SNPs produced novel disease associations of two types: (1) with SNPs that in the original reporting populations were in high LD with the reported variant but were not in LD in with the index variant in African populations and (2) with SNPs that were not in LD with the previously reported variant either in the original or in the African population. They produced a revised score that included both these novel associations (4 of each type were tentatively identified). While it will be important to replicate the revised score in both African and non-African ancestry women before it can be fully accepted, the revised score was highly predictive of risk in their sample.

Domination of trait variance by either gene × gene interactions or gene × exposure interactions would greatly reduce the overall heritability that can be explained by simple gene-risk summaries such as the score described above [20]. Use of multiple ethnic groups in meta-analysis not only has the potential to refine the effects of each allele included in such a summary but also can yield information about the predominance of interactive effects versus simple additive genetic effects on disease risk or trait mean. If interactive effects predominate, then it would be expected that many associations would fail to replicate in other populations and that additional fine mapping of risk associations would not be enough to find more robust associations. On the other hand, if it can be verified that most risk loci replicate in all populations, then interactive effects may be less important than sometimes feared. Large-scale attempts to replicate associations in other ethnic groups which were found originally in European samples are currently ongoing (as of this writing) in such studies as the PAGE consortium [14].

8.8 Fine Mapping of Single-SNP Associations: Conditional Analyses

Densely genotyping markers around SNPs that have been well replicated in a search for markers that are more associated with the outcome of interest than the *index signal*, i.e., the previously reported SNP association, requires us to judge whether any associations found this way either underlie or enhance the reported signal. A simple approach guiding such a judgment is to first include the index signal in a baseline model and perform a likelihood ratio test of whether the newly discovered allele passes an appropriate significance threshold when added to the baseline model; and then second to perform the reverse analysis, the new allele is forced into the baseline model, and a test for the significance of the index signal, conditional on the new allele, is constructed. Possible results of this analysis are:

1. The new association enters the model significantly in the first test, and the index signal does not enter in the second test.
2. The new association fails to enter the model significantly in the first test, but the index signal also fails to enter in the second test.
3. The new association enters the model significantly in the first test, and the index signal also enters in the second test.
4. The new association fails to enter the model significantly in the first test, while the index signal does enter the model in the second test.

The (tentative) conclusion from result (1) is that the new association is more strongly associated with the same causal allele than is the index signal; from result (2) we might conclude that the new allele and the index signal are equivalently associated with the same causal allele; from result (3) we would tend to conclude that there is more than one causal allele at work in the region being fine-mapped and these are not highly correlated with each other; from result (4) the conclusion would be the index signal remains the most closely associated allele.

The strength of our confidence in these conclusions depends upon the significance level used in the test and the power of detecting conditional associations. There have been some suggestions made concerning appropriate significance levels to use in fine mapping. It is generally agreed that requiring genome-wide significance (p-values of 5×10^{-8} or so) for the results of the fine mapping is too stringent since there is a very high prior probability that a causal variant exists in the region and a high prior probability is an accepted rationale for accepting reduced p-value [36]. A seemingly more reasonable criterion would be for a fine-mapping study to use the Bonferroni test according to the number of associations investigated during the fine mapping exercise, so that a level of significance of $0.05/n$, where n is the number of alleles used in the fine mapping, is required. For example, in the paper described above, Chen et al. [32] used a modification of this criteria when fine-mapping associations and searching for new alleles in regions surrounding 19 risk loci for breast cancer. They used a more stringent criterion to accept that a new allele was an independent risk predictor (i.e., pointing to a new risk allele not associated with original index signal), i.e., to accept result 3 they required a Bonferroni correction for all the SNPs genotyped in all regions considered, whereas to accept that the new allele was a better predictor of the same underlying causal allele (result 1) required only Bonferroni correction for the SNPs genotyped in each specific (of 19) region. Here the onus is on the new allele to pass the appropriately Bonferroni-adjusted criteria during the first test, the significance criteria for the second test (when the index allele is competing against the new allele) arguably could be much more relaxed since the index allele already has been judged to be globally significant in other analyses.

Clearly the confidence in the conclusions when either result 2 or result 4 is seen depends upon the power to detect conditional associations. An approximation to the sample size needed to detect the influence of a causal variable X (the test SNP) when another noncausal but correlated variable Z (the index SNP) is already in the model is to divide the sample size computed with only variable X in the model by $(1 - R_{xz}^2)$ with R_{XZ}^2 being the squared correlation between the two variables. This approximation follows because one of the primary determinants of the power of detecting an effect of X is the variance of X in the population; when computing the power of a test of whether X is influential in the presence of Z, we may replace the variance of X with the variance of X conditional on Z which is $\mathrm{Var}(X)(1 - R_{XZ}^2)$. Since needed sample size is inversely proportional to the variance of the predictor, we can use standard sample size programs to compute conditional power for a fixed sample size, n, by using an effective sample size of $n_{eff} = n(1 - R_{XY}^2)$ in the place of n when running these programs.

8.9 Fine Mapping in Admixed Populations

In Chap. 4 the use of global ancestry estimated by principal components is described for the purpose of control of false-positive rates due to recent or incomplete admixture. We now consider issues related to fine mapping in admixed populations; to simplify matters, only admixed populations having two ancestral populations are discussed. We also assume that the true effect of the underlying causal variant of interest on phenotype mean or risk is the same in both mixing populations. At the outset, it is important to understand that studying an admixed population can provide more power to detect the effect of a large range of variants than can studies that are restricted either to a single ancestry or to a combination of single ancestry studies reflecting the source populations of the admixed population. If we only study one ancestry source, then a study of the admixed population will have greater power to detect the influence of any allele that is more common in the other (unstudied) ancestral population. Of course, power is lost for study of alleles that are less common in the other unstudied source population. However, now consider a comparison of the power of an admixed study to an equally sized study (in combination) of the two source populations. Moreover, we will also require that the number of subjects being studied in each of the two source populations is proportional to each populations' contribution to the admixed population. In this case for any allele, A, with different allele frequencies in the two source populations, one can show that $Var(n(A))$ in the admixed population will be greater than in the two source populations, after stratification for population source, even after adjusting for global ancestry, G. For constant effect size (increase in phenotype mean or disease log odds ratio per allele), the power to detect the effects of allele A on phenotype mean or disease risk is largely determined by the variance of $n(A)$; therefore, it is expected that in general, admixed populations will provide more power for the same number of subjects under study than would a stratified study of the source populations. This power gain is especially noticeable for alleles which are greatly differentiated in the two source populations.

As described in Chap. 7, Sect. 7.7.2, we expect that more recently admixed populations will pay a greater penalty in power than will less recently admixed populations for having to correct for global ancestry because the paucity of recombination will mean there is much more variance in global ancestry in recently admixed populations than in older admixed populations. Nevertheless, even for very recently admixed populations, correcting for global ancestry has less of an effect on power than does correcting for population membership in a stratified un-admixed study; again, this holds especially true for highly differentiated risk alleles.

There is a flip side however of studying very recently admixed populations, which is that haplotypes tend to be longer than in the ancestral populations. In particular, alleles that are unlinked but highly differentiated in frequency between the two source populations will tend to be linked in the admixed population. A risk allele that is highly differentiated may have higher power to be detected in the admixed study but will also be linked with other highly differentiated alleles. Correction for global ancestry will eliminate "cross-chromosome" associations due to very recent admixture, as well as associations between variants at different ends of the same chromosome, but will not eliminate the associations between highly differentiated SNPs riding on as yet un-recombined haplotypes. Therefore, a differentiated risk allele will have greater power to be detected in a recently admixed population but will be more difficult to localize, i.e., to distinguish from associations with other differentiated markers.

8.9.1 The Role of Local Ancestry Adjustment

Since localization of risk alleles is an important aspect of post-GWAS analyses there has been much recent discussion of the role of local ancestry adjustment in association-based studies of admixed populations [37–41]. The ancestry of a particular genomic sequence containing an allele of interest can be traced back to one of the mixing ancestral populations and estimation of local ancestry has been of long interest [38, 42] for several reasons, notably for admixture mapping [43, 44]. The interest here is not on how well local ancestry can be estimated in practice or on the use of local ancestry estimates to perform admixture mapping but rather on whether or not local ancestry should be routinely adjusted for in association studies in admixed groups, assuming that local ancestry at each allele of interest can indeed be estimated with precision.

The hope is that adjusting for local ancestry, L, coded as 0, 1, or 2, copies from one of the two source populations, will allow for better localization of the signal because after adjusting for local ancestry, differentiated SNPs not linked in the source populations will no longer appear to be linked in the admixed population. This is true but it should also be noted that adjusting for local ancestry is expected to reduce power of association tests especially for highly differentiated SNPs, this follows because it can be shown that the expected value of $Var(n(A)|L)$ is less than or equal to $Var(n(A)|G))$ with equality only when the allele frequencies are equal in the two populations. Therefore, adjusting for local ancestry is two-faced; while it eliminates admixture-based LD, it also tends to reduce power. Moreover, it only improves localization ability for differentiated variants; these are exactly the ones for which the difference between expected $Var(n(A)|L)$ and $Var(n(A)|G)$ is the greatest, i.e., where the power loss for correcting for local ancestry is greatest.

In summary, it appears unreasonable to always require local ancestry adjustment before declaring that a significant association is detected in an admixed population. Local ancestry adjustment while reducing artificial admixture-based LD, something which is undoubtedly needed for localization, is at best an imperfect tool for localization because it also reduces power and, for example, may not be as useful for localizing alleles as would be the inclusion of other unrelated populations in multiethnic analyses.

Finally, we must consider the extent to which large modern-day admixed groups actually do show longer LD after correction for global admixture than is seen in relatively non-admixed populations. In the study of the HapMap 3 populations and of data from the Multiethnic Cohort Study (personal communication J Zhang), only relatively modest increases in LD in the large admixed populations could be detected relative to unmixed source populations.

8.10   Polygenes and Heritability

It has been assumed for a very long time that there are traits which must be influenced by the effects of many genes each contributing relatively small amounts to phenotypic variance. Fisher [45] pointed out that this was the reason that genes which are inherited in a Mendelian fashion could explain the heritability of continuous phenotypes such as height, a point of controversy in the early history of modern genetics. For the time being, we consider a simplified situation wherein the only genetic effect on a phenotype of interest is through the (weighted) sum of the alleles of many independent associated SNPs.

8.10.1   Fraction of Familial Risk Explained by a Polygene Under a Multiplicative Model

Suppose that the probability of a binary outcome of interest can be approximated as $\log \Pr(D_i = 1 | v_i) = \alpha + \beta v_i$ (e.g., this is often used to approximate a logit model when D denotes a rare disease). Here v_i is a normally distributed polygene with mean zero and variance set to equal one so that the variance of the risk variable βv_i is equal to β^2. We can show that under this model that in order to explain a simple family relative risk of FRR (relative risk of disease in a relative of an individual with disease) for a coefficient of relationship equal to k solely on the basis of the polygene, then β must be equal to $\sqrt{\frac{\log(FRR)}{k}}$. Here our polygene may be thought of as the sum of many weighted normalized (to mean zero) alleles with the weights, w_k, proportional to the log relative risks, $\log RR_k$, associated with the allele but scaled so that total polygene variance $\mathrm{Var}(v_i) = \sum_k 2p_k(1 - p_k)w_k^2$ equals 8. Notice that under these assumptions, a number of other relevant observations fall out as well. For example, in order to explain a familial risk coefficient of two between first-degree relatives (e.g., similar to that seen for many cancers), the variance β^2 of individual relative risk associated with the polygene should equal 8.39. If this is the case, then individuals in the top quintile of risk will have average risk which is about 6.9-fold that of the remainder of the population. Perhaps more realistically (see below), if only half this FRR can be explained by a simple polygene, then the upper quintile will still be at 4.4-fold increased risk of the outcome compared to the lower 80 % of the population. Higher familial risks require larger β in this simple polygenic model.

8.10.2   Synergies Between Polygenes and Environmental Variables

It is seen above that in order to explain a large fraction of familial risk with a simple combination of genetic variants, i.e., a polygene, this polygene must be highly predictive of individual risk. Identification of such high-risk individuals could be important for many reasons, with application of focused screening being one often discussed example. In certain occupational settings, interaction of genetic risk and risk due to exposures from the job is of potential concern. For example, if the individuals who are most susceptible, based on their polygenes, v_i, are also the most susceptible to exposures on the job, then it could be that protection schemes should be modified for those individuals. For example, if exposures and genetic risk synergize in a multiplicative fashion, i.e., the relative risk associated with v_i holds for all levels of the exposure of interest, then it can be readily shown that the fraction of excess cases due to exposure is higher in the genetically exposed. In the example above (where the most genetically susceptible 20 % have a risk 6.9-fold the remainder of the population), about 63 % of total cases occur among the most susceptible quintile; moreover, the same fraction of the excess cases due to exposure (those that would not be seen in the absence of exposure) would also occur among the most genetically susceptible quintile. In this setting one could imagine a system of personalized standards that would try to hold down each individual's absolute excess risk of an adverse event or disease to some permissible level by modifying the individual exposure amounts allowed according to genetic risk and the synergism between genetic risk and exposure.

At present, these question are far more hypothetical than real, since the genetic basis for very few complex diseases is well understood to date, and for most diseases, only a fraction (such as carriers of BRCA mutations) of high-risk individuals can be identified on the basis of current knowledge. Nevertheless, as the polygenic component of risk is identified and quantified, the evaluation of the joint impact of polygenes and other exposures is likely to become increasingly important.

8.11   GWAS Heritability Analysis

At present, there is controversy about the overall contribution of additive genetic risk to heritability. In an interesting series of papers, Yang, Visscher, and colleagues [46–49] have used GWAS studies to estimate the overall polygenic contribution of common variants to complex phenotypes without actually identifying the specific genes that contribute to the polygene. (A similar effort using different methods has been described in Purcell et al. [50]). Here we go over the basics of what they are attempting and also discuss the behavior of these estimates in the presence of population stratification.

The original analyses of Yang et al. [46] discussed estimation of the heritability of height. Their analysis is closely related to the use of random effects models to correct for population stratification and relatedness described in Chap. 4, Sect. 4.2.3. In their original analysis of height, for example, they fit essentially the same variance components model as does the EMMAX program [51] which we display as

$$E(Y_i) = X'_i\beta \qquad (8.16)$$

and

$$\text{Var}(Y) = \sigma^2 I + \gamma^2 K, \qquad (8.17)$$

where $Y = (Y_1, Y_2, \ldots, Y_N)$ is the vector of observations of height and where we estimate K using SNP data by constructing the $N \times N$ Balding-Nichols relationship matrix $\hat{K}$ (see Chaps. 2 and 4) with components

$$\hat{k}_{ij} = 1/M \sum_{l=1}^{M} \frac{(n_{il} - 2\hat{p}_l)(n_{jl} - 2\hat{p}_l)}{2(\hat{p}_l)(1 - \hat{p}_l)},$$

where $\hat{p}_l$ for $l = 1, \ldots, M$ are the estimated allele frequencies of each genotyped SNP. (Actually Yang et al. replaced the diagonal elements $\hat{k}_{ii}$ with a revised version having better sampling properties when rare SNPs are used in the analysis.) Unlike in Kang et al. [51] who used the variance model (8.17) to adjust for population stratification when SNP allele counts, n_{il}, are included in the mean model (8.16), the interest in the heritability analysis is not in the effect of individual SNPs; rather, the estimates of the variance components γ^2 and σ^2 are examined and reinterpreted. Yang et al. interpret the variance component γ^2 as being related to the polygenic effect of all the measured SNPs combined (including the effects of those that are in close LD with the measured SNPs), and they estimate the fraction of the overall trait variance that is due to the effects of a polygene as equal to $h^2 = \frac{\gamma^2}{\sigma^2 + \gamma^2}$.

The interpretation of the variance components as indicative of the total variance due to SNPs was based on an underlying model

$$Y_i = \mu + g_i + e_i \quad \text{and} \quad g_i = \sum_{l=1}^{M} z_{il} u_l, \qquad (8.18)$$

with z_{il} a normalized version of n_{il} and u_l proportional to the effect (e.g., linear regression slope parameter) of this normalized variant (here g_i is equivalent to the polygene v_i above multiplied by the polygene effect β). It is also assumed that e_i is independent of $e_{i'}$ for $i \neq i'$.

Treating the effects, u_l, of each normalized SNP as an independent mean zero random variables with variance equal to $\frac{\gamma^2}{M}$ gives the random effects version of model (8.18) as

$$E(Y_i) = \mu \quad \text{and} \quad \text{Var}(Y) = \sigma^2 \mathbf{I} + \gamma^2 \frac{1}{M} \mathbf{Z}\mathbf{Z}'. \tag{8.19}$$

Note that $\frac{1}{M} \mathbf{Z}\mathbf{Z}'$ is equivalent to the estimated relationship matrix $\hat{\mathbf{K}}$ discussed previously.

In their initial paper, Yang et al. used this method to estimate that 45 % of the variability of height can be explained by considering all SNPs simultaneously, i.e., the estimate $\hat{\gamma}^2$ was equal to 45 % of total estimated variance $\hat{\sigma}^2 + \hat{\gamma}^2$; note that this is far greater than the 10 % of variance explained by the SNPs in the "mega-analysis" of Lango Allen et al. using many more participants than in the Yang et al.'s paper. A later paper from the same group [48] went on to apportion this overall trait variance into components that are due to certain types of SNPs, such as all SNPs on given chromosomes and all "genic" versus "intergenic" SNPs (i.e., SNPs close to or within the transcribed region of known genes and SNPs outside of these transcribed regions), by restricting the SNPs used in $\mathbf{Z}$. They also used liability models [19] to extend these methods to binary (case–control) outcomes.

8.11.1   Heritability Estimation in the Presence of Population Stratification

It is striking that the model used by Kang et al. [52] is essentially identical to that used by Yang et al. [46] but that the focus is so different. For Kang et al. the SNPs that are used in the estimate, $\hat{\mathbf{K}}$, are of no special interest themselves, other than to capture hidden structure and relatedness and the SNPs that are used are not interpreted as necessarily being in close LD with causal SNPs; the parameter γ^2 is a nuisance parameter which is assumed to capture the effects of hidden population structure and relatedness. On the other hand, Yang et al. basically assume that all related individuals have been removed from the analysis and that gross population structure and admixture is either absent or accounted for (by use of principal components or similar methods) so that γ^2 can be interpreted as the direct effect of the portion of the measured SNPs that either are causal or are in close LD with causal SNPs.

It is clear that in a number of instances the resulting heritability estimates $h^2 = \frac{\gamma^2}{\sigma^2 + \gamma^2}$ may be biased estimates of the inherent predictive capacity of the measured SNPs [52]. For example, Browning and Browning [53] have shown that severe hidden population stratification (i.e., the presence of several different non-mixing groups) can bias GWAS heritability estimates, even after adjusting for principal components, as can the presence of unknown close relatives in the data [52].

More precisely, consider an expansion of model (8.18)

$$Y_i = \mu + g_i + g_i^{\,U} + e_i, \tag{8.20}$$

where again $g_i = \sum_{l=1}^{M} z_{il} u_l$ and the additional effect g_i^U refers to unmeasured causal variants, z_{il}^U; with $g_i^U = \sum_{l=1}^{M^U} z_{il}^U u_l^U$, we assume that the effects, u_l^U of the unmeasured SNPs are distributed with mean zero and variance γ_U^2 / M_U. If this is the correct model, then writing this in terms of the induced variance components we have

$$E(Y_i) = \mu \quad \text{and} \quad \mathrm{Var}(Y) = \sigma^2 \mathbf{I} + \gamma^2 \frac{1}{M} \mathbf{Z} \mathbf{Z}' + \gamma_U^2 \frac{1}{M_U} \mathbf{Z}^{\mathbf{U}} \mathbf{Z}^{\mathbf{U}\prime}. \tag{8.21}$$

Finally, suppose that we fit the variance model (8.19) rather than the true model (8.21). If the matrices $\frac{1}{M}\mathbf{Z}\mathbf{Z}'$ and $\frac{1}{M_U}\mathbf{Z}^{\mathbf{U}}\mathbf{Z}^{\mathbf{U}\prime}$ are similar to each other, then it can be shown that the estimate of γ^2 from fitting (8.19) will be biased upward, towards $\gamma^2 + \gamma_U^2$. Remembering from Chaps. 2 and 4 that a consequence of population stratification and cryptic relatedness is that all variants will tend to have a similar covariance matrix structure, reflecting the hidden structure in the sample, we would expect $\frac{1}{M}\mathbf{Z}\mathbf{Z}'$ and $\frac{1}{M_U}\mathbf{Z}^{\mathbf{U}}\mathbf{Z}^{\mathbf{U}\prime}$ to be similar to each other when hidden stratification is present; hence, the estimation of γ^2 could be confounded with γ_U^2. See Chen et al. [54] for considerable further discussion of this phenomenon in the context of an analysis of the heritability of height in an African American sample.

8.12 Analysis of Rare Variants

GWAS studies to date have largely focused upon the discovery of common variants that are related to diseases and other phenotypes. There is increasing interest in rare variants as causes of complex diseases and phenotypes. It part this may be attributed to disappointment with the failure (in most instances) of GWAS studies to find common variants that explain a large fraction of phenotype heritability or of familial risk [55, 56]. Some researchers (based on analyses such as those of Yang et al. and Purcell et al.) call for additional scrutiny of common variants already accessible by standard technologies, but using very large sample sizes, however, many others [18, 57–60] are drawn to models in which rare variants play a more prominent role in disease susceptibility.

Coinciding with the maturation of high-throughput sequencing technologies (refs) interest in DNA sequencing as the primary or sole source of information about upon genetic variation for large-scale association studies. High-throughput sequencing can be used for selected regions (such as in numerous candidate gene and fine-mapping studies) and is increasingly being applied to interrogate all coding variation, as in the National Heart Lung and Blood Institute's exome sequencing project, ESP [61], and in some studies the entire genome.

There are many statistical issues in the construction of data usable for association analyses from the massive amounts of raw sequence reads generated by these technologies (reference). Of note here [62] is the topic of using haplotype and genotype imputation methods discussed earlier in this book to improving variant calling by imputation across site. However, the primary problem to be considered directly here is in describing and evaluating methods for relating rare and very rare variation to disease risk.

8.13   Contribution of Rare SNPs to Phenotypic Variance and Heritability Under a Polygenic (Additive) Model

For a continuous trait with variability determined by additive effects of individual (statistically independent) causal alleles, the contribution to trait variance of a single given variant, j, with frequency p_j and effect on the mean of β_j per allele in the population of interest is $2p_j(1 - p_j)\beta_j^2$.

In order that rare variation plays an important role in disease heritability, it should be obvious that either phenotype effects and risk or odds ratios need to be much larger for rare alleles or that the fraction of rare alleles that are causal variants should be higher than for common alleles. Chapter 2 introduced the Wright formulae [57, 63, 64] for distribution of allele frequencies under an assumption of constant population size; we revisit that formula here. The Wright formula is

$$f(p) = kp^{(\beta_S-1)}(1 - p)^{(\beta_N-1)}e^{\sigma(1-p)}, \tag{8.22}$$

where p is the allele frequency, β_S is the (scaled see Chap. 2) mutation frequency, β_N is the scaled reversion frequency, σ is the scaled selection rate, and k is a normalization constant. When risk alleles are reproductively neutral ($\sigma = 0$), as can be expected for most late-onset disease alleles, and when the mutation rates are small, this function is almost equal to $\frac{k}{p(1-p)}$ which is a symmetric U-shaped curve. The contribution to the variance of phenotype Y of a causal (additive) allele is

$$2p(1 - p)\beta^2, \tag{8.23}$$

where β is the effect parameter. If we assume that all effects are additive and that the effect size, β, is constant for all risk alleles, then the contribution to phenotypic variance of risks alleles with frequency between p_0 and p_1, found by multiplying equation (8.23) by (8.22) and integrating, simply reduces to $2k\beta^2(p_1 - p_0)$. This implies that the relative contribution of rare alleles (say $p < 0.01$, or $p > 0.99$) to phenotype variance is very small compared to the common alleles (p between 0.05 and 0.95 frequency). As described in Chap. 2, arguments like this motivate the *complex disease common variant* hypothesis that underlies array-based GWAS studies.

There are several arguments in favor of a more important role for rare variants in disease risk; these include:

1. The detection through large-scale DNA sequencing of considerably more rare variation than expected under the constant population size model, presumably due to recent explosive world population growth. Recent large-scale sequencing in the *1000 Genomes Project* shows that there is a surfeit of SNP alleles with frequency less than 0.5 % compared to that expected under the constant population size model [65].
2. The clear role that rare variants, and especially protein-modifying rare risk alleles, play in high-penetrance genes for Mendelian disorders c.f. the *Online Mendelian Inheritance in Man* (OMIM) database [66].
3. Some evidence that risk alleles for certain complex human diseases are more likely to occur in evolutionarily highly conserved regions, when the DNA sequences of different species are considered [67], implying that such genes are under selective pressure.

Point 1 indicates that rare variants, simply by being more numerous, may play a less limited role in disease heritability, even if risk allele magnitudes are not greater than for common variants. If one assumes that risk alleles are associated with reduced reproductive fitness ($s > 0$), then the allele frequency from the Wright formula shifts to the left considerably. For example, if disease alleles are associated with negative selection that decreases reproductive fitness by as little as 0.03 % (scaled selection coefficient $\sigma \equiv 4N_e s = 12$ assuming the commonly accepted value of 10,000 for N_e), then the U shape of the variant distribution becomes much closer to an "L" (see Fig. 8.1a), and therefore the relative contribution to phenotype variance and heritability due to rare alleles is larger than that due to common alleles (Fig. 8.1b, d). In addition, it is unrealistic that all risk variants have the same effect size β. It is sometimes assumed [57, 68] in discussions of the contribution of rare variants to disease risk that there is a link between the effect size of a variant and the selection coefficient σ. If σ increases with the magnitude of β, then larger effect sizes will be restricted to rare risk alleles so that the relative contribution of rare variants is increased even further. This link is certainly reasonable for risk alleles for fatal diseases with nontrivial incidence during reproductive lifespan, as well as for nonfatal diseases of early adulthood or before with very severe social effects, e.g., autism and schizophrenia.

In the remainder of this section, we discuss the practical implications of assuming that rare alleles explain a large portion of phenotype variance.

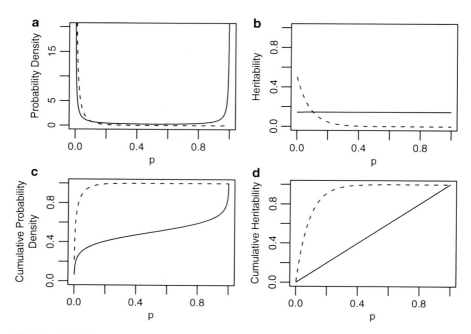

Fig. 8.1 Allele frequency distributions (**a**) and fraction of genetic variance (**b**) under a neutral model (*solid lines*) and under a mild selection model (*dotted line*) with $4N_e = 12$; also shown are cumulative frequencies (**c**) and cumulative heritability (**d**) under the same models

8.14   Moderately Rare Single-SNP Analysis

As described in Chap. 7, in order to be detectable in single-SNP analysis, rare variants must have higher effects than common SNPs in order to be detectable using the types of tests described in Chap. 3. When SNPs are very rare, several different types of breakdown in the asymptotic distribution of test statistics may be expected. We first consider the Wald test in a very simple setting, that of a case–control study, where a rare SNP count is the only predictor in the model, and in addition we assume (to simplify the treatment but with no loss of generality) that the SNP is rare enough so that there are no study participants who carry two copies of the rare allele. The expected data can be displayed as a two-by-two table.

		Disease status	
		0	1
SNP risk allele count	0	n_{00}	n_{01}
	1	n_{10}	n_{11}

Here n_{00} and n_{01} (the noncarriers) are many more than n_{10} and n_{11} (the carriers). For a two-by-two table such as above, the ML estimate of the log odds ratio,

denoted as b below, can readily be shown to be equal to $\hat{b} = \log(n_{00}) + \log(n_{11})$
$-\log(n_{10}) - \log(n_{01})$ and the estimated variance, $\text{Var}(\hat{b})$, of this estimate equal to
$\frac{1}{n_{00}} + \frac{1}{n_{11}} + \frac{1}{n_{10}} + \frac{1}{n_{01}}$. Now consider what happens when there is a very strong positive
effect on risk of a rare SNP. In fact let us assume that in a given dataset the minor
allele for the rare SNP is only seen among the cases so that n_{10} is 0. In this case, the
estimate of the odds ratio is infinite as is the estimate of the variance so that a Wald
test is undefined. Moreover, it can be shown that when applying the Fisher's scoring
procedure to such data that if a Wald test, $\hat{b}^2/\text{Var}(\hat{b})$, is calculated using the
estimates given at the end of each iteration, then this quantity goes to zero as the
iterations proceed (see Homework).

In practical implementations of iterative logistic regression procedures as in
PLINK and SAS, the programs will stop when the changes in log likelihood
decrease beyond some point; noting that the parameter estimates are still changing,
SAS will insert a missing value for the Wald test (and for the p-value for testing the
null hypothesis), whereas PLINK or glm in R will generally substitute a value near
0 for the Wald test and near 1 for the p-value.

Let us consider instead the likelihood ratio test and score test. The likelihood for
these data (assuming an unmatched case–control study) is

$$n_{01}\log\frac{\exp(a)}{1 + \exp(a)} + n_{00}\log\frac{1}{1 + \exp(a)} + n_{11}\log\frac{\exp(a + b)}{1 + \exp(a + b)}$$
$$+ n_{10}\log\frac{1}{1 + \exp(a)}. \tag{8.24}$$

The score test for the hypothesis $b = 0$ (b is the $\log(OR)$) is obtained by first
maximizing (8.24) with respect to a with $b = 0$, which gives $\hat{a}_0 = \log\left(\frac{n_{01}+n_{11}}{n_{00}+n_{10}}\right)$
(i.e., the log of the number of cases/number of controls). We then calculate the 1st
derivative of (8.24) with respect to b (call it D_b) and matrix of second derivates
with respect to (a, b) (call the elements D_{aa}, D_{ab}, and D_{bb}) and evaluate them all at
$b = 0$, and $a = \hat{a}_0$ to form the score test (see Chap. 3) for $b = 0$, as $- D_b^2/(D_{bb} -
D_{ab}^2/D_{aa})$. This test can be easily seen to equal

$$\frac{(n_{00}n_{11} - n_{10}n_{01})^2(n_{01} + n_{11} + n_{10} + n_{00})}{(n_{00} + n_{10})(n_{01} + n_{00})(n_{10} + n_{11})(n_{01} + n_{11})}. \tag{8.25}$$

Note that when n_{10} is zero, the score has value equal to

$$\frac{n_{00}n_{11}(n_{01} + n_{11} + n_{00})}{(n_{01} + n_{00})(n_{01} + n_{11})}.$$

This can be seen to increase with n_{11} so that this test, unlike the Wald test, remains
sensitive to very strong effects of rare variants. Because of this type of behavior the

score test is generally considered to be more powerful than the Wald test for rare variants, the failures of the Wald test are described more generally in Huack [69].

Note however that the score test still relies upon asymptotic approximations to provide p-values. In the example above, the score test can be further seen to be identical to the (uncorrected) Pearson χ^2 for independence of the rows and columns of a 2×2 table. When expected cell sizes (expected values of the n given marginal totals) are small, the chi-square approximation is poor and is often overly liberal, i.e., rejecting the null hypothesis much more often than desired. This behavior can be quite serious for "unbalanced" case–control studies, for example, when there are many more controls than cases, the expected value of n_{11} can become very small for rare variants. The use of exact logistic regression [70] may be needed to provide believable p-values for very rare variants especially in unbalanced designs. For example, in an analysis of exonic variation (almost 200,000 protein coding SNPs) in relation to breast and prostate, Haiman et al. [71] found that the score test produced hundreds of nominally globally significant p-values (all for very rare SNPs) when examining ER breast cancer cases which used approximately 10 times as many controls as cases. None of these rare-SNP associations remained globally significant when exact logistic regression was applied.

For continuous phenotypes, similar problems occur. If phenotype residuals are truly normally distributed, then the usual regression tests are exact, but when normality is not perfect, the apparent effects of rare variants can be extremely distorted. This is especially true when interest is in the tails of the distributions of parameter estimates. Violations of normality that are not very important when tests are conducted at $p = 0.05$ may be very important for values at the levels for global significance (approximately $p = 5 \times 10^{-8}$) appropriate for GWAS studies. Moreover, as the number of rare variants that can be tested increases (through large-scale sequencing or by further GWAS SNP array development), these GWAS p-values (defined for the analysis of common SNPs) may be much too large to guard against global type I errors when testing many rare variants.

8.15 Burden and Pathway Analysis

The application of sequencing technology rather than genotyping known variants allows for the simultaneous discovery and testing of exceedingly rare variants. However, individual testing of SNPs reaches a point of vanishing returns even if (because of effects on reproductive fitness) large effect sizes are expected to be restricted to rare alleles. One hope is that numerous rare phenotype or risk-altering alleles will cluster in identifiable regions of the genome such as within or near known genes or known pathways of genes or in regions involved in the control of such genes. If candidate genes or gene combinations or other well-defined genomic regions can be identified a priori, then cumulative testing of the effects of all rare variation found within these genes or pathways can be approached from a variety of angles. We consider two here.

8.15.1 A Weighted Sum Statistic

Madsen and Browning [68] propose a weighted sum method applicable to case–control studies in which mutations are grouped according to function (e.g., gene/pathway) and each individual is scored by a weighted sum of the minor allele counts in each component group (e.g., each gene or pathway). In order that this sum not be dominated by common variants, they suggest weighting each minor allele according to its frequency in unaffected individuals with smaller weights given to more frequent mutations. More specifically, they suggest

$$\text{burden}_i = \sum_j \frac{1}{\gamma_j} n_{ij}, \tag{8.26}$$

where n_{ij} is the number of copies of the minor allele for mutation j carried by subject i and the sum is over all n_j individuals with data for mutation j. The (inverse) weight γ_j is equal to $\sqrt{2\hat{p}_j(1-\hat{p}_j)}$ where p_j is an estimate of allele frequency of mutation j in controls adjusted to avoid zeros as $\hat{p}_j = (m_j^U + 1)/(2n_j^U + 2)$ where m_j^U is the total count of mutation j in the unaffected individuals and n_j^U is the number of unaffected individuals with data for mutation j. Madsen and Browning then perform a Wilcoxon test for whether the distribution of burden$_i$ differs between cases and controls and finally use a permutation procedure (permuting affection status) to assign p-values to the results. This final permutation step is needed because the weights are calculated using only the unaffected individuals; otherwise, this procedure would show many false-positive risk scores since null alleles that by chance are more common in the controls are down-weighted, while those that are by chance less common in the controls are up-weighted in the calculations. In power calculations (accomplished through simulations), Madsen and Browning show that this testing procedure works well in simulations in which disease risk alleles are rare and are weakly selected against (with σ in the Wright formulae set to 12) but where there is a strong non-probabilistic inverse relationship between the effect (odds ratio) of a given variant and the frequency, p, of the risk alleles in unaffected individuals (the assumed relationship is $r = c/p + 1$ with c a constant determined by the total amount of population risk explained by a particular "gene").

There are a number of important questions about this procedure including its behavior and power (1) when not all alleles affect risk and (2) when not all risk alleles are the minor alleles (i.e., when there are rare protective alleles along with the rare risk alleles).

The first of these questions is partially answered in simulations but these restricted to (seemingly quite permissive) situations when there are an equal number of causative and non-causative loci (and with the non-causative alleles all having the same direction of effect).

8.15.2 Omnibus Tests, Variance Components, and Kernel Machines

A natural alternative to burden-based tests which assume directionality of effect are tests of the form $\beta_1 = \beta_2 = \cdots = \beta_M = 0$ where β_k is the effect of the kth variant, i.e., a simultaneous test of the composite null hypothesis that all genetic effects are zero (here we are assuming an additive model in the counts, n_k, of the kth allele; for rare variants, very few homozygotes for the minor allele will be observed so that there is no ability to distinguish between dominant, additive, or codominant models). When modeling the effects of each variant using a GLM, tests of equality can be performed as score tests with the number of degrees of freedom for the score test being equal to the number, M, of SNPs (unless some of these are redundant, i.e., are in perfect LD with other SNPs, in which case the rank is reduced by the number of redundant). There are a host of other omnibus tests (see [72] for a review) that have been proposed; here we focus on those that are related to variance component methods. We start here by assuming that the outcome of interest is a quantitative trait which we model as Gaussian with mean equal to

$$E(Y) = \mathbf{X}\beta + Z_1 b_1 + Z_2 b_2 + \cdots + Z_M b_M \qquad (8.27)$$

and variance matrix $\sigma^2 \mathbf{I}$. Here we are distinguishing between adjustment variables (such as age, sex, principal components), which are included in the covariate matrix $\mathbf{X}$, and the SNP variables Z (each Z_k is a $N \times 1$ vector containing the counts n_{ik} of the number of the kth SNP allele carried by the ith individual). Model (8.27) is a fixed effects model, but we are free to consider an alternative model in which each b_k is regarded as a random variable (independent of the others) with mean zero and variance σ_k^2. In this case our model becomes

$$\begin{aligned} E(Y) &= \mathbf{X}\beta \\ \mathrm{Var}(Y) &= \sigma^2 \mathbf{I} + \sigma_1^2 Z_1 Z_1{}' + \sigma_2^2 Z_2 Z_2{}' + \cdots + \sigma_M^2 Z_M Z_M{}'. \end{aligned} \qquad (8.28)$$

So far we have not really gained anything in terms of model parsimony since this model has just as many parameters as does model (8.27) (fewer mean terms but more variance components). For rare SNPs where there are few or no homozygotes for the minor allele, so that each element of Z_k is either 0 or 1, fitting model (8.28) is equivalent to fitting a very unbalanced $2 \times 2 \times 2 \ldots \times 2 = 2^M$ random effects ANOVA model with no interaction terms. In perfectly balanced designs of this type, the F statistics for testing that each of the β_k parameters is zero are identical to the F statistics for testing that each of the σ_k^2 parameters is zero so that we would expect no differences in performance (type I error or power) between fixed and random effects model when testing whether all (fixed or random) parameters are equal to zero. For unbalanced designs (where each cell size is not equal), models such as (8.28) can be fit using maximum likelihood or restricted maximum likelihood methods and again we would expect little or no differences in the performance of the two models.

Note that here (when all the SNPs are rare) there is comparatively little information available that can distinguish σ_1^2 from σ_2^2, or σ_2^2 from σ_3^2, especially if each variant has only relatively modest effects. We can introduce parsimony by using a model for the variances such as $\sigma_k^2 = w_k^2 \sigma_g^2$ where we chose various forms for weights w_k. For example, if we assume that all σ_k^2 are equal to each other (e.g., all $w_i^2 = 1$), then the model for the variance matrix of Y is now

$$\mathrm{Var}(Y) = \mathbf{I}\sigma^2 + \sigma_g^2 \mathbf{Z}\mathbf{Z}' \qquad (8.29)$$

with $\mathbf{Z}$ equal to the $N \times M$ matrix with columns equal to $Z_1 \ldots Z_M$. (For convenience in our further discussion but without loss of generality, we also assume that columns of $\mathbf{Z}$ sum to zero, i.e., the means have been subtracted from each Z_k) The model (8.29) replaces M unknown variance components in model (8.28) with 1 unknown component σ_g^2. In this situation then we can expect performance to improve, especially if the model for w_k^2 is "correct" (i.e., that $w_k^2 \sigma_g^2$ is close to the true σ_k^2); essentially, we are (hoping) to trade some loss in estimating each β_k correctly (e.g., increased bias if the modeled σ_k^2 differs from the true value) with increased power (decreased variance) to detect joint effects of the whole set of SNPs. This basic idea, of trading some bias for decrease in variance or increase in predictive power, underlies a very large body of statistical research starting with Stein shrinkage [73] and ridge regression [74] in the 1960s and early 1970s and including the shrinkage and variable selection methods such as the Lasso [75]; the connection between variance components models and shrinkage methods of each of these is very strong [76].

For the general model (8.28), the $\mathrm{Var}(Y)$ can be rewritten as

$$\mathrm{Var}(Y) = \sigma^2 \mathbf{I} + \sigma_g^2 \mathbf{Z}\mathbf{D}\mathbf{Z}', \qquad (8.30)$$

with $\mathbf{D}$ equal to a diagonal matrix, $\mathrm{diag}(w_1^2, w_2^2, \ldots, w_M^2)$, with the weights on the diagonal. Note that if the $\mathbf{Z}$ matrix is centered at zero by subtracting the column means from each column and if the weights are equal to $w_k = 1/\sqrt{2p_k(1 - p_k)}$ with p_k the allele frequency of the kth SNP, then this model is equivalent both to the model discussed above for estimating heritability and to the variance model used for adjustment for population structure in the EMMAX program [51]. Since under the general model, the genetic variance for a given SNP is equal to $2p_k(1 - p_k)\sigma_k^2$, it follows that taking $w_k = 1/\sqrt{2p_k(1 - p_k)}$ is equivalent to assuming that all SNPs (no matter how rare) tend to explain the same amount of phenotypic variance. While this may be an appropriate model to use for correction for population stratification (since then $\frac{1}{M}\mathbf{Z}\mathbf{D}\mathbf{Z}'$ estimates the relationship matrix when we have a very large number of SNPs included), it seems like a very strong assumption to use in actual analysis of the heritability of a given set of SNPs. (Note however that this is in fact the model advocated by [68] discussed above.)

Modeling the (squared) weights, w_k^2, can involve other features than simply allele frequency. For example, one can consider the use of "prior covariates" in the sense of [77] to characterize the appropriate weight for the kth SNP as a function of features such as pathway membership and predicted functionality (e.g., as is assessed for coding variants by Polyphen [78] or SIFT [79]).

In general it is expected that if the weights used in model (8.30) are reflective of the true contribution of the normalized SNP variable Z_k to trait variance, then tests of the null hypothesis that $\sigma_g^2 = 0$ will be more powerful than when other (inappropriate) weights are used. For example, a simulation ([80], Ph.D. Thesis) when the true weights were equal for each SNP but the data was analyzed using $w_k = \frac{1}{\sqrt{2p_k(1-p_k)}}$, then the variance attributable to the SNP counts in Z (i.e., the "heritability" estimate) was underestimated by approximately 1/3.

Fisher's scoring algorithms for maximizing the likelihood in the general linear structured covariance matrix problem (of which the above is a special case) are discussed by many authors starting with [81]. The score test statistic, assuming multivariate normality of Y and using formulas from [81], for testing $\sigma_g^2 = 0$ in (8.30) can be computed as

$$T^2 = N \frac{\left[\frac{(Y-\mathbf{X}\hat{\beta})'\mathbf{ZDZ}'(Y-\mathbf{X}\hat{\beta})}{\hat{\sigma}^2} - \mathrm{tr}(\mathbf{ZDZ}') \right]^2}{N \, \mathrm{tr}(\mathbf{ZDZ}'\mathbf{ZDZ}') - \mathrm{tr}(\mathbf{ZDZ}')^2}. \tag{8.31}$$

Asymptotically this will have a central χ_1^2 distribution under the null hypothesis that $\sigma_g^2 = 0$. (Here $\hat{\sigma}^2$ and $\hat{\beta}$ are estimated under the null hypothesis using OLS regression.)

8.15.2.1 Sequence Kernel Association Test

One of the most influential recent papers on testing for the composite effects of rare variants, by Wu et al. [82], introduced what is known as the sequence kernel association test (SKAT). This test picks up on the themes introduced above and greatly extends them. The simplest sequence kernel association test is based on properties of the statistic $Q = (Y - \mathbf{X}\hat{\beta})'\mathbf{ZDZ}'(Y - \mathbf{X}\hat{\beta})$ which appears above as well. A little thought shows Q is a measure of the covariance (or similarity) computed over all pairs of individuals (i, i') between the pairs of residuals $(Y_i - X'_i\hat{\beta})$ and $(Y_i - X'_{i'}\hat{\beta})$ of the regression on $\mathbf{X}$ and the genetic similarities (captured by the (i, i')th element of $\mathbf{ZDZ}'$) between the same pairs. Notice that the assumption that the score test is distributed (under the null) as a central χ_1^2 statistic is essentially assuming that $\frac{Q}{\hat{\sigma}^2}$ is normally distributed with mean $\mathrm{tr}(\mathbf{ZDZ}')$ and variance $\frac{N}{N \text{ tr}(\mathbf{ZDZ'ZDZ'}) - \text{tr}(\mathbf{ZDZ'})^2}$. The paper by Wu et al. [82] replaces this assumption with a more sophisticated representation of the behavior of Q as a mixture of χ_1^2 random variables with the weights corresponding to the eigenvalues of the matrix $\mathbf{RZDZ'}$ $\mathbf{R}$ where $\mathbf{R}$ is the matrix $(I - X(X'X)^{-1}X')$. Note that applying this matrix $\mathbf{R}$ to Y (i.e., computing $\mathbf{R}Y$) gives the residuals $(Y - \mathbf{X}\hat{\beta})$ and that the variance–covariance matrix of the residuals $(Y - \mathbf{X}\hat{\beta})$ is $\sigma^2\mathbf{R}$ (since $\mathbf{R}$ is symmetric and idempotent, i.e., $\mathbf{RR} = \mathbf{R}$). This representation can readily be shown to be exact when Y is distributed as multivariate normal and so is not reliant on large sample approximations in this case. Next [82] extends the methods to logistic regression by replacing $(Y - \mathbf{X}\hat{\beta})$ in Q with the residuals $Y - \text{logit}^{-1}(\mathbf{X}\hat{\beta})$ and replacing the matrix $\mathbf{R}$ with a matrix $\mathbf{P}^{1/2}$ where $\mathbf{P}$ is an approximation to the variance–covariance matrix for the logistic residuals, i.e., the eigenvalues of $\mathbf{P}^{1/2}\mathbf{ZDZ'}\,\mathbf{P}^{1/2}$ are used in place of the eigenvalues of $\mathbf{RZDZ'}$ $\mathbf{R}$ to compute the null distribution of Q.

The sequence kernel method can make use of other similarity matrices besides $\mathbf{ZDZ'}$ to define Q; for example, to capture quadratic and first-order interactions as well as main effects, the quadratic kernel function $K(Z_i, Z'_1) = \left(1 + \sum_{k=1}^{M} w_k^2 Z_{ik} G_{i'k}\right)^2$ is used to provide the (i, i') element of the similarity matrix (replacing $\mathbf{ZDZ'}$ in Q). Other versions of the kernel function can be constructed to assess gene $\times$ environment interactions (see Homework) on a mass basis, etc.

8.16 Final Remarks

The elephant in the room of genetic association studies at the time this is written is the role that next-generation whole genome sequencing (WGS) will play in future association studies. Next-generation sequencing's impact so far has been almost entirely on variant discovery as in the exome sequencing project [62] and the 1KG project [66]. To date, no large association studies have been based on using whole genome sequencing as the primary technology for variant assessment for all individuals in the study. This is only now beginning to change in candidate gene studies, with exploratory efforts underway within such US NIH led projects as the GAME-ON consortium (Genetic Associations and Mechanisms in Oncology). Sequencing has the potential of identifying regions of the genome either that harbor extremely high risk but very rare alleles or which are rife with rare variants which individually do not make much of an impact (and may in fact be seen only once in a particular study) but which collectively are important. Finally, sequencing has the potential (when DNA for parents as well as affected and unaffected offspring are available) to determine the role of de novo variation in particular genes as a cause of sporadic disease [83].

At present, it is still not known whether rare variation in most common diseases plays an important role in overall disease heritability. The advent of WGS sequencing has provided the rationale for the development of the burden and omnibus tests that are described in Sect. 8.15; however, the main issue of how to group regions of the genome together in order improve the power of these tests is unsolved at this point. Right now, there are still many hurdles for the use of WGA sequencing in large association studies; these include:

1. Sheer cost issues, with WGA sequencing dropping in cost but still far above that of SNP array-based technology.
2. Sequencing quality. Quality of sequencing varies over the genome both randomly (as the coverage, i.e., number of molecules actually read at a given location varies according to chance) and according to features of the genome such as the existence of repetitive DNA sequences and pseudo genes.
3. Bioinformatics issues as the degree of processing in order to turn sequence reads into genotype calls that can be used in statistical analyses require intensive computing and massive data manipulation and storage.
4. Annotation requirements, the burden and omnibus tests described in Sect. 8.15, are much better motivated and much more powerful if the genetic regions or types of variants that they are applied to have a high prior probability of including rare variants affecting disease risk or phenotype mean. At present is in only for the 1–2 % of the genome that is coded into protein for which good annotation exists.
5. Database issues. Each sequencing study is likely to identify new variants not seen before in any previous individuals; the logistics of keeping track of them, i.e., their base position, alleles, and strand, will itself be a nontrivial task.
6. Meta-analysis issues. There is a need to expand meta-analysis methods to include the summarization of the results of burden and omnibus tests over large numbers of studies, in order to enhance the power to detect modest effects of such summaries.
7. Reuse of control data. Because of the expense of WGS, it is very attractive to consider using publically available sequences as controls in case–control studies while reserving study resources to sequence only cases. This can be extremely problematic, partly for reasons described in Chap. 7, Sect. 7.7.3.1, related to small ethnicity differences, but also because of variation in sequencing quality. For example, if $40\times$ coverage is available for the cases (meaning that on average, each DNA locus has had 40 DNA molecules sequenced), but if only $10\times$ is available for the controls (or vice versa), then there is a potential for an increase in false-positive associations since sequencing errors will be differential, affecting cases differently than controls.

Because of cost considerations, it makes sense to restrict WGS sequencing to a subset of individuals in the study, perhaps those with extreme phenotypes (very early age at onset or high level of family history), and develop a much shorter list of regions for which targeted sequencing will be applied to the remainder of the study. This involves many of the same elements as the two-staged genotyping designs described in Chap. 7, Sect. 7.6.

Ultimately, however, it is the unknown state of nature that will determine whether variants that are so rare that they require sequencing to detect even in large studies will play an important role in disease etiology and prediction. If the first few studies that really give WGS a chance to shine (i.e., are large enough to be able to cast light upon the fundamental issue about the role of rare relative to common variation) are positive, then rapid spread of WGS studies can be expected, especially if costs fall quickly. On the other hand, early null results for rare variants will be likely to slow enthusiasm for this avenue of investigation. The most likely (to this author) scenario for the future is that neither profoundly positive nor profoundly negative results will appear quickly, leading to much controversy about the value of WGS for association testing over the next few years.

8.17 Chapter Summary

This chapter has focused on analyses that typically take place after GWAS for a particular study has been analyzed using standard single-SNP analyses, such as meta-analysis, replication of results in other populations, and multiethnic fine mapping of associations. Heritability estimation using GWAS data has also been discussed. In addition, it has discussed several issues that are motivated by the attempts to assess the role of rare rather than common variation in association studies. This later topic is motivated by the advent of whole genome sequencing technology.

Homework

1. Behavior of Wald tests for rare events. Consider the following data table

		Disease status	
		0	1
SNP risk allele count	0	1000	994
	1	0	6

We can fit a logistic regression model to these data as

```
> N<-c(1000,0,994,6) # cell sizes
> n<- c(0,1,0,1) # Snp count
> D<-c(0,0,1,1) # case control status
> summary(glm(D~n,weights=N,family=binomial()))
```

which gives
Coefficients:

	Estimate	Std. Error	z value	Pr(>|z|)
(Intercept)	-0.00602	0.04479	-0.13	0.89
n	13.68889	231.72630	0.06	0.95

Notice that (as described in Sect. 8.14) that the estimate of the effect of SNP count variable n is very large but so is its standard error.

(a) Run these same data in SAS. What does SAS report as the significance of the genotype count variable?
(b) In R it is possible to control the number of iterations that are performed in Fisher's scoring in the glm function through the parameter maxit. Write an R program that will run 1 iteration, then print out the parameter estimates and z value, and then run 2 iterations and print out the parameter estimates, z value, etc. What is happening to the numerator, and the denominator, as we increase maxit? Which seems to be going to infinity faster, the numerator or the denominator?
(c) Use a chi-square test to test whether there is any dependence between the rows and columns of the above table.
(d) Perform a Fisher's exact test of the same hypothesis.

What is your conclusion about:

(i) Which tests are most reliable?
(ii) Whether there is an association between genotype count and disease risk.

2. The program METAL (see links below) is a widely used program for meta-analysis of genome-wide association data. It implements most or all of the meta-analysis methods described in Sect. 8.1. In addition, it keeps track of allele and strand differences. If the first study reports counting the C allele of a C/T SNP when it computed a logistic regression slope estimate for this SNP and the next study reports counting the T allele, a third study reports counting (on the other strand) a G allele, and a fourth study reports counting an A allele, METAL will adjust the estimates appropriately, as if they were all counting the C allele. This feature alone saves the users considerable work when dealing with a diverse number of platforms. Now suppose, as in Sect. 8.6.3, that the score test rather than the Wald test is to be used as the test reported by each study. It turns out that there is still a way to use METAL to compute the combined test (8.15), thereby retaining all of the usual benefits of METAL. The following procedure will work.

(i) Fit the null model containing all terms but the SNP allele of interest.
(ii) Add the SNP allele to the alternative model but constrain the fitting algorithm to:

(a) Use as starting values the parameter estimates of the previous fit + 0 as the starting value for the SNP effect β_1.
(b) Perform only 1 step of the Fisher's scoring procedure.

This can be accomplished in R as

```
> M0<- glm(y~z,family=binomial())
> M1<- glm(y~z+n,family=binomial(),maxit=1,start=c(m0$coefficients,0))
```

Here Z is an $N \times p$ matrix of adjustment variables needed in the null model, and n is the SNP count to be added to the model.

Then we can compute the score statistic as follows:

```
> betahat<-summary(m1)$coefficients[p+2,1]
> Varbetahat<- summary(m1)$coefficients[p+2,2]^2
> score <- betahat^2/Varbetahat
```

And Fisher's information as

```
> info<-1/std1^2
```

Now the score test is

```
> score^2/info
```

Which is identical to

```
> Betahat^2/Varbetahat
```

(a) Justify this procedure for calculating the score test. Hint, start with Fisher's scoring that can be written as (as in Chap. 3, Sect. 3.4.5)

$$\theta_1 = \theta_0 + i^{-1}(\theta_0)U(\theta_0; Y),$$

where $\theta = (\lambda, \beta)$ with λ the $p + 1$ vector of nuisance parameters. If we set θ_0 to the parameter estimates under the null hypothesis (as done in model M1), then after 1 iteration, $\hat{\beta}$ will be equal to $i^{\beta_0 \beta_0} U(\beta_0, \hat{\lambda}, Y)$. The estimated $\text{Var}(\hat{\beta})$ will be equal to $i^{\beta_0 \beta_0}$.

(b) Show that if there are L studies to be analyzed as above, then (8.6) equals (8.15).

3. Show that for logistic regression with $\mu_i = \text{logit}^{-1}(\alpha' X_i)$, the variance of the vector of residuals $Y - \hat{Y}$ can be approximated as $V - VX(X' VX)^{-1}X' V$ where V is a diagonal matrix with diagonal elements equal to $\mu_i(1 - \mu_i)$. Hint: express (in vector matrix form) $Y - \hat{Y} = Y - \mu - (\hat{Y} - \mu)$ and then use a first-degree Taylor expansion to approximate $(\hat{Y} - \mu)$ as $VX(\hat{\alpha} - \alpha)$. Use Fisher's scoring (3.12) to approximate $(\hat{\alpha} - \alpha)$ as $\hat{\alpha} - \alpha = -i^{-1}(\alpha)U(\alpha; Y)$. This together with expressions for i and U approximates $Y - \hat{Y}$ as a known matrix times Y uses matrix formula to determine its variance; see also reference [82].

Links

METAL—Meta Analysis Helper

http://www.sph.umich.edu/csg/abecasis/metal/

References

1. Glass, G. V. (1976). Primary, secondary, and meta-analysis of research. *Educational Researcher, 5*, 3–8.
2. Armitage, P. (1984). Controversies and achievements in clinical trials. *Controlled Clinical Trials, 5*, 67–72.
3. DerSimonian, R., & Laird, N. (1986). Meta-analysis in clinical trials. *Controlled Clinical Trials, 7*, 177–188.
4. Stram, D. O. (1996). Meta-analysis of published data using a linear mixed-effects model. *Biometrics, 52*, 536–544.
5. Begg, C. B., & Pilote, L. (1991). A model for incorporating historical controls into a meta-analysis. *Biometrics, 47*.
6. Torri, V., Simon, R., Russek-Cohen, E., Midthune, D., & Friedman, M. (1992). Statistical model to determine the relationship of response and survival in patients with advanced ovarian cancer treated with chemotherapy. *Journal of the National Cancer Institute, 84*, 407–414.
7. Lindstrom, M., & Bates, D. (1990). Nonlinear mixed effects models for repeated measures data. *Biometrics, 46*, 673–687.
8. Borenstein, M., Hedges, L. V., Higgins, J. P. T., & Rothstein, H. R. (2009). *Introduction to Meta Analysis*. West Sussex, UK: Wiley.
9. Kavvoura, F. K., & Ioannidis, J. P. (2008). Methods for meta-analysis in genetic association studies: A review of their potential and pitfalls. *Human Genetics, 123*, 1–14.
10. Hirschhorn, J. N., Lohmueller, K., Byrne, E., & Hirschhorn, K. (2002). A comprehensive review of genetic association studies. *Genetics in Medicine, 4*, 45–61.
11. Hirschhorn, J. N., & Altshuler, D. (2002). Once and again-issues surrounding replication in genetic association studies. *The Journal of Clinical Endocrinology and Metabolism, 87*, 4438–4441.
12. de Bakker, P. I., Ferreira, M. A., Jia, X., Neale, B. M., Raychaudhuri, S., & Voight, B. F. (2008). Practical aspects of imputation-driven meta-analysis of genome-wide association studies. *Human Molecular Genetics, 17*, R122–128.
13. Cornelis, M. C., Agrawal, A., Cole, J. W., Hansel, N. N., Barnes, K. C., Beaty, T. H., et al. (2010). The gene, environment association studies consortium (GENEVA): Maximizing the knowledge obtained from GWAS by collaboration across studies of multiple conditions. *Genetic Epidemiology, 34*, 364–372.
14. Matise, T. C., Ambite, J. L., Buyske, S., Carlson, C. S., Cole, S. A., Crawford, D. C., et al. (2011). The Next PAGE in understanding complex traits: Design for the analysis of population architecture using genetics and epidemiology (PAGE) study. *American Journal of Epidemiology, 174*, 849–859.
15. Altshuler, D., Brooks, L. D., Chakravarti, A., Collins, F. S., Daly, M. J., & Donnelly, P. (2005). A haplotype map of the human genome. *Nature, 437*, 1299–1320.
16. 1000 Genomes Project Consortium. (2010). A map of human genome variation from population-scale sequencing. *Nature, 467*, 1061–1073.
17. Wang, Z., Jacobs, K. B., Yeager, M., Hutchinson, A., Sampson, J., Chatterjee, N., et al. (2011). Improved imputation of common and uncommon SNPs with a new reference set. *Nature Genetics, 44*, 6–7.
18. Dickson, S. P., Wang, K., Krantz, I., Hakonarson, H., & Goldstein, D. B. (2010). Rare variants create synthetic genome-wide associations. *PLoS Biology, 8*, e1000294.
19. Falconer, D. S., & Mcackay, T. F. C. (1996). *Introduction to quantitative genetics*. Harlow, England: Longman.
20. Zuk, O., Hechter, E., Sunyaev, S. R., & Lander, E. S. (2012). The mystery of missing heritability: Genetic interactions create phantom heritability. *PNAS, 1–6*.
21. Lango Allen, H., Estrada, K., Lettre, G., Berndt, S. I., Weedon, M. N., Rivadeneira, F., et al. (2010). Hundreds of variants clustered in genomic loci and biological pathways affect human height. *Nature, 467*, 832–838.

22. Hedges, L. V., & Olkin, I. (1985). *Statistical methods for meta-analysis*. London: Academic.
23. Mosteller, F. (1995). The Tennessee study of class size in the early school grades. The future of children. *Critical Issues for Children and Youths, 5*, 113–127.
24. Zaykin, D. V. (2011). Optimally weighted Z-test is a powerful method for combining probabilities in meta-analysis. *Journal of Evolutionary Biology, 24*, 1836–1841.
25. Won, S., Morris, N., Lu, Q., & Elston, R. C. (2009). Choosing an optimal method to combine P-values. *Statistics in Medicine, 28*, 1537–1553.
26. Fisher, R. A. (1932). *Statistical methods for research workers*. Edinburgh: Oliver and Boyd.
27. Self, S., & Liang, K.-Y. (1987). Asymptotic properties of maximum likelihood estimators and likelihood ratio tests under nonstandard conditions. *Journal of the American Statistical Association, 82*(398), 605–610.
28. Chen, Z. (2011). Is the weighted z-test the best method for combining probabilities from independent tests? *Journal of Evolutionary Biology, 24*, 926–930.
29. Lancaster, H. O. (1961). The combination of probabilities: An application of orthonormal functions. *Australian Journal of Statistics, 3*, 20–33.
30. Cai, Q., Long, J., Lu, W., Qu, S., Wen, W., Kang, D., et al. (2011). Genome-wide association study identifies breast cancer risk variant at 10q21.2: Results from the Asia Breast Cancer Consortium. *Human Molecular Genetics, 20*, 4991–4999.
31. N'Diaye, A., Chen, G. K., Palmer, C. D., Ge, B., Tayo, B., Mathias, R. A., et al. (2011). Identification, replication, and fine-mapping of Loci associated with adult height in individuals of African ancestry. *PLoS Genetics, 7*, e1002298.
32. Chen, F., Chen, G. K., Millikan, R. C., John, E. M., Ambrosone, C. B., Bernstein, L., et al. (2011). Fine-mapping of breast cancer susceptibility loci characterizes genetic risk in African Americans. *Human Molecular Genetics, 20*, 4491–4503.
33. Haiman, C. A., Chen, G. K., Blot, W. J., Strom, S. S., Berndt, S. I., Kittles, R. A., et al. (2011). Characterizing genetic risk at known prostate cancer susceptibility loci in African Americans. *PLoS Genetics, 7*, e1001387.
34. Haiman, C. A., & Stram, D. O. (2010). Exploring genetic susceptibility to cancer in diverse populations. *Current Opinion in Genetics and Development, 20*, 330–335.
35. Udler, M. S., Meyer, K. B., Pooley, K. A., Karlins, E., Struewing, J. P., Zhang, J., et al. (2009). FGFR2 variants and breast cancer risk: Fine-scale mapping using African American studies and analysis of chromatin conformation. *Human Molecular Genetics, 18*, 1692–1703.
36. Wacholder, S., Chanock, S., Garcia-Closas, M., El Ghormli, L., & Rothman, N. (2004). Assessing the probability that a positive report is false: An approach for molecular epidemiology studies. *Journal of the National Cancer Institute, 96*, 434–442.
37. Kang, S. J., Larkin, E. K., Song, Y., Barnholtz-Sloan, J., Baechle, D., Feng, T., et al. (2009). Assessing the impact of global versus local ancestry in association studies. *BMC Proceedings, 3*(Suppl 7), S107.
38. Pasaniuc, B., Sankararaman, S., Kimmel, G., & Halperin, E. (2009). Inference of locus-specific ancestry in closely related populations. *Bioinformatics, 25*, i213–i221.
39. Qin, H., Morris, N., Kang, S. J., Li, M., Tayo, B., Lyon, H., et al. (2010). Interrogating local population structure for fine mapping in genome-wide association studies. *Bioinformatics, 26*, 2961–2968.
40. Wang, X., Zhu, X., Qin, H., Cooper, R. S., Ewens, W. J., Li, C., et al. (2010). Adjustment for local ancestry in genetic association analysis of admixed populations. *Bioinformatics, 27*, 670–677.
41. Liu, J., Lewinger, J. P., Gilliland, F. D., Gauderman, W. J., & Conti, D. V. (2013). Confounding and heterogeneity in genetic association studies with admixed populations. *American Journal of Epidemiology, 177*, 351–360.
42. Patterson, N., Hattangadi, N., Lane, B., Lohmueller, K. E., Hafler, D. A., Oksenberg, J. R., et al. (2004). Methods for high-density admixture mapping of disease genes. *The American Journal of Human Genetics, 74*, 979–1000.

43. Freedman, M. L., Haiman, C. A., Patterson, N., McDonald, G. J., Tandon, A., Waliszewska, A., et al. (2006). Admixture mapping identifies 8q24 as a prostate cancer risk locus in African-American men. *Proceedings of the National Academy of Sciences of the United States of America, 103*, 14068–14073.

44. Cheng, C. Y., Kao, W. H., Patterson, N., Tandon, A., Haiman, C. A., Harris, T. B., et al. (2009). Admixture mapping of 15,280 African Americans identifies obesity susceptibility loci on chromosomes 5 and X. *PLoS Genetics, 5*, e1000490.

45. Fisher, R. A. (1918). The correlation between relatives on the supposition of Mendelian inheritance. *Transactions of the Royal Society of Edinburgh, 52*, 399–433.

46. Yang, J., Benyamin, B., McEvoy, B. P., Gordon, S., Henders, A. K., Nyholt, D. R., et al. (2010). Common SNPs explain a large proportion of the heritability for human height. *Nature Genetics, 42*, 565–569.

47. Yang, J., Lee, S. H., Goddard, M. E., & Visscher, P. M. (2011). GCTA: A tool for genome-wide complex trait analysis. *The American Journal of Human Genetics, 88*, 76–82.

48. Yang, J., Manolio, T. A., Pasquale, L. R., Boerwinkle, E., Caporaso, N., Cunningham, J. M., et al. (2011). Genome partitioning of genetic variation for complex traits using common SNPs. *Nature Genetics, 43*, 519–525.

49. Yang, J., Weedon, M. N., Purcell, S., Lettre, G., Estrada, K., Willer, C. J., et al. (2011). Genomic inflation factors under polygenic inheritance. *European Journal of Human Genetics, 19*(7), 807–812.

50. Purcell, S. M., Wray, N. R., Stone, J. L., Visscher, P. M., O'Donovan, M. C., Sullivan, P. F., et al. (2009). Common polygenic variation contributes to risk of schizophrenia and bipolar disorder. *Nature, 460*, 748–752.

51. Kang, H. M., Sul, J. H., Service, S. K., Zaitlen, N. A., Kong, S. Y., Freimer, N. B., Sabatti, C., et al. (2010). Variance component model to account for sample structure in genome-wide association studies. *Nature Genetics, 42*, 348–354.

52. Zaitlen, N., & Kraft, P. (2012). Heritability in the genome-wide association era. *Human Genetics, 131*(10), 1655–1664.

53. Browning, S. R., & Browning, B. L. (2011). Population structure can inflate SNP-based heritability estimates. *The American Journal of Human Genetics, 89*, 191–193.

54. Chen, F., Chen, G. K., Thomas, V., Ambrosone, C. B., Bandera, E. V., Berndt, S. I., Bernstein, L., et al. (2013) Methodological considerations related to a genome-wide assessment of height heritability among people of African Ancestry, *In review*

55. Manolio, T. A., Collins, F. S., Cox, N. J., Goldstein, D. B., Hindorff, L. A., Hunter, D. J., et al. (2009). Finding the missing heritability of complex diseases. *Nature, 461*, 747–753.

56. Nielsen, R. (2010). Genomics: In search of rare human variants. *Nature, 467*, 1050–1051.

57. Pritchard, J. K. (2001). Are rare variants responsible for susceptibility to complex diseases? *The American Journal of Human Genetics, 69*, 124–137.

58. Fearnhead, N. S., Winney, B., & Bodmer, W. F. (2005). Rare variant hypothesis for multifactorial inheritance: Susceptibility to colorectal adenomas as a model. *Cell Cycle, 4*, 521–525.

59. Bodmer, W., & Bonilla, C. (2008). Common and rare variants in multifactorial susceptibility to common diseases. *Nature Genetics, 40*, 695–701.

60. De La Vega, F. M., Bustamante, C. D., & Leal, S. M. (2011). Genome-wide association mapping and rare alleles: From population genomics to personalized medicine – Session introduction. *Pacific Symposium on Biocomputing, 74–75*.

61. Fu, W., O'Connor, T. D., Jun, G., Kang, H. M., Abecasis, G., Leal, S. M., et al. (2013). Analysis of 6,515 exomes reveals the recent origin of most human protein-coding variants. *Nature, 493*, 216–220.

62. Li, Y., Willer, C. J., Ding, J., Scheet, P., & Abecasis, G. R. (2010). MaCH: Using sequence and genotype data to estimate haplotypes and unobserved genotypes. *Genetic Epidemiology, 34*, 816–834.

63. Wright, S. (Ed.). (1949). *Adaptation and selection*. Princeton, NJ: Princeton University Press.

64. Ewens, W. J. (1979). *Mathematical population genetics*. New York, NY: Springer.

65. Abecasis, G. R., Auton, A., Brooks, L. D., DePristo, M. A., Durbin, R. M., Handsaker, R. E., et al. (2012). An integrated map of genetic variation from 1,092 human genomes. *Nature, 491*, 56–65.

66. Hamosh, A., Scott, A. F., Amberger, J. S., Bocchini, C. A., & McKusick, V. A. (2005). Online Mendelian inheritance in man (OMIM), a knowledgebase of human genes and genetic disorders. *Nucleic Acids Research, 33*, D514–517.

67. Huang, H., Winter, E. E., Wang, H., Weinstock, K. G., Xing, H., Goodstadt, L., et al. (2004). Evolutionary conservation and selection of human disease gene orthologs in the rat and mouse genomes. *Genome Biology, 5*, R47.

68. Madsen, B. E., & Browning, S. R. (2009). A groupwise association test for rare mutations using a weighted sum statistic. *PLoS Genetics, 5*, e1000384.

69. Hauck, W., & Donner, A. (1977). Wald's test as applied to hypotheses in Logit analysis. *JASA, 72*, 851–853.

70. Hirji, K. F., Mehta, C. R., & Patel, N. R. (1987). Computing distributions for exact logistic regression. *JASA, 82*, 1110–1117.

71. Haiman, C. A., Han, Y., Feng, Y., Xia, L., Hsu, C., Sheng, X., et al. (2013). Genome-wide testing of putative functional exonic variants in relationship with breast and prostate cancer risk in a multiethnic population. *PLoS Genetics, 9*(3), e1003419.

72. Basu, S., & Pan, W. (2011). Comparison of statistical tests for disease association with rare variants. *Genetic Epidemiology, 35*, 606–619.

73. James, W., & Stein, C. (1961). Estimation with quadratic loss. *Proceedings of the Fourth Berkeley Symposium on Mathematical Statistics and Probability, 1*, 361–379.

74. Hoerl, A. E., & Kennard, R. W. (1970). Ridge regression: Biased estimation for nonorthogonal problems. *Technometrics, 42*, 80–86.

75. Tibshirani, R. (1996). Regression shrinkage and selection via the Lasso. *Journal of the Royal Statistical Society, Series B, 58*, 267–288.

76. Greenland, S. (2000). Principles of multilevel modelling. *International Journal of Epidemiology, 29*, 158–167.

77. Lewinger, J. P., Conti, D. V., Baurley, J. W., Triche, T. J., & Thomas, D. C. (2007). Hierarchical Bayes prioritization of marker associations from a genome-wide association scan for further investigation. *Genetic Epidemiology, 31*, 871–882.

78. Ramensky, V., Bork, P., & Sunyaev, S. (2002). Human non-synonymous SNPs: Server and survey. *Nucleic Acids Research, 30*, 3894–3900.

79. Kumar, P., Henikoff, S., & Ng, P. C. (2009). Predicting the effects of coding non-synonymous variants on protein function using the SIFT algorithm. *Nature Protocols, 4*, 1073–1081.

80. He, J. (2013). Polygenes and Estimated Heritability of Prostate Cancer in an African American Sample using GWAS data, PhD Thesis, Preventive Medicine, University of Southern California, Los Angeles

81. Anderson, T. W. (1973). Asymptotically efficient estimation of covariance matrices with linear structure. *The Annals of Statistics, 1*, 135–141.

82. Wu, M. C., Lee, S., Cai, T., Li, Y., Boehnke, M., & Lin, X. (2011). Rare-variant association testing for sequencing data with the sequence kernel association test. *The American Journal of Human Genetics, 89*, 82–93.

83. O'Roak, B. J., Deriziotis, P., Lee, C., Vives, L., Schwartz, J. J., Girirajan, S., et al. (2011). Exome sequencing in sporadic autism spectrum disorders identifies severe de novo mutations. *Nature Genetics, 43*, 585–589.

Index

Printed by Publishers' Graphics LLC
FMRO140211.15.17.4